Competency Based

Textbook of Psychiatry

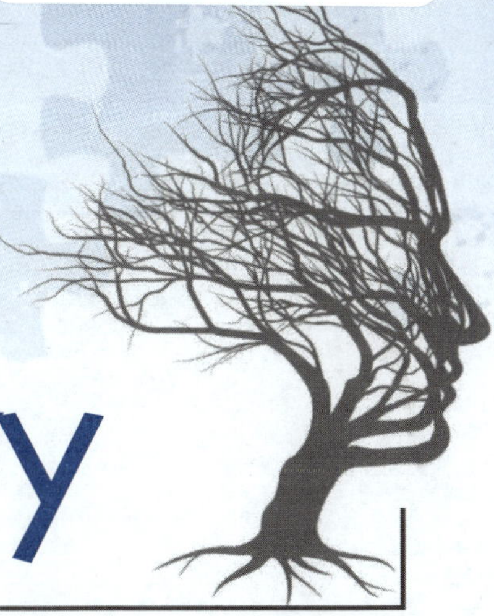

As per the latest CBME Guidelines |
Competency based Undergraduate Curriculum for the Indian Medical Graduate

Competency Based

Textbook of Psychiatry

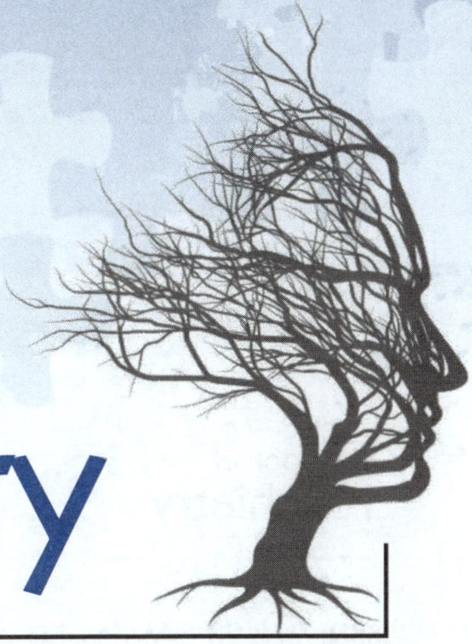

As per the latest CBME Guidelines |
Competency based Undergraduate Curriculum for the Indian Medical Graduate

RK Meher MD (Psychiatry)
Assistant Professor
Department of Psychiatry
VSS Institute of Medical Sciences and Research (VIMSAR)
Burla, Odisha

CBSPD

CBS Publishers & Distributors Pvt Ltd

New Delhi • Bengaluru • Chennai • Kochi • Kolkata • Lucknow • Mumbai
Hyderabad • Jharkhand • Nagpur • Patna • Pune • Uttarakhand

Competency Based

Textbook of

Psychiatry

As per the latest CBME Guidelines | Competency based Undergraduate Curriculum for the Indian Medical Graduate

ISBN: 978-93-5466-694-0

First Edition 2024

Published by Satish Kumar Jain and produced by Varun Jain for

CBS Publishers & Distributors Pvt Ltd

4819/XI Prahlad Street, 24 Ansari Road, Daryaganj, New Delhi 110 002, India

Ph: 011-23289259, 23266861, 23266867 Fax: 011-23243014

Website: www.cbspd.com e-mail: delhi@cbspd.com

Corporate Office: 204 FIE, Industrial Area, Patparganj, Delhi 110 092, India

Ph: 011-49344934 Fax: 011-49344935

e-mail: publishing@cbspd.com; publicity@cbspd.com

Branches

- **Bengaluru:** Seema House 2975, 17th Cross, K.R. Road, Banasankari 2nd Stage, Bengaluru 560 070, Karnataka, India
  Ph: +91-80-26771678/79 Fax: +91-80-26771680 e-mail: bangalore@cbspd.com
- **Chennai:** 7, Subbaraya Street, Shenoy Nagar, Chennai 600 030, Tamil Nadu, India
  Ph: +91-44-26680620, 26681266 Fax: +91-44-42032115 e-mail: chennai@cbspd.com
- **Kochi:** 42/1325, 1326, Power House Road, Opposite KSEB, Power House, Ernakulum 682018, Kochi, Kerala, India
  Ph: +91-484-4059061–67 Fax: +91-484-4059065 e-mail: kochi@cbspd.com
- **Kolkata:** 147, Hind Ceramics Compound, 1st Floor, Nilgunj Road, Belghoria, Kolkata 700056, West Bengal, India
  Ph: +91-33-25330055/56 e-mail: kolkata@cbspd.com
- **Lucknow:** Basement, Khushuma Complex, 7 Meerabai Marg (behind Jawahar Bhawan), Lucknow 226001, UP, India
  Ph: +91-522-4000032 e-mail: tiwari.lucknow@cbspd.com
- **Mumbai:** PWD Shed, Gala No. 25/26, Ramchandra Bhatt Marg, Next JJ Hospital Gate No. 2, Opp. Union Bank of India, Noorbaug, Mumbai 400009, Maharashtra, India
  Ph: +91-22-66661880/89 e-mail: mumbai@cbspd.com

Representatives

- **Hyderabad** 0-9885175004
- **Jharkhand** 0-9811541605
- **Nagpur** 0-8692091830
- **Patna** 0-9334159340
- **Pune** 0-9664372571
- **Uttarakhand** 0-9716462459

Printed at: Rashtriya Printers, Dilshad Garden, Delhi, India

to

my late father

Narahari Meher

Preface

I feel great pleasure in presenting this book *Competency Based Textbook of Psychiatry* to the beloved students. There is a general perception among undergraduate students that a comprehensive textbook in psychiatry with conceptual understanding is lacking. With the commencement of a competency-based curriculum for Indian medical graduates by National Medical Commission (NMC), there was a need for a textbook on psychiatry covering all these competencies. Furthermore, because of the unfamiliarity of undergraduate students with various aspects of psychiatry, a concept-based textbook that makes psychiatry simple yet interesting is the need of the hour. All these needs of undergraduate students have been kept in mind during the course of the preparation of the book. Constructive comments and suggestions are always welcome from the readers of this book.

I am deeply obliged to Dr HR Phookun, former Head of the Department of Psychiatry, Gauhati Medical College, Guwahati, Assam, who inspired me to pursue an academic career and to write this book. I also took great inspiration from dedicated teachers like Dr Deepesh Bhagabati, Dr Suresh Chakravarty, Dr Deepanjali Medhi, Dr Mythily Hazarika and Dr Bishnu Bashyal during my postgraduate study at Gauhati Medical College. I am also thankful to my friend Dagindra Meher for helping me out with the illustrations.

RK Meher

Preface

Chapter 1

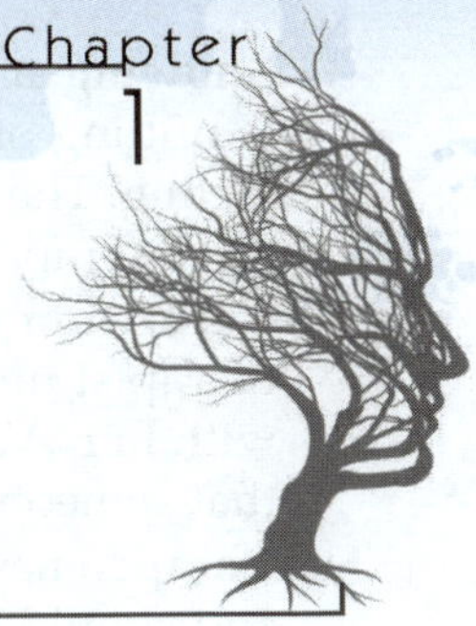

Doctor–Patient Relationship

> **Competency achievement:** The students should able to
> 1. **PS1.1** Establish rapport and empathy with patients
> 2. **PS1.2** Describe the components of communication
> 3. **PS1.3** Demonstrate breaking of bad news in a simulated environment
> 4. **PS1.4** Describe and demonstrate the importance of confidentiality in patient encounters.

INTRODUCTION

A healthy doctor–patient relationship is the cornerstone of patient evaluation and treatment in psychiatry and establishing rapport with the patient is the prerequisite step in psychiatric evaluation and care. To establish a good rapport, it is important to acquire good communication skills for undergraduates and also for postgraduates. Another important aspect of psychiatry is to know about confidentiality and its importance. In this chapter, we will discuss these important preliminary aspects in psychiatry such as rapport establishment, communication skills, breaking of bad news, and confidentiality.

ESTABLISHING RAPPORT WITH THE PATIENT

A healthy rapport between the patient and the therapist is the cornerstone of psychiatric evaluation and care. Rapport is the development of empathy for the patient's cause or in simple words putting oneself in the shoes of the patient to feel what he or she is going through. Rapport includes trust and the dynamic empathetic relationship shared between the patient and the therapist. Rapport is established by showing genuine interest in the patient through active listening, remembering, and showing true empathy.

How to build rapport?

The establishment of a healthy rapport with the patient involves the following components:

1. **Active listening:** Actively engaging the patient by showing genuine interest is the cornerstone of rapport establishment. Positive body language, reassuring gestures such as head nodding, and positive comments during the conversation help build a healthy rapport. Repeating the patient verbatim and asking for clarification from time to time reassures the patient that the therapist is actively listening and is genuinely showing interest.
2. **Showing respect:** The patient is a human being sitting across the table and should be treated with respect. Showing respect makes the patient more comfortable which helps in opening up. The therapist should avoid doing any kind of judgment and should accept the patient for who they are.

3. **Showing empathy** is the most important aspect of rapport establishment. Empathy is putting oneself in the shoes of the patient and feeling what he or she might be feeling. The therapist should feel from the patient's perspective instead of showing mere sympathy toward the patient's suffering.
4. **Validation of the patient's cause:** Validation means telling the patient that the therapist understands what he is going through and it is okay to share the details with him. Validation helps the patient in sharing information as he comes to know that someone genuinely understands his suffering.
5. **Competency:** Competency means the therapist should be true about his capability and should understand to what extent he can help the patient. In case of a lack of confidence about taking the case, the therapist should make a proper referral which helps gain the genuine trust of the patient.

COMPONENTS OF COMMUNICATION IN PSYCHIATRY

Good communication skills are necessary to build a good doctor-patient relationship in the medical profession, especially in psychiatry. Good communication skill is imperative in rapport establishment and patient evaluation in psychiatric practice. Medical graduates should be familiar with the components of good communication which helps them in clinical evaluation and effective management of patients. Good communication should have the following basic components as suggested by **S Priebe et al**.

1. **Focus on the patient's concern:** Patients' concerns and wishes should be the cornerstone of communication in psychiatry and given primary importance above all. Patient-centered communication and care involve understanding the patient's suffering, wishes, and well-being, showing empathy toward his cause, and maintaining confidentiality.
2. **Positive regard and personal respect:** The patient should be accepted as a person and not as a case and should be dealt with due respect. The patient should be allowed to express his emotion, thought, and perception without any fear of negative judgment. Expressed emotions such as rejection, criticism, and critical judgment regarding the illness are associated with bad prognosis and negative outcomes, and poor compliance, especially in psychotic illnesses such as schizophrenia.
3. **Involvement of the patient in decision making:** This is of particular importance in the treatment of neurotic illnesses such as depression, anxiety, and OCD. The psychiatrist should discuss the nature of the illness in detail and present all possible treatment modalities with associated pros and cons. The patient should take the lead in decision-making after getting the proper information regarding his illness and possible treatment approaches, with the psychiatrist acting as a guide to choose the best treatment for him. However, this approach may not be feasible in treating psychotic illnesses and in emergency settings.
4. **Genuineness:** A psychiatrist should be genuine, warm, and open in his approach to the patients. Genuineness on the part of the psychiatrist built a long-lasting trustworthy patient–doctor relationship. While treating a patient a psychiatrist should be aware of his capabilities and genuinely disclose his competency, field, and scope of therapy and make a proper referral if the case is beyond his competency. Such approaches help build a trustworthy reputation for the physician.
5. **Using a psychological approach:** It is beneficial to employ a psychotherapeutic approach in the treatment of psychiatric patients. Any one of the standard

therapeutic models such as client-centered therapy, supportive psychotherapy, or cognitive behavioral therapy may be employed. This helps in building a good doctor-patient relationship as many patients come for counseling and talk therapy. Even if medications are necessary in a case, including a psychotherapeutic approach helps rapport building and treatment compliance.

BREAKING OF BAD NEWS: SPIKES PROTOCOL

Many healthcare providers, be it physicians or nursing personnel, find it difficult to break the bad news to patients or their family members, mostly because of a lack of proper communication skills. Breaking bad news from time to time is inevitable in day-to-day healthcare practice and healthcare providers find it difficult to handle these situations. Effective and empathetic communication skills are necessary to communicate bad news to patients or their loved ones.

The bad news is defined as any information which hurts the future life course of a patient and/or his loved ones. Healthcare providers have to convey bad news to the patient or the family members especially in the emergency department, ICU, cancer units, cardiology, or nephrology unit. While sharing bad news the caregiver must adopt an empathetic approach with proper knowledge of the information and its impact on the psychological well-being of the party involved. Several structured formats have been developed to help healthcare providers in this regard. The SPIKES approach is most commonly adopted by healthcare staff across the world while breaking bad news to patients. This format was developed by **Walter Baile et al**.

The SPIKES Format

The SPIKES format is an acronym for a stepwise strategy of breaking bad news consisting of the following components:

1. Setting-up
2. Perception
3. Invitation
4. Knowledge
5. Empathetic approach and
6. Strategy for future actions

Setting-up

Bad news which is capable of evoking negative emotion in the patient or family members should be conveyed in a proper setup. It is desirable to mentally rehearse what should be told and how it should be told using proper kind and empathetic words which convey the information. The set-up should be relaxing with the practitioner sitting on a chair and maintaining an open posture. The message should be delivered confidently without hesitation in kind and empathetic words while maintaining strong eye contact.

Perception

The depth of perception of the patient regarding the unexpected news should be assessed with subtle questioning regarding their expectations and possible negative outcomes. What they know regarding the illness so far, what they expect about the report and possible outcomes etc should be assessed carefully.

Invitation

After breaking the bad news, the caregiver must listen to the quarries patiently and answer them. Many patients or family members after hearing about the bad news enquire about the seriousness of the illness and any possible treatment or cure available. These quarries must be answered properly.

Knowledge

Many times a warning signal may help in embracing the bad news of the patient. Such phrases as 'I am sorry the reports are not so good' or 'the results are not as we expected' may set the stage for the breaking of bad news. The news should be delivered slowly with patience, allowing the strained situation to calm down a little bit before delivering the final negative information. Sharing the information in chunks can greatly help in calming down the situation and making the patient ready to embrace negative emotions associated with the bad news. The information should be delivered in a non-technical way, in a language the patient can understand clearly.

Empathy

After hearing about the bad news, emotion runs high. Many start crying and sobbing which can make the situation awkward for the caregiver. The health professional must be aware of these and must know how to stay calm and show empathy toward their emotional outburst.

One of the important aspects in this regard is possible denial by the patient or family members after hearing the bad news. It must be understood that in these situations denial is used as a defense mechanism to deal with overwhelming emotions. The health professional should not outrightly negate this state of denial and must give them time to come and embrace the truth.

Strategy for Future Action

Lastly, the patient and family members must be involved to adopt a plan of action. Before discussing anything about future action, the therapist must make sure that they understand the nature of the disease and its possible outcomes. Any pending investigation that is necessary to plan for future action must be conveyed. Lastly, it is necessary to know whether the party wants to discuss future activities and is willing to go through possible treatment strategies.

CONFIDENTIALITY AND ITS IMPORTANCE

In psychiatry, the communication between the therapist and the patient is very private. The patient puts a great deal of faith in the therapist and discloses lots of personal information to him. It is unethical for the part of the therapist to disclose this personal information shared with him to others. This ethical obligation is known as confidentiality.

The concept of confidentiality is universal in the medical field and is not limited to psychiatric practice. This personal information shared by a patient to the caregiver should not be disclosed unless the patient gives consent to do so. However, there are certain special circumstances where personal information can be shared with or without the consent of the patient. These are described below under the heading 5 Cs of confidentiality.

5 Cs of Confidentiality

1. **Consent:** A clinician may share information about a patient after obtaining valid consent from the patient or legal guardian (or nominated representative). These situations generally arise when information regarding the patient is needed to be shared while making publications or other academic activities such as teaching.

2. **Court order:** A competent judiciary may direct the treating physician to release some confidential information about the patient. In these cases, the therapist should share only information needed upon receiving a written order from the competent judiciary.
3. **Continued treatment:** While making a referral, the clinician may release certain minimum information about the disease condition of the patient which helps in better management of the patient's condition.
4. **Complying with the law:** It is necessary to share confidential information under certain circumstances prescribed by the law, e.g. mandatory reporting of child abuse under the POCSO act, complying with the investigation department, etc.
5. **Communicating a threat:** It is of particular importance in psychiatry. Sometimes a patient may disclose his intentions to harm others. In these cases, the treating psychiatrist must make the possible victim aware of these facts or he may communicate these kinds of violent intentions to the law enforcement authority. The Tarasoff case is a famous example in this regard.

It should be remembered that these circumstances to breach confidentiality vary from jurisdiction to jurisdiction and the treating physician must be aware of the prevalent laws of the state in this regard.

SUMMARY

1. Rapport is defined as the understanding of the patient's feelings by developing true empathy for the patient's cause. A healthy rapport between the patient and the therapist is the cornerstone of psychiatric evaluation and treatment.
2. Rapport is established by actively listening to what the patient says, showing respect, and showing empathy for the patient.
3. Good communication skill is needed to establish rapport, smooth evaluation, and management of the patient by focusing on the patient's concerns, showing genuine interest in the patient's cause, and involving the patient in decision-making.
4. One of the important skills for medical graduates to acquire is the skill to break the bad news to patients and their relatives.
5. The six-step SPIKES protocol developed by Walter Baile and colleagues is widely used for effective communication during breaking bad news in clinical settings which includes setting-up, perception, invitation, knowledge, empathetic approach, and strategy for future actions.
6. Confidentiality is an obligation for the physician under which it is considered unethical to disclose anything shared by a patient with others without the consent of the patient. However, there are certain special circumstances where confidentiality may be breached with or without the consent of the patient. These are known as the 5 Cs of confidentiality: consent, court order, continued treatment, compliance with the law, and communicating a threat.

BIBLIOGRAPHY

1. Norfolk, Tim and Birdi, Kamal and Walsh, Deirdre. The role of empathy in establishing rapport in the consultation: A new model. Medical education, 2007;41:690–7.
2. S Priebe, S Dimic, C Wildgrube, J Jankovic, A Cushing, R McCabe. Good communication in psychiatry—a conceptual review, European Psychiatry, 2011. Volume 26, Issue 7, pp 403–7.
3. Baile WF, Buckman R, Lenzi R, Glober G, Beale EA, Kudelka AP. SPIKES-A six-step protocol for delivering bad news: application to the patient with cancer. Oncologist, 2000;5(4):302–11.
4. Rosenzweig MQ. Breaking bad news: a guide for effective and empathetic communication. Nurse Pract. 2012 Feb. 12;37(2):1–4.
5. Merideth P. The Five C's of Confidentiality and How to DEAL with Them. Psychiatry (Edgmont), 2007 Feb;4(2):28–9.

Chapter 2

Mental Health

Competency achievement: The students should able to

1. **PS2.1** Define stress and describe its components and causes
2. **PS2.2** Describe the role of time management, study skills, balanced diet, and sleep-wake habits in stress avoidance
3. **PS2.3** Define and describe the principles and components of learning, memory, and emotions
4. **PS2.4** Describe the principles of personality development and motivation
5. **PS2.5** Define and distinguish normality and abnormality

INTRODUCTION

Mental health and well-being is gaining tremendous importance in recent times. Everyone is concerned about how to avoid or cope with stress in day-to-day activities to maintain good mental health. In this topic, we will learn about the definition and characteristics of stress, coping skills, and the importance of sleep, a healthy diet, and time management in avoiding stress. Furthermore, we will also learn some basic concepts regarding memory, emotion, and motivation which also contribute to our mental health and well-being.

STRESS: COMPONENTS AND ITS CAUSES

Definition

Stress is defined as any change, either positive or negative, that evokes **psychological, physical, and/or emotional reactions** in an individual. In day-to-day life, all of us are exposed to life events that catch our attention and demand our efforts. These events and situations which **demand our attention and efforts** impart variable levels of stress on our psychological well-being. People employ various coping skills to smoothly handle these stressful events. Stress only becomes problematic when it is **significant enough in terms of intensity and/or duration**; so that the individual's coping mechanisms fail to handle it.

Types of Stress

Stressful events are generally classified based on the **timing of their occurrence and duration of persistence** into the following types:

1. **Acute stress:** Any sudden change in the smooth running of the life of an individual result in acute stress. These changes can be negative such as the death of a loved one, accidents, loss of job, etc. or can be positive such as marriage, the birth of a child,

traveling, etc. Acute stresses are an intricate part of our daily life and no one can completely avoid them.

2. **Chronic stress:** These are situations that are continuously impacting the life of an individual negatively. These include ongoing marital problems, financial problems, job stress, etc. Any long-standing chronic stress can ultimately cause debility and ultimately leads to the development of psychiatric illnesses such as depression.
3. **Episodic stress:** Some individuals are periodically exposed to stressful events at regular intervals. These include regularly transferable jobs, people exposed to periodic calamities such as floods and droughts, etc. Individuals exposed to episodic stress gradually develop coping skills to deal with them.

Signs of Stress

When an individual is exposed to some significant stress, he shows certain psychological, emotional, and physical changes. These are known as signs of stress and are described below.

1. **Psychological signs** include apprehension, excessive worry, impairment in attention and concentration, and impairment in memory.
2. **Emotional signs** include irritability, frustration, and being touchy.
3. **Physical signs** of stress are muscle tension, headache, somatic symptoms such as pain, tingling, poor immunity with frequent infections, etc. Other measurable physical signs of stress are rapid pulse, high blood pressure, weight loss, and so on.
4. **Behavioral features** of stress are loss of interest in pleasurable activities, sleep disturbances, impaired self-care, indulgence in substance abuse behavior, etc.

Neurobiology of Stress

Exposure to stress leads to a slew of neurochemical changes in the body known as a stress reaction. **Stress reaction** involves following 3 phases:

1. **The alarm phase** is characterized by hypervigilance, autonomic hyperactivity, and sleep disturbance, due to sympathetic hyperactivity and subsequent secretion of noradrenaline.
2. **The phase of resistance** is characterized by activation of the HPA axis and increased secretion of corticosteroids (Fig. 2.1). Steroid soothes the mind with a general feeling of well-being and helps the patient cope with stress. However, long-standing stress ultimately gives rise to the phase of exhaustion.
3. **The phase of exhaustion** is characterized by prolonged secretion of steroids which results in poor immunity, impaired insulin resistance, increased vulnerability to infection, and development of depression.

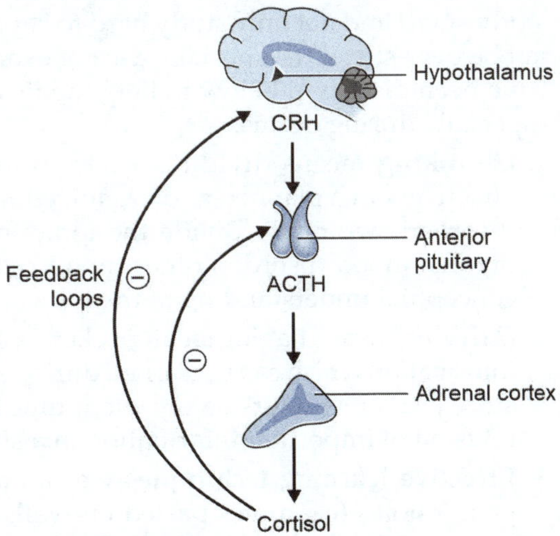

Fig. 2.1: Components of the hypothalamic-pituitary axis.

COPING MECHANISM

Coping mechanisms or coping skills are **thought and behavioral patterns** employed voluntarily by an individual to handle stress. Coping mechanisms can be **proactive** when they are in place before the impact of stress **or reactive** when they are employed only after the impact of stress. Proactive coping skills make the life of a person smooth while reactive coping skills make it more flexible.

Coping mechanisms are commonly classified into the following types.

1. **Problem-focused**, in which the problem causing the distress is actively addressed with proper planning, finding possible solutions, or restraining or withdrawing from the competition.
2. **Emotion-focused coping skills** help mitigate the psychological impact of stress with a positive mental attitude, acceptance, or humor.
3. **Social coping skills** employ social support systems such as help from family and friends to deal with stressful situations.

Commonly used coping mechanisms that can help in mitigating the negative psychological, physical, and emotional ill effects of stressful events are:

1. **Positive self-care** such as making the bed, cleaning the room, grooming, and spending time with nature.
2. **Engaging oneself** in an enjoyable hobby such as art, music, and sport.
3. Regular **physical exercise** like walking, cardiac exercise, swimming, etc.
4. Using **relaxation strategies** like deep breathing, JPMR (Jacobson progressive muscle relaxation techniques), and aromatherapy.
5. Practicing regular **meditation and mindfulness.**

IMPORTANCE OF STUDY SKILLS, TIME MANAGEMENT, AND SLEEP–WAKE CYCLE IN STRESS MANAGEMENT

Effective Study Skills

The undergraduate medical syllabus is very vast and difficult to memorize. One should study smart and not only study hard to cope with such a vast and difficult syllabus and not be over-stressed, especially during exams. Some evidence-based study techniques have been discussed below to help medical graduates learn how to study effectively, especially during exams.

1. **Chunking** means dividing a large topic into smaller ones that can be learned effectively in a planned and organized manner. For example, while studying mood disorders, we might divide the topic into depressive disorders, bipolar disorder, organic mood disorder, other mood disorders, etc. to make a more effective and conceptual understanding of the topic.
2. **Carrying** means having small pocketbooks, notes, etc. containing important relevant information which can be learned during spare time and also before exams. Especially, since just a few hours before exam time is scarce for revision, carrying helps in the revision of important information in a short duration of time.
3. **Effective learning techniques** we can employ to memorize better are flashcards, post-it notes (e.g. notes pasted on walls), discussing in a group, reading the same topic at different locations, etc. These techniques help in revising important topics without repeatedly going through textbooks which are time-consuming.

4. **Alternative resources** mean seeking alternative resources apart from textbooks for effective preparation and learning. These include solving past exam papers, question banks, YouTube videos, audiobooks, Mobile apps, etc. These alternative sources help in clearing basic concepts and also help in memorizing texts better within a reasonable period.

Time Management Strategy

Time is limited for all; however, as doctors, our duties and responsibilities are never-ending. We, as doctors, have to study, perform clinical duties, have family responsibilities, and also have to socialize, and give time for personal growth (keep some time for hobbies and passion). Effective time management strategies are necessary to smartly allocate our limited time for various important tasks in our day-to-day life. Some effective time management strategies are described below.

1. **Prioritization:** Prioritizing our work is the most important aspect of time management. It is often seen that we spend a good amount of time on nonsignificant tasks and at the end of the day little time remains for important tasks. We can follow the 80/20 rule which suggests giving 80% of the time to important work and 20% to nonsignificant and casual aspects of life. This rule saves a good amount of time to be invested in important productive work which helps in personal growth.
2. **Making a 'to-do' list:** It is always wise to make a list of works to be done on a priority and urgency basis which guides us on which work to be completed first. One of the widely used listing methods prioritizes works in the following order.
   A. Urgent and Important
   B. Not urgent but important
   C. Urgent but not important
   D. Neither urgent nor important.
3. **Delegating responsibilities**, one of the wisest time management skills is to distribute work and responsibilities among those in contact (family, friends, and subordinates). This skill prevents us from being overwhelmed with work and responsibilities and helps in completing tasks within a reasonable time. Another important skill is to say 'no' to certain requests and orders which are not that important in improving our personal growth and productivity.
4. **Starting with time**, if a task is important then we should invest time as early as possible to complete it within a reasonable time. Delaying to start on a task leads to piling up of a lot of important tasks to be done and will make us nervous and confused. This may lead to disorganization and multitasking which is often inefficient and detrimental. To avoid multitasking we should invest our valuable time in important tasks as early as possible.
5. **Not procrastinate**, procrastination is prevalent among medical professionals because of a lack of effective time management skills and a gradual loss of interest. Procrastination is a bad habit and hinders our personal and professional growth to a great extent. Once we start investing time in an important task, we should not leave it without completing it which gives meaning to our efforts and gives a sense of completion.

Balanced Diet

Stress is multiplied by continuous or intermittent anxiety states. Hence, managing anxiety is imperative in managing stress in day-to-day life. Our diet also contributes significantly to managing anxiety in our day-to-day life. We must have a comprehensive idea regarding various food items which can either increase or improve anxiety.

Foods Contributing to Anxiety and Stress

1. **Caffeine:** Many medical professionals frequently consume tea and coffee to stay alert in their busy work schedules. Moderate consumption of caffeine-containing beverages is part of professional life. However, it should be kept in mind that caffeine can stimulate the fear circuit and can cause or aggravate anxiety which can lead to stress. Furthermore, caffeine can significantly impair sleep which further aggravates anxiety and stress. So, it is prudent to limit our dependence on caffeine to stay alert, especially during evening hours.
2. **Alcohol:** Many medical professionals often consume alcohol on the weekend to get relaxation from a heavy work schedule throughout the week. However, alcohol consumption is relaxing only on a short-term basis. Regular intake of alcohol can significantly impair sleep quality and enhance anxiety during drug-free periods (when one is not intoxicated). Alcohol can also negatively impair the cognitive abilities and work capacity of an individual. Alcohol addiction causes significant distress to the individual and the family members and has a tremendous negative impact on the professional life of a doctor.
3. **Artificial sweeteners:** Artificial sweeteners, especially those derived from glutamate and aspartate, can significantly increase anxiety and stress. They don't have any dietary value and can alter gut bacteria leading to stomach upset and loss of appetite which significantly increases stress.

Foods Improving Anxiety and Stress

1. **Dietary fibers** have significant anti-inflammatory properties and also restore the health of gut microbiota. It is found that stress and anxiety are associated with substantial CNS and peripheral inflammation. Consumption of dietary fibers helps reduce inflammation and subsequently improves stress and anxiety.
2. **Polyunsaturated fatty acids** found in fish, seafood, and certain vegetables can also improve CNS inflammation, significantly improving stress and anxiety.
3. **Aged or fermented foods** such as yogurt are rich sources of probiotics that restore the gut microflora. There is significant evidence that the gut and CNS are intricately connected and mutually affect each other. Maintenance of healthy gut microbiota can significantly improve stress and anxiety which can be achieved with frequent consumption of aged and fermented foods such as yogurt.

Sleep Quality and Stress

Poor quality of sleep causes tremendous psychological and physical stress which impairs study and academic performance in medical students. Sleep problems may present with either increased latency time, frequent awakening from sleep, or poor subjective quality of sleep. Adoption of sleep hygiene can significantly improve sleep quality.

Sleep hygiene is defined as a set of behavioral modifications that improves sleep quality. Some do's and don't aspects of good sleep hygiene are described below.

1. **Use the bed for sleeping only** and don't use it for any other work, especially stressful work. Doing work full of stress such as thesis work, note taking, etc. while sitting in

bed can make stress get associated with bed (classical conditioning) which can make the bedroom environment non-relaxing that can affect sleep.

2. **Maintain a good sleep–wake cycle** by going to bed and waking in the morning on a stipulated schedule. An irregular sleep-wake cycle can disrupt the sleep cycle and impact the quality of sleep.
3. **Limit screen time** before going to bed and falling asleep. Blue light emitted by mobile and TV screens can disrupt the circadian rhythm and can delay the onset of sleep.
4. **Reading a storybook** to bed can relax the mind and help to fall asleep. Listening to an audiobook is even better in this gadget-oriented world.
5. **Practice relaxation**. Doing meditation, deep breathing, and other relaxing activities can cool the mind and body before going to sleep and helps in falling asleep quickly. However, doing strenuous exercise before bedtime can delay the onset of sleep and should be avoided.
6. **Limit tea and coffee before bedtime**. Stimulating substances such as caffeine in tea and coffee and tobacco in cigarettes can activate the mind and delay the onset of sleep and can negatively impact the quality of sleep. These stimulating substances should be avoided in the evening hours for a good night's sleep.

PRINCIPLES AND COMPONENTS OF LEARNING, MEMORY, EMOTION AND MOTIVATION

Principles of Learning

Principles of learning are based on the findings of experiments by **Ivan Pavlov**, **BF Skinner,** and **Albert Bandura** which are described below.

1. Classical Conditioning

Classical conditioning or respondent conditioning is also known as Pavlovian conditioning after the Russian physiologist Ivan Pavlov, who experimentally showed classical conditioning for the first time. After observing that the dog he was experimenting with (for the mechanism of digestion) starts salivating just seeing the experimenters even before the food was presented, he considered showing it experimentally. It is natural that when food is presented the dog starts salivating. He rang a bell before presenting food to the dog for a few days and observed that the dog now starts salivating upon hearing the ringing sound of the bell, even before the food was presented. He drew the following conclusion from this experiment.

A. Food is a natural stimulus that stimulates salivation and is known as an **unconditioned stimulus** (UC)

B. The ringing sound of a bell does not elicit any response by itself and is known as a **neutral stimulus**.

C. After **pairing** a neutral stimulus (ringing of a bell) with an unconditioned stimulus (food), the response (salivation) can be elicited by the neutral stimulus only, now the neutral stimulus is called a **conditioned stimulus**.

The theoretical aspect underlying classical conditioning is that there is an occurrence of **associative learning** on pairing Unconditioned stimulus with neutral stimulus for a few days. On exposure to the conditioned stimulus (after conditioning) the animal expects the natural stimulus and starts the response reflexly (expectation).

Classical conditioning can explain the development of some illnesses in psychiatry such as phobic disorder. In **phobic disorders,** a harmless stimulus gets associated with a harmful or threatening stimulus and subsequently elicits the fear response by itself (after conditioning). The urge to take an addictive substance (**craving**) when exposed to some cues (wine shop, friends, bottles, etc) is also thought to be due to classical conditioning.

2. Operant Conditioning

Apart from classical conditioning, associative learning can occur in some other ways which are known as operant conditioning. The conceptual framework on operant conditioning was developed by **Edward Thorndike** and subsequently expanded by **BF Skinner** with his famous experiments. Operant conditioning is nothing but a modification of the behavior of an animal by presenting them with rewards or punishments after the behavior. BF Skinner showed using rats, and pigeons as experimental animals, and a device known as Skinner's box that targets behavior (opening of the door of the box) can be encouraged or discouraged by giving a reward or punishment (respectively) after performing the behavior. For example, if the animals were presented with food (rewarding stimulus) after opening the door of the box, the probability of occurrence of the target behavior (opening of the door) is increased considerably. Similarly, if they are presented with some punishment (electric shock) on opening the box, the target behavior is seldom performed thereafter.

From this experiment, Skinner concluded that most of the behavior shown by an animal is learned through experiences. Behaviors get modified (increased or decreased) over time depending upon whether their performance leads to rewards or punishments.

A. **The reward** can be the addition of some pleasant stimulus (food) that reinforces the behavior, in which case it is known as **positive reinforcement**, or by removing some unpleasant stimulus, in which case it is known as **negative reinforcement**. Both positive and negative reinforcement encourages the target behavior, one under addition (positive) and another by subtraction (negative) respectively.

B. On the other hand, target behaviors can be discouraged by giving **punishment** just after the performance of the behavior. Punishment can be an addition of unpleasant stimuli (**positive punishment**) or the removal of pleasant stimulation (**negative punishment**). According to Skinner, any target behavior of an animal (or human) can be encouraged or discouraged by presenting them with rewards or punishments.

3. Social Learning Theory

Albert Bandura argued that learning all behaviors via personal experience is either not possible during a lifetime or too risky sometimes. He theorized that many of our behaviors are also learned by observing others in different situations which are known as social learning. He showed experimentally how children learn behavior by observing adults performing some action with his famous **'bobo doll'** experiment.

Application of Learning Theories

Principles of learning theories are widely applied in the treatment of various neurotic illnesses collectively known as **behavioral therapies**. These include **systematic desensitization**, **applied behavioral analysis,** and **contingency management** which are described in **Chapter 20.**

PRINCIPLES OF MEMORY

Definition

Memory is the **psychological process** of acquisition, storage, and retrieval of information. Memorizing events related to oneself and facts related to the outer world is an important aspect of one's life and gives special meaning to the life of an individual. Memories about various incidents in the life of an individual are sewn together to form a personal **mental autobiography** for the individual. Memory problems can have a tremendous impact on one's personal and social life as seen in cases of dementia.

Types of Memory

Memory can be classified into **different categories** based on the types of information stored or based on the period of its persistence.

Types of Memory Based on Types of Information Stored (Fig. 2.2)

1. **Implicit or procedural memory:** Procedural memory involves the acquisition and storage of **skilled motor activities** such as swimming, riding a bicycle, playing musical instruments, etc. Procedural memory is a function of the **cerebellum**, although, frequently modulated by inputs from the basal ganglia and cerebral cortex. One of the core characteristics of procedural memory is that once acquired it becomes **unconscious** and lasts for life.
2. **Explicit or declarative memory:** Declarative memory involves the acquisition and storage of memories about **personal events and real-world facts** and figures which can be **consciously recalled** from time to time. Declarative memory is a highly complex process and involves various steps such as encoding, storage, and retrieval, each of which is managed by various specialized regions of the brain. Declarative memory can be grouped into
   A. **Episodic or autobiographical memory** involves the acquisition and storage of **information related to oneself** such as birthdays, marriage anniversaries, days of personal achievement, etc. Episodic memories are sewn one after another to form a mental autobiography of a person and are one of the most important parts of the life of a person.
   B. **Semantic memory** involves the acquisition and storage of **information related to the real world** such as important facts and figures. Examples of semantic memory are memorizing when India got her independence, the highest mountain peak in the world, the value of pi, etc.

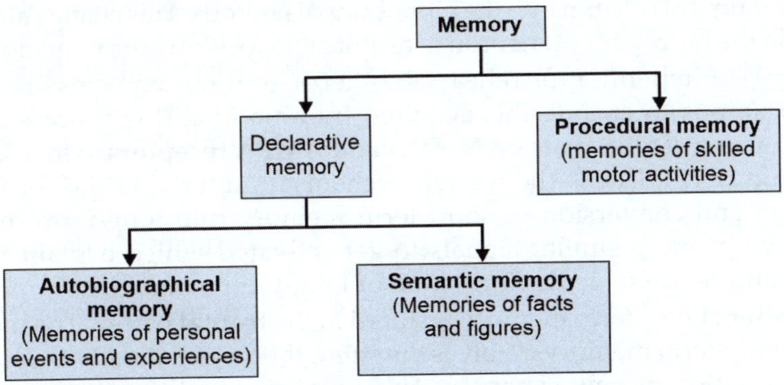

Fig. 2.2: Types of memory based on types of information stored

Types of Memory Based on the Duration of Persistence

Memory can also be grouped into the following three categories depending upon the period of storage of acquired information:

1. **Sensory memory:** Just after its bombardment, the sensory information (visual, auditory, or tactile) is retained almost in detail for a brief period. This retention of sensory information just for a brief period which is often vivid is known as sensory memory. Depending upon the sensory modality, sensory memory can be **iconic** (visual), **echoic** (auditory), or **haptic** (tactile). Sensory memory can only become short-term memory when we pay attention to it.
2. **Short-term memory:** Sensory memory can be retained for a **few seconds to a few minutes** when attention is focused on specific information. This form of memory which is retained for a few seconds to a few minutes is known as **short-term memory**. Short-term memory can be converted into long-term memory by a **deliberate rehearsal** of the information acquired.
   Working memory is a special type of short-term memory that helps us retain the required information on hand and carry out intended activities. Working memory also involves the manipulation of information. Remembering a phone number and dialing the numbers to call a friend is an example of working memory.
3. **Long-term memory:** Some memories are retained for months to years or for life and fall in this category. Short-term memory can be converted into long-term memory with **repetition or rehearsal.** Some emotionally loaded information can be directly converted into long-term and is known as **emotional memory**.

Memory Processes

Formation and use of memory involve following basic steps:

1. **Registration:** Registration involves the acquisition of information through special senses and their subsequent processing in the cerebral cortex. Information from special sense organs goes to the primary sensory cortices (parietal, occipital, and temporal cortices) and is then processed in the sensory association cortex. This processing of acquired information in the cerebral cortices is the basic neurological mechanism for sensory memory. From there, information now flows to the **hippocampus** where further encoding and consolidation occur.
   Information flowing from the sensory association cortex is further processed in the hippocampus which involves some molecular changes inside the hippocampal neurons such as the inflow of calcium into the hippocampal neurons. This change at the molecule level inside the hippocampal neuron is responsible for short-term memory.
2. **Encoding:** With repetition or rehearsal, other neural mechanisms are recruited in the hippocampus to encode this acquired information. This process involves the sequential action of glutamate on **NMDA and AMPA receptors** to invoke **long-term potentiation (LTP)**. LTP is the neural mechanism underlying the consolidation of information and conversion of short-term memory into long-term memory. LTP requires two or more similar signals to get activated which explain the need for repetition and rehearsal in the formation of long-term memory.
3. **Consolidation:** Long-term memory is stored in the **frontal cortex**. The mechanism of storage of long-term memory involves the strengthening of already existing synapses and the formation of new synapses. This involves repetitive rehearsal of already acquired information which invokes LTP in the hippocampal-frontal circuit which helps in the expression of genes involved in protein synthesis. These genes and their protein products result in the formation of new neuronal connections in the frontal cortex which stabilizes the stored information.

4. **Retrieval:** Retrieval is the process of reactivation of stored memory making it conscious from time to time. Retrieval is necessary for making use of stored memory and without retrieval memory has no useful purpose. Retrieval of a specific memory can occur without any clue (**free recall**) or after presentation with certain clues related to the memory (**cued recall**).

LTP: Neurobiological Basis of Memory

Long-term potentiation or LTP is a neurological phenomenon considered the biological basis of memory. LTP has been demonstrated extensively in the **hippocampal areas** associated with the encoding of memory.

LTP starts with a perceptual signal that activates the NMDA receptor in a neuron. However, for completion, LTP requires a second similar signal that activates the AMPA receptor on the same neuron. This sequential bombardment of two similar signals can lead to full-fledged LTP which results in the activation of genes leading to protein synthesis. This process of gene activation and subsequent protein synthesis is necessary for the strengthening of already existing neuronal connections and the formation of new connections among the neurons which are the biological basis of long-term memory.

PRINCIPLES OF EMOTION

Definition

Emotion is the inner feeling in response to some external events or stimuli that can color our perceptions, thoughts, and behaviors. Emotion has a subjective tonal quality (the inner feeling) and some objective physiological responses such as changes in heartbeats, respiration, muscle tension, etc.

Types of Emotion

Psychologist **Paul Eckman** identified 6 types of **basic emotions**: **Happiness, sadness, disgust, fear, surprise, and anger**. These basic types of emotions are similar across human societies and cultures. Another psychologist, **Robert Plutchik**, proposed that more complex or **synthetic emotions** can be generated by blending basic emotions. For example, the blending of happiness and surprise can form the emotion of joy. Other examples of synthetic emotions are love, affection, compassion, etc.

Theories of Emotions

Various theories of emotions try to explain both the subjective feelings and objective bodily changes associated with emotion. Some well-known theories of emotions are

1. **James–Lange theory:** This theory was developed independently by **William James and Carl Lange**. According to this theory, on exposure to an emotion-provoking situation, an individual experiences physiological reactions such as increased heart rate, perspiration, tremor, etc and it is the interpretation of these physiological changes by the individual that determines the specific emotion. For example, when an individual sees a bear in the woods he experiences palpitations, tremors, and perspiration; the individual interprets these changes as fear. According to this theory, different emotions elicit different bodily physiological changes, the interpretation of which results in specific emotional experiences. The James–Lange theory is particularly applicable in cases of panic attacks and phobias in which physiological changes occur without any stimulus but it is the interpretation of the physiological reaction as fearful that leads to panicky feelings.

2. **Cannon–Bard theory: Walter Cannon**, an American physiologist, criticized James-Lange's theory of emotion and stated that it is not the interpretation of bodily physiological changes that determine emotion as both emotional experience and bodily changes occur simultaneously and not one after the other. Along with his doctoral student **Philip Bard**, he developed a theory of emotion based on the activation of brain structures during emotion. According to this theory, whenever an individual is exposed to an emotion-provoking situation, there is an activation of the thalamus. Once the thalamus is activated, it sends signals to the cerebral cortex which is responsible for the subjective experience of emotion. Similarly, another signal is also sent to the body via a sympathetic pathway which is responsible for bodily changes associated with emotion such as palpitation, tremor, perspiration, etc. So, it is the activation of the cerebral cortex that primarily determines the emotion and bodily changes merely accompany them.
3. **Schachter–Singer two-factor theory: Schachter and Singer** put forward the first cognitive theory of emotion which is similar to the James–Lange theory. According to this theory, the physiological response to any emotion-provoking situation is the same and it is the individual's perception of the situation that determines the emotion. For example, both fearful and exciting situations evoke palpitation and tremor but it is the fearful situation (a bear in the wood) or exciting situation (seeing the same bear in a zoo) that determines the specific type of emotion felt by the individual. It should be noted that although Schachter-Singer's theory seems similar to James–Langes theory, the fundamental difference lies whether the interpretation of bodily sensations as in James–Langes theory or the interpretation of the situation as in Schachter–Singer theory which determines the emotional experience.

Neurobiology of Emotion

Emotion in humans is regulated by structures of the **limbic system**. Cortical limbic structures such as the **orbitofrontal cortex** are associated with the subject sensation of emotion. The **amygdala** is the primary center of emotional regulation and its extensive connection with other structures of the brain results in the full-fledged expression of emotions. Brain stem structures such as the locus coeruleus and parabrachial nucleus etc control the physiological response of emotions such as palpitation, tremor, and perspiration. These structures are stimulated by the amygdala in response to an emotional stimulus.

PRINCIPLES OF MOTIVATION

Definition

Motivation is the driving force that **activates specific behaviors**. It is the motivation that forces us to indulge in certain activities that define our behavior. Motivation is often modified by the biological, emotional, and social tendencies of an individual.

Types of Motivation

1. **Intrinsic vs extrinsic motivation:** Intrinsic motivation comes from the inside of an individual such as reading a book to gain knowledge only. On the other hand, extrinsic motivation comes from the outside environment such as taking part in a running competition to win a trophy.
2. **Conscious vs unconscious motivation:** Motives about which we are well aware and the reason behind is clear are known as conscious motivations, e.g. taking part in a

competitive exam. On the other hand, unconscious motivations are hidden and we are not always aware of them and the reason behind them is unclear, e.g. choosing a life partner.

Components of Motivation

Motivation had the following three basic components:

1. **Initiation** is the decision an individual makes to indulge in a particular behavior.
2. **Persistence** is the continuous efforts put by the individual to remain indulged in that particular behavior initiated by him despite various obstacles faced.
3. **Intensity** is the amount of effort put in by the individual to achieve a specific goal.

Theories of Motivation

Theories of motivations are categorized as content theories and process theories and are described below.

A. Content Theories

1. ***Maslow's hierarchy of needs:*** In the year 1943, American psychologist Abraham Maslow put forward one of the best-known theories of motivation, famously known as Maslow's hierarchy of needs. According to his theory, motivation arises from an animal's endeavor to fulfill certain needs which progress from basic needs to complex needs as described below (Fig. 2.3).

   a. **Physiological needs** are basic needs that are essential for the survival of the individual. These include food, water, air, etc. which are needed for the maintenance of bodily homeostasis.

   b. **Safety and security needs** are a bit more complex than physiological needs. These needs are not essential but are generally needed for the survival of the individual in adverse environmental conditions. These include safety against predators, financial security, maintenance of good health, etc.

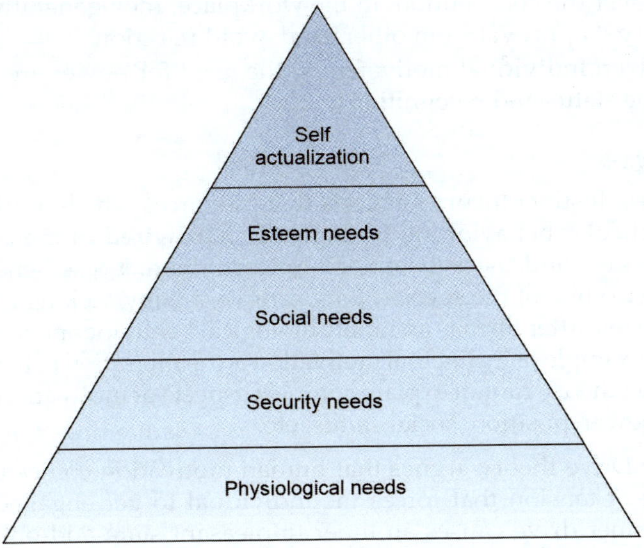

Fig. 2.3: Maslow's hierarchy of needs.

c. **Social needs** include friendship, romantic relationships, family relationships, community belongingness, etc. These needs are pursued for finding love, acceptance, and belongingness.
d. **Esteem needs** are more complex and are pursued only after meeting the basic needs described above. This includes professional and academic achievement, involvement in philanthropic activities, pursuing passion and hobbies, etc. Fulfillment of these needs gives a sense of self-satisfaction and a sense of contribution to society leading to appreciation by others. These needs increase the self-esteem and personal worth of an individual.
e. **Self-actualization needs** are the highest level of needs and are pursued by a few individuals only. It involves the full exploitation of one's potential, capabilities, and opportunities for personal growth and the betterment of humankind.

2. ***Aldefer's ERG theory:*** **Clayton Alderfer** further elaborated Maslow's theory of need and categorized all these needs into three domains: existence, relatedness, and growth. The existence domain includes basic physiological and safety needs, the relatedness domain includes social and relationship needs and the growth domain includes esteem needs and self-actualization.

3. ***McClelland's need theory:*** Psychologist David McClelland argued that motivation for human behaviors comes from the will to fulfill three needs. These needs as described by him are:
a. **Need for achievement:** Individuals motivated by a need for achievement are practical and put a great deal of faith in their performance and hard work. They are generally consistent with their work and indulge in activities associated with the promotion and personal growth. They generally prefer to get involved in work with moderate risk as they believe work with low risk is less desirable and work with high risk is a matter of luck rather than hard work.
b. **Need for affiliation:** Individuals motivated by a need for affiliation get themselves involved in socialization, group activities, and collaboration. They prefer collaborative group work over the competition. In the workplace, they generally adhere to rules and norms to get approval from others and avoid rejection.
c. **Need for power:** Individual motivated by the need for power are competitive and always pursue status and recognition.

B. Process Theories

1. ***Instinct theory:*** Instinct theory suggests that the forces which motivate a person to engage in a particular behavior are **biologically hardwired** in the person under the evolutionary process and there is no need to learn them. These behaviors are innate and ensure the survival of the species. For example, a baby seeking a mother's nipple for nourishment just after birth is an innate biological behavior and is not learned from others. Another example of instinctual motivation is the migration of birds before winter. However, instinct theory cannot explain complex aspects of motivation in humans such as striving for power, position, social status, etc.

2. ***Drive theory:*** Drive theory argues that human motivation comes from some inner drive or feeling of tension that forces the individual to get engaged in a particular behavior. This inner drive causes an inner unpleasant state and only after fulfilling the need initiated by the drive, the person feels satisfied. For example, when a person

feels hungry he engages in eating behavior to satiate. Almost all basic human behaviors such as eating, drinking, mating, etc. and some complex behaviors such as the need for power and status can be explained by drive theory. However, drive theory cannot explain such behavior as riding a roller coaster. Why are individuals interested in riding a roller coaster although it does not fulfill any inner drive?

3. ***Arousal theory:*** According to arousal theory, individuals are engaged in specific behaviors to maintain an optimum level of **physiological arousal**. This optimum state of arousal varies from person to person. Whenever a person feels low, he engages himself in some exciting activities like going out, partying, riding a roller coaster, etc. On the other hand, if the person feels overstimulated, he engages in some relaxing activities like taking a nap, sitting calmly on a chair, listening to music, etc. So, people are engaged in activities to maintain an optimum physiological arousal state which determines the motivation to engage in a specific behavior. As we see, this theory nicely explains why we go for a roller coaster ride!

Neurobiology of Motivation

The reward circuit which projects from **VTA** (ventral tegmental area) to **NAc** (nucleus accumbens) in the limbic system is primarily concerned with motivation (*see* Fig. 5.1). Dopamine is the chemical secreted in this circuit and the action of dopamine on the NAc results in the sensation of pleasure. Any kind of activity which activates this reward circuit with the secretion of dopamine is desirable due to the pleasure sensation associated with it and makes the animal indulge in such activities.

CONCEPT OF NORMALITY AND ABNORMALITY

There is ongoing fierce debate on deciding what is normal and what is abnormal, especially in psychiatry. What may appear normal in certain situations may be regarded as abnormal in another situation. For example, in a normal civilized society, cruelty toward animals and aggression in adolescents may be considered abnormal; however, in certain African nomadic tribes, these traits are considered perfectly normal and desirable. Another example is the maintenance of the low body weight which may be considered abnormal in the community; however, is highly desired and praised in the modeling profession.

It is quite difficult to assess and decide what is normal. In a broader term, a normal individual maintains a consistent level of functioning over a while and must:

1. Be able to experience the existence of self and the world around him.
2. Be able to perceive the environment and react accordingly
3. Be able to communicate with the use of language, gestures, and symbols
4. Be able to make and carry out social and personal relationships
5. Be able to empathize and can see the world from other's perspectives
6. Be able to understand the values, norms, and ethics of the society

There is much debate in deciding when normality ceases to exist and abnormality sets in. **DSM-5** has devised an ingenious criterion of '**significant impairment in socio-occupational functioning of the individual**' as a trademark to distinguish abnormality from normal behavior and it is included in every diagnosis mentioned in DSM-5. According to DSM-5, nothing is abnormal unless it causes significant impairment in the socio-occupational well-being of an individual.

In psychiatry, it is very difficult to draw a line between normality and abnormality causing widespread controversy regarding various psychiatric diagnoses. Many activists involved in the antipsychiatry movement are rejecting psychiatric illnesses arguing them as normal variations in human behavior. For example, according to these activists, hyperactivity and impulsivity in ADHD and poor socialization in Autism is regarded just as normal variations in childhood development and should not be considered illnesses and there is no need for treatment. However, it should be remembered that psychiatric conditions are real and are causing tremendous problems in the life of the sufferers, and treating these illnesses can significantly improve the quality of life of these individuals.

SUMMARY

1. Stress is defined as any change which evokes psychological, physical, and/or emotional reactions in an individual. Stress can be classified as acute, chronic, or episodic stress.
2. When an individual is exposed to stress he develops certain psychological, emotional, physical, and behavioral changes collectively known as stress reactions.
3. Positive coping skills such as self-care, following a passion or hobby, physical exercise, practicing relaxation, etc can help effectively handle stress in life.
4. Memory is the psychological process of acquisition, storage, and retrieval of information and is classified as sensory, short term and long-term memory. Furthermore, procedural memory involves the acquisition of motor skills while declarative memory involves consciously memorizing facts and figures.
5. The neurobiology of memory involves encoding, consolidation, stabilization, and retrieval processes. Hippocampus is the most important brain area involved in memory formation.
6. Emotion is the inner feeling in response to some external stimuli which color our perception, thought, and behavior. Emotions can be primary (fear, happiness, anger, etc) or synthetic emotions such as love and compassion.
7. Theories of emotion include the James-Lange theory, the Cannon-Bard theory, and the Schachter-Singer theory. According to Schachter-Singer's theory, which is the most accepted one, it is the individual's perception of the situation which determines the emotion.
8. Motivation is the driving force underlying the specific behavior shown by an organism. Various theories of motivation are Maslow's hierarchy of needs, Alderfer's ERG theory, McClelland's need theory, intrinsic theory, drive theory, and arousal theory
9. The concept of normality in psychiatry is a bit controversial and is widely debated. As per DSM-5, nothing is considered a disorder unless it causes significant impairment in the socio-occupational functioning of an individual.

BIBLIOGRAPHY

1. Anisman H, Merali Z. Understanding stress: characteristics and caveats. Alcohol Res Health. 1999;23(4):241–9.
2. Algorani EB, Gupta V. Coping Mechanisms. [Updated 2022 Apr 28]. In: StatPearls [Internet]. Treasure Island (FL): StatPearls Publishing; 2022 Jan.
3. Fowler A, Whitehurst K, Al Omran Y, Rajmohan S, Udeaja Y, Koshy K, Gundogan B. How to study effectively. Int J Surg Oncol (N Y). 2017 Jul;2(6):e31.
4. Porta CR, Anderson MR, Steele SR. Effective time management: surgery, research, service, travel, fitness, and family. Clin Colon Rectal Surg. 2013 Dec;26(4):239–43.
5. Naidoo U. Eat to Beat Stress. Am J Lifestyle Med. 2020 Dec 8;15(1):39–42.
6. Irish LA, Kline CE, Gunn HE, Buysse DJ, Hall MH. The role of sleep hygiene in promoting public health: A review of empirical evidence. Sleep Med Rev. 2015 Aug;22:23–36.

7. Rossiter, J. Learning Theory Principles for Psychotherapy. *Psychology*, 2022;**13**:743–66.
8. Camina E and Guell F. The Neuroanatomical, Neurophysiological, and Psychological Basis of Memory: Current Models and Their Origins. *Front. Pharmacol*, 2017;8:438.
9. Šimi G, Tkal i M, Vuki V, Mulc D, Špani E, Šagud M, Olucha-Bordonau FE, Vukši M, R Hof P. Understanding Emotions: Origins and Roles of the Amygdala. Biomolecules. 2021 May 31;11(6):823.
10. Izard CE. Emotion theory and research: highlights, unanswered questions, and emerging issues. Annu Rev Psychol. 2009;60:1–25.
11. Morgan CT and King RA. Introduction to psychology, 1966. (3rd ed.). McGraw-Hill.
12. Oyebode F. Sims' symptoms in the mind: Textbook of descriptive psychopathology. (2015). (6th ed.). Elsevier Saunders.

Chapter 3

Introduction to Psychiatry

Competency achievement: Students should be able to

1. **PS3.1** Describe the growth of psychiatry as a medical specialty, its history, and its contribution to society
2. **PS3.12** Describe, discuss and distinguish psychotic and non-psychotic (mood, anxiety, stress-related) disorders
3. **PS3.2** Enumerate, describe, and discuss important signs and symptoms of common mental disorders
4. **PS3.3** Elicit, present and document history in patients presenting with a mental disorder
5. **PS3.4** Describe the importance of establishing rapport with patients
6. **PS3.5** Perform, demonstrate, and document a mental status examination
7. **PS3.6** Describe and discuss biological, psychological and social factors and their interactions in the causation of mental disorders

INTRODUCTION

An introduction to psychiatry seems lame without discussing the history of psychiatry and its growth. Furthermore, understanding the basic concept of neurosis and psychosis is a prerequisite before learning about major psychiatric illnesses such as schizophrenia, mania, and depression. It is also important to have some idea about prevalent classification systems in psychiatry as preliminary learning.

HISTORY OF PSYCHIATRY

The earliest mentions of mental illnesses can be found in **Indian Ayurvedic texts** such as ***Charaka Samhita***. As early as the 4th century BCE, **Hippocrates** theorized that mental illnesses could be due to physiological disturbances in the body. Such philosophical ideas are considered breakthroughs in an age when mental illnesses were considered as acts of evil spirits and possession. In those days, proper medical treatment for mental illnesses was lacking and patients were treated via religious ways such as exorcism.

The earliest history of **the institutional treatment** of psychiatric patients can be traced back to 9th century **Baghdad** where psychiatric wards were attached to general hospitals known as ***Bimaristan***. The first **psychiatric asylum** was opened in **Bethlehem in England** in the early fifteenth century. Psychiatric asylums were relatively humane institutions for psychiatric patients as they were free to roam around within its boundary and were provided with good food and living conditions. Still, some patients were chained and proper medical treatment was virtually absent. With the start of the **renaissance movement**, more humane treatments, similar to treatment for patients of other medical illnesses, were demanded for patients by intellectuals. With this comes the concept of opening **psychiatric wards in general hospitals** and asylums were gradually closed.

Emil Kraepelin was among the first to propose a **classification of psychotic illnesses** into ***dementia praecox* and *manic depressive insanity*. A modern classification system** of psychiatric illnesses came into being in the form of **DSM**-1 (Diagnostic and Statistical Manual for mental disorders) in **1952** published by the **American Psychiatric Association**. The first criteria-based diagnostic formulation was introduced in **DSM-III** in **1980**. A chapter on the classification of mental and behavioral disorders was first added to **ICD-6 published in 1949 by WHO**.

In the late nineteenth and early twentieth century, an **induced seizure** was the treatment of choice for psychotic illnesses such as schizophrenia. Before the advent of ECT, a seizure was induced by **camphor injection** or insulin-induced hypoglycemia, both of which were dangerous. **Electrically induced** seizure in the form of **ECT** was developed by **Lucio Bini** and **Ugo Cerletti** in the year **1938**. ECT was both safe and effective for psychotic illnesses but its response is short lasting. In those days, **psychoanalysis** was the treatment of choice for **neurotic illnesses.**

A breakthrough in the pharmacological treatment of psychiatric illnesses, especially schizophrenia, and mania, occurred **in the year 1951** with the discovery of the antipsychotic properties of **chlorpromazine**. Following this, other antipsychotic agents differing from one another in their potency and side effects were subsequently developed. The **first atypical antipsychotic 'clozapine'** was introduced in **1970** followed by other atypical antipsychotics such as risperidone, olanzapine, and amisulpride.

With the advent of antipsychotic medications, gradually their mechanism of action was elucidated paving the way for the **neurotransmitter hypothesis** of psychiatric illnesses. First, the **dopamine hypothesis** was proposed followed by the serotonin and glutamate hypothesis for schizophrenia. The neurotransmitter hypothesis was extrapolated and similar hypotheses were also proposed for other psychiatric illnesses such as the **serotonin hypothesis** for depression and anxiety disorders.

NEUROSIS VS PSYCHOSIS

Psychiatric illnesses are broadly classified into two categories: psychoses and neuroses. The term neurosis was coined by English physician William Cullen to denote a group of illnesses which arise due to unequal state of excitement or collapse of the nervous system. He also included mental illnesses in this category. However, Karl Friedrich Constatt coined the term psychosis as an abbreviation for 'psychic-neurosis' for illnesses that affect the mind which were previously included under the broader category of neuroses, to distinguish them from illnesses of the brain. Subsequently, diseases of the CNS arising due to some pathology such as dementia and seizure disorders were removed from neurotic spectrum leaving only psychiatric illnesses arising due to stress or emotional disturbances in this category. Even if the dichotomy of psychoses and neuroses is controversial, still it is a very basic concept to learn in psychiatry.

Psychosis is the principal defining feature of psychiatric illnesses grouped under psychoses such as schizophrenia, mania, delusional disorders, etc. Psychosis is defined by following three **characteristic features:**

1. **Lack of insight**
2. **Loss of reality contact** and
3. **Loss of ego boundary**

Insight

Insight is defined as **awareness about one's illness**. The patient must understand the nature of the illness and must understand that the symptoms are because of the illness he is suffering from. A mere enumeration of symptoms does not signify the presence of insight. For example, a patient with schizophrenia may complain about hearing voices and suspecting others of malevolent intentions; however, this is not considered intact insight. For the insight to be considered intact, he must understand that these symptoms are because of some mental illness and there is a need for treatment. Insight can be **graded as**

1. **Grade I or No insight** (patient altogether denies having any illness).
2. **Grade II or Some insight** (sometimes accepts having some illness and sometimes denies).
3. **Grade III** (Attributing symptoms to **physical illness** or **outside factors** such as acts of spirits).
4. **Grade IV or Intellectual insight** (understands the illness and the need for treatment).
5. **Grade V or True emotional insight** (fully understands the illness, its impact on personal well-being, and its ramification on near and dear ones).

Reality Contact

Reality contact is maintained through the processes of **perception, cognition,** and **conation**. Various stimuli from the surrounding environment are gathered via sense organs through the process of **perception**. This information obtained via sense organs is processed in the CNS which is known as **cognition. Conation** is the process of reacting to external stimuli appropriately.

Any disturbance in perception, cognition, or conation is considered an **impairment in reality contact. Hallucination**, which is defined as perception without any stimulus, is a **disturbance of sensory perception**. Likewise, **delusions** defined as false and firm belief arises from **information misprocessing** fall within the domain of **distorted cognition. Disorganized behaviors** are examples of **disturbance in conation**. Therefore, the presence of hallucinations, delusions, and/or disorganized behavior signifies impairment in reality contact.

Ego Boundary

The ego boundary is defined as the perceived boundary of the **subjective self.** Every individual has a subjective idea of self, regarding what is **'me'** and what is **beyond me**. Claims of being possessed by a spirit or thought insertion and withdrawal are considered as a breach in the ego boundary of the individual.

The presence of any one of the characteristic features of psychosis is sufficient for a psychiatric illness to be labeled as a psychotic illness. In **neurotic illnesses** such as anxiety disorders, phobias, OCD, etc. insight is generally present and there is no impairment in reality contact and ego boundary.

INDIAN SYSTEM OF PSYCHIATRIC CLASSIFICATION

A system of classification of psychiatric illness has been proposed by various authors **(Wig and Singh)** to suit the Indian context. However, it has only academic and historical significance as current systems of classification mentioned in **ICD-10** (international classification of diseases for mental and behavioral disorders, 10th edition) and **DSM-5** (diagnostic and statistical manual of mental disorders, 5th edition) are in widespread use.

The Indian System of Classification

A. Psychoses

1. Functional
   a. Schizophrenia
      - Simple schizophrenia
      - Paranoid schizophrenia
2. Affective
   a. Mania
   b. Depression
3. Organic
   a. Acute
   b. Chronic

B. Neuroses

1. Anxiety neurosis
2. Depressive neurosis
3. Hysterical neurosis
4. Obsessive compulsive neurosis
5. Phobic neurosis

C. Special Disorders

1. Childhood disorders
   a. Conduct disorder
   b. Emotional disorders
2. Personality disorders
   a. Sociopath
   b. Psychopath
3. Substance abuse
   a. Alcohol abuse
   b. Other drugs abuse
4. Psychophysiological disorders
   a. Asthma
   b. Psoriasis

D. Mental Retardation

1. Mild
2. Moderate
3. Severe
4. Profound

PSYCHIATRIC INTERVIEW

Introduction

Psychiatric evaluation generally covers two important domains: history taking and mental status examination. Psychiatric history is the subjective information obtained directly from the patient or the person accompanying him (a family member, a friend, a co-worker, etc.). The mental status examination or MSE is the psychiatric counterpart of the physical examination carried out in other branches of medicine. MSE is often considered the jewel of psychiatric interviews. MSE is the objective tool used by the interviewer to obtain information about the current psychiatric illness.

A good psychiatric history has the following parts.

1. **Patient's particulars** include such personal information as name, age, sex, marital status, religion, ethnicity, locality, etc. After knowing the name, the patient should be called by his/her name throughout the interview period. Marital status, religion, ethnicity, etc have special bearings on the development of psychiatric illnesses and should be noted meticulously.
2. **Informant:** Reliability and adequacy of the information.

   As psychotic patients seldom reveal the symptoms themselves, detailed history regarding the evolution of symptoms should be taken from the persons accompanying the patient who is known as informants in psychiatric terminology. Close family members such as parents, spouses, and siblings generally give the most reliable and adequate information.
3. **Chief complaints:** The symptoms for which the patient has been brought to psychiatric care are known as chief complaints. Evaluation of chief complaints should be with open-ended questions such as 'what brings you here or 'how can I help you'. Open-ended questions involving what, how, when, etc. should be the standard for the evaluation of psychiatric symptoms. Subsequently, closed-ended questions may be asked to probe further into the detail of the symptoms. Unlike in other medical specialties in which chief complaints are very few, in psychiatry, all chief complaints should be mentioned in chronological order which can be many.
4. **History of present illness:** The onset of the symptoms and their gradual evolution over the period should be evaluated in detail. Aggravating and relieving factors are also to be evaluated. The course of an illness whether it is continuous or episodic, gradually deteriorating or relapsing-remitting in nature should be carefully elucidated. History of any kind of treatment taken for the current illness and response to it is to be assessed.

   It should be remembered that impairment in a patient's biological functions should be asked and noted which are frequently missed by the informant. **Biological functions** are evaluated in the following context.

   A. Sleep
   B. Appetite
   C. Bowel and bladder functions
   D. Self-care and
   E. Sexual functions
5. **History of past psychiatric illness:** The occurrence of the same psychiatric illness or any other psychiatric illnesses in the past must be enquired about. Some psychiatric illnesses such as BPAD are episodic in nature and the patient becomes completely

symptom-free in between the episodes. The circumstances in which the past episode occurred, duration of the illness, psychiatric treatment taken and period for which medications were taken are also needed to be asked.

Apart from the history of similar illnesses, the history of any other psychiatric illnesses and the circumstances surrounding them are also useful.

6. **History of medical illness:** It comes under the purview of current medical history. Any non-psychiatric illnesses the patient is suffering from must be enquired about. Such long-standing illnesses as diabetes mellitus, hypertension, chronic kidney disease, chronic heart ailments, etc have special places in the occurrence of certain psychiatric illnesses and for treatment decision-making. For example, depression and anxiety are more common in patients with comorbid long-standing illnesses such as diabetes mellitus. Similarly, the presence of DM and hypertension are contraindications for use of some second-generation antipsychotics such as clozapine and olanzapine.
7. **Family history:** Most psychiatric illnesses are genetically determined to a good extent. Hence, the presence of the same psychiatric illness in other family members adds to diagnosing a case and also helps in deciding a management plan as a response to treatment is also genetically determined. The presence of other medical illnesses such as DM and HTN is also helpful in prudent treatment decision-making.

   Family history also includes information about family members, the closeness between family members, economic and living conditions, knowledge and attitude about the illness among the family members, etc.
8. **Birth and early developmental history:** A good birth history includes a history of any risk factor during pregnancy, time and term of birth, place of delivery, the procedure of delivery (normal or instrumental), birth cry and any complication during delivery, any illness during infancy, etc. All these factors have special implications for the development of psychiatric illnesses, especially neurodevelopmental disorders such as intellectual disability, autism, ADHD, and schizophrenia.

   Timing and acquisition of developmental milestones in the following domains should be meticulously evaluated.

   a. Gross motor development
   b. Fine motor development
   c. Language development and
   d. Social development
9. **Sexual history:** A proper sexual history should encompass attainment of puberty (starting of menstruation in girls and acquisition of secondary sexual characters in boys), personal reaction to first menstruation in girls, source of acquisition of sexual knowledge, sexual identity and orientation, any sexual contact (both penetrative and non-penetrative) and reaction to first sexual experience, the general attitude toward sexuality, etc.
10. **Personal history:** Personal history includes the educational status of the patient, source of income, Job satisfaction, marital status, marital relationship, relation with children, etc.
11. **History of substance abuse:** History of substance abuse is very crucial in psychiatry as many substances of abuse can induce psychiatric illnesses and the presence of psychiatric illness makes the patient prone to develop substance abuse behavior. The type of substance being abused, duration of abuse, whether the patient has developed dependence, etc. should be enquired about.

12. **Premorbid personality:** The overall personality of the patient before the development of the illness is known as premorbid personality. The most important aspect of personality is whether the person is an extrovert or an introvert. Extrovert persons are more prone to develop mood disorders such as depression and BPAD while introverts are more prone to develop schizophrenia and anxiety disorders. Other aspects of premorbid personality are the ways of handling stress, coping skills of the individual, socialization, religiousness, belief in god, etc.

MENTAL STATUS EXAMINATION

The mental status examination is the equivalent of a physical examination in other medical specialties and is considered the jewel **of a psychiatric interview**. MSE starts as soon as the patient enters the interview room starting with observing the attire, gait, and behavior of the patient. MSE has the following headings:

General Appearance

General appearances such as dressing and attire, body build and gait, and the presence of abnormal movements should be carefully noted. The attire or dressing of the patient may be appropriate or inappropriate, adequate or inadequate. Psychotic patients tend to wear inappropriate clothes; for example, manic patients wear fancy and stylish clothes while schizophrenic patients generally wear dirty worn out, or baggy clothes.

The body build and gait of the patient should be observed as soon as the patient enters the room. Built can be of three types such as **ectomorphic** (thin built), **endomorphic** (floppy built), and **mesomorphic** (muscular built). Ectomorphic individuals are more prone to develop anxiety neurosis and schizophrenic psychosis while endomorphic people are prone to develop mood disorders such as depression and bipolar disorder.

Another important aspect to be noticed during the initial evaluation is whether the patient is maintaining good **eye-to-eye contact** or not. Good eye-to-eye contact helps in building **rapport** with the patient. Poor eye-to-eye contact and poor rapport establishment indicate a diagnosis of psychotic disorders such as schizophrenia.

Psychomotor activity is another important point to be noted during an initial evaluation. Patients with increased psychomotor activity are often restless and inattentive which is seen in anxiety, delirium, and mania. The decreased psychomotor activity makes the patient lethargic and slow as seen in depression.

The presence of abnormal movements such as stereotyped movements, mannerisms, tremors, dyskinetic movements, and features of EPS (extrapyramidal symptoms), etc. should be noted. **A stereotype** is defined as purposeless repetitive movement (abnormal wrist movement) while **mannerism** is a repetitive movement that is apparently purposeful (waving of hands, saluting, etc.). **Extrapyramidal symptoms** such as resting tremor, bradykinesia, akinesia, etc. arise as side effects of antipsychotic treatment. **Echolalia** (patient repeating words spoken by the interviewer), **palilalia** (patient repeating his own words again and again), and **echopraxia** (patient imitates the movements and gestures of the interviewer) may be seen in schizophrenia and organic mental illnesses such as dementia.

Mood and Affect

The mood is defined as the **persistent emotional feeling tone** perceived by the person himself and is subjective in nature. Mood can be sad, happy, irritable, etc. Persistent feeling of sadness (depressed mood) is the characteristic feature of depressive disorders while a euphoric or irritable mood is seen in manic episodes.

Affect is the external manifestation of subjective mood via **facial expressions**. Affect can be appropriate to the mood state or inappropriate to the mood state. The inappropriate affect is generally seen in patients with schizophrenia and other psychotic disorders. Another important aspect of affect is its range of expression. When the patient can express all the repertoire of affects, the range is said to be normal. In the case of restricted affect the patient can express only a limited range of emotions. Restricted affect can be restricted toward depression (as seen in depressive disorders) or elation (as seen in mania). Blunt or flat affect is a lack of facial expression and is usually seen in cases of schizophrenia.

Speech

Speech is assessed in terms of coherence, relevance, spontaneity, reaction time, volubility, and prosody of speech.

When speech is not understandable, it is known as **incoherent speech**. Incoherent speech is mainly found in delirium but can be a feature of disorganized schizophrenia. When speech is understandable but is not in the context of the question asked, it is known as irrelevant speech which is a feature of schizophrenia (**loosening of association**).

Another important aspect of speech is **reaction time** which signifies how promptly the patient is replying to the queries. Reaction time is decreased in manic patients while it is increased in cases of depression.

The prosody of speech means the presence of melody in speech and the loss of prosody can make the speech monotonous. Monotonous speech is generally found in depression.

Thought

A Patient's thought process can be inferred from the speech of the patient. Thought disturbance can be grouped into the following headings

1. ***The flow of thought*** is the speed at which words are expressed while speaking. Disturbances in the flow of thought can be present as

a. **Flight of ideas** is seen in manic patients as ideas and thoughts come into the mind at a rapid pace in these patients. This results in speech production at a tremendous speed as if coming with pressure (**pressure of speech**) with high volubility. The patient may jump rapidly from one topic to another but the topics are interrelated (either via theme or via clang association). **Prolixity** is a less severe variation of flight of ideas and is seen in patients with hypomania.

b. **Thought blocking** is the sudden break in the train of thought and the patient explains it as if his mind went blank without any ideas coming into it. Thought blocking is characteristically seen in schizophrenia.

c. **Circumstantiality** is the over-inclusion of minor details of every aspect of a topic while speaking, making it elaborate and boring. It is seen in patients with OCD and OC personality disorder.

d. **Tangentiality** is often confused with circumstantiality. However, in tangentiality, the patient just touches the relevant topic once and deviates away never to return to the original topic. (Analogous to a tangent touching a circle just at the point of origin only).

e. **Perseveration** is defined as failure to proceed beyond the initial response to changing stimuli with repetition of the initial response again and again. For example, the patient answers correctly when his name is asked but tells his name only to every question asked thereafter.

2. ***Content of thought:*** Delusion is included in the disturbance of the content of thought. Delusion is defined as a false and firm belief that persists even after there is evidence to the contrary and it is not shared by people from the same sociocultural background. Delusion is seen in psychotic disorders such as schizophrenia, mania, delusional disorders, etc. Some common delusions seen among psychiatric patients are:

a. **Delusion of persecution**, the patient believes that people are conspiring against him. Persecutory delusion is the most common type of delusion in schizophrenia.
b. **Delusion of reference**, the patient believes that people are talking about him which is also commonly seen in schizophrenia.
c. **Delusion of grandiosity**, most commonly seen in manic patients, a delusion of grandiosity may involve following themes.
   - Power
   - Possession or value
   - Position or identity and
   - Relation
d. **In the delusion of guilt**, the patient believes that he has done an unpardonable sin. Delusion of guilt is seen commonly in depressive disorders.
e. **Delusion of theft**, the patient believes that people are trying to snatch his property. It is seen commonly in patients with dementia.
f. **Delusion of morbid jealousy**, the patient believes that one's spouse is being unfaithful to him/her. It is commonly found in patients with paranoid schizophrenia, delusional disorder, and alcohol-induced psychosis.
g. **Delusion of nihilism**, the patient believes that he is dead or dying, the world has come to end or a part of him is dead and rotting. It is commonly seen in patients with psychotic depression and organic psychosis.
h. **Bizarre delusions**, logically impossible beliefs. Bizarre delusions are characteristic of schizophrenia. (Once a schizophrenic patient refused to pass urine even if his bladder was painfully distended, as he believed that he may cause a severe flood and devastation just by passing urine!)

   The presence of **hopelessness, helplessness, worthlessness, and suicidal ideas** as seen in cases of depression are also categorized as disturbances of the content of thought.

3. ***Possession of thought:*** Thought insertion thought withdrawal and thought broadcasting are disturbances of possession of thought commonly seen in schizophrenia. In **thought insertion**, the patient claims that his thoughts are not his thoughts and are being inserted by an outside agent or force. In **thought withdrawal,** the patient claims that his thoughts are being withdrawn from him and are coming to be known by others. In **thought broadcasting**, the patient claims that his ideas and thoughts are being known by everyone and are also being broadcasted on radio, television, and via print media.

Obsessive thoughts also fall within the disturbances in the possession of thought. Obsessive thoughts are defined as repetitive intrusive thoughts that come into the mind even if there is resistance to prevent them and cause distress or discomfort. However, these thoughts are recognized by the patient as his thoughts and have not been inserted by any outside agent or force. Obsessive thoughts are characteristic features of obsessive-compulsive disorder.

4. ***Form of thought*:** Disturbance in the form of thought is known as formal thought disorder and is commonly seen in schizophrenia and organic brain disorders. In schizophrenia, the thought is concrete and lacks abstract quality.

According to Schneider, a healthy thought has the following qualities.

a. **Constancy:** A healthy thought should be complete by itself and does not change its context unless consciously done so.
b. **Organization:** Healthy thinking is well organized with all its components logically related to one another.
c. **Continuity**: There must be a sense of continuity in the expression of a healthy thought

Schneider identified 5 formal thought disorders frequently seen in patients with psychosis

a. **Derailment:** In a derailment, the thought slides on another thought which is not logically related to the former one.
b. **Substitution:** In substitution, a major thought is substituted by a subsidiary thought making the expression concrete.
c. **Omission:** Characterized by the senseless omission of a thought or a part of it.
d. **Fusion:** In fusion, heterogeneous elements of thought are fused making the speech incoherent.
e. **Driveling**: There is a distorted intermixture of constituent parts of a complex thought making the expression understandable but irrelevant.

Neologism (novel words) is also considered a formal thought disorder in which the patent invents new words and terms for already existing things which is sensible to him only. Neologism is usually seen in schizophrenia.

Perceptual Disturbances

1. **Illusion** is the false interpretation of a real stimulus (interpreting a rope as a snake due to poor visibility). Illusion has no psychopathological importance.
2. **Pareidolia** is suddenly seeing forms and images in ambiguous stimuli (seeing a face in the clouds). Pareidolia also has no psychopathological importance.
3. **Hallucination** is defined as perception occurring without any stimulus and is perceived outside the subjective space as vividly as a real stimulus. Hallucination can occur in any sensory modalities and is accordingly categorized as visual, auditory, gustatory, olfactory, and tactile hallucinations. Auditory hallucinations are commonly seen in schizophrenia and other functional psychoses. The presence of visual hallucination indicates organicity (e.g. dementia or delirium) and should be evaluated accordingly.
4. **Pseudohallucination** is perception emanating from inside the subjective space of the individual. A patient complaining of hearing voices inside his head is considered to have pseudohallucination.

Assessment of Cognitive Functions

Cognitive functions are **higher mental functions** that fall under the purview of cortical functions. Following cognitive functions should be assessed during the psychiatric interview

1. **Orientation** is assessed by checking the orientation of the patient to person, place, and time and the sequence should be maintained.
2. **Attention and concentration** are assessed together by **digit forward and digit backward tests**. The digits are presented in groups of 2, 3, and 4…digits, and the patient is asked to recall them either in the same order (**digit forward test**) or in reverse order (**digit backward test**). Certain rules must be followed while doing digit forward or digit backward tests.
3. **Intelligence** is assessed in terms of the **general fund of knowledge,** simple **arithmetic ability,** and reading and writing abilities. However, it depends upon the educational background of the individual.
4. **Abstract ability** is assessed by **similarity testing**. The patient may be asked to tell the similarity between varied objects such as a bus and a train, a table and a chair, etc. The answer should be at the level of abstraction for example when asked about similarities between a train and a bus the answer should be that they are motor vehicles and modes of transportation and answers such as both having wheels, engines, etc. do not signify intact abstract ability.
5. **Assessment of reasoning** is done by presenting imaginary situations in various contexts and assessing the explanations given for his supposed action. For example, the patient may be asked what he will do if he sees a fire burning at the corner of a cinema hall he is in. The normal response is when he tells you that he will alert others and cry for help and if the fire is big enough then he will call the fire brigade. A depressive patient may say that he will be unable to do anything, no help will come, etc. A schizophrenic patient may present an ambivalent response.
6. **Assessment of memory** involves assessment of **immediate, recent, and remote memory.** Immediate memory is assessed by three object recall tests; recent memory is assessed by asking what he had for breakfast, how did he reach the hospital, and so on? Remote memory is assessed by enquiring about past personal events such as marriage date and year, name of his school, year of passing, etc.

Insight

Insight is defined as **awareness about one's illness.** A mere enumeration of symptoms does not signify the presence of insight. For example, a patient with schizophrenia may complain about hearing voices and suspecting others of malevolent intentions, but this is not considered intact insight. For the insight to be considered intact, he must understand that these symptoms are because of some mental illness. Insight can be **graded as:**

a. **Grade 1: No insight,** patient altogether denies having any illness.
b. **Grade 2: Some insight** sometimes accepts having some illness and sometimes denies it.
c. **Grade 3**: Attributing symptoms to **physical illness or outside factors** such as acts of spirits.
d. **Grade 4: Intellectual insight,** understanding the illness, and the need for treatment.
e. **Grade 5: True emotional insight,** fully understanding the illness, its impact on personal well-being, and its ramification on near and dear ones.

Physical Examination

A complete physical examination including pulse rate, blood pressure, heart sounds and respiratory function should be done. A thorough neurological examination is mandatory in all cases of psychiatric illnesses.

Diagnostic Formulation

After complete history taking, mental status examination, and physical examination a **provisional diagnosis** is made based on commonly used diagnostic criteria. Currently, diagnostic criteria mentioned in **ICD-10** are widely used in India and abroad excluding North America where that of **DSM-5** is primarily used. In cases of confusion, one or more **differential diagnoses** should be made depending on the assessment; however, making a differential diagnosis is not mandatory in all cases.

Treatment Plan

A pragmatic treatment plan should be formulated after making the diagnosis. A healthy treatment plan should take into account the **presenting symptoms, and patient profile such as age, sex, weight, etc. presence of any medical illness, personality profile,** etc. Previous medication, if any, to which the patient has responded should be considered as a first choice or the medication to which a blood-related family member, if any, has responded can also be considered as the first choice. Usually, psychotropic medications are started at low doses and the dose is gradually increased to reach an optimum dose. In all cases, polypharmacy should be avoided as far as possible.

EXPLANATORY MODELS IN PSYCHIATRY

Psychiatric illnesses have been a matter of concern for the human race since antiquity. Many have attempted to explain the possible causation for the characteristic symptoms of psychiatric illnesses. The followings are some of the prevalent explanations given for the causation of psychiatric illnesses:

1. **The moral model** explains psychiatric illnesses as occurring due to an individual's deviation from morality such as selfishness.
2. **The religious model** explains psychiatric illnesses as forms of punishment for religious transgression.
3. **The spiritual model** suggests that psychiatric illnesses occur due to the action of malevolent spirits (and because of sorcery or witchcraft). These beliefs are still prevalent in some countries like India, Sri Lanka, and Bangladesh and in other developing countries.
4. **The biopsychosocial model** suggests that psychiatric illnesses arise from the complex interaction between biological, psychological, and social factors.

The biopsychosocial model was first proposed by George Engel in 1977 and is the most widely accepted model since then. This model emphasized **biological factors, psychological build, and the social milieu** of an individual in the development of psychiatric illnesses. These factors and their contribution toward the development of a psychiatric illness are described under the following headings.

Biological Factors

The human brain consists of around 1 billion neurons and close to 1 trillion connections between them. These neurons connect to form neural circuits and communicate with each other via neurotransmitters to carry out certain meaningful actions underlying brain functions: perception, cognition, emotion, and conation. Any defect in the structural aspect of neural circuitry or impairment in the underlying information-sharing process can lead to abnormality in psychiatric illnesses. These structural or functional abnormalities in the neural circuitry can arise from the following factors.

1. **Genetic factors**, it has been widely observed that most psychiatric illnesses run in families, suggesting a genetic contribution to the causation of the illness. However, these genetic factors only increase the probability of developing psychiatric illnesses and are not fully responsible for the causation. Furthermore, no single gene is responsible for developing any psychiatric illness and the inheritance pattern is polygenic with each gene contributing to some extent toward the development of the illness. These genetic factors interact with other psychological and social factors in a complex way ultimately leading to the onset of the illness.
2. **Infections,** certain infections also lead to damage or dysfunction of neural circuitry leading to the development of the disease. For example, Herpes Simplex infection during childhood can increase the probability of developing schizophrenia in adulthood.
3. **Brain damage or injury** especially during the neural development phase can contribute to the development of psychiatric illnesses. For example, cerebral hypoxia during childbirth can contribute to the development of autism in children and schizophrenia in adulthood.
4. **Substance abuse** for prolonged periods can result in long-lasting dysfunction of the brain leading to paranoia, anxiety neuroses, and depression.
5. **Other factors** such as poor nutritional status, and exposure to heavy metals (e.g. lead) can also contribute toward the causation of psychiatric illnesses.

Psychological Factors

An individual's emotional or psychological state and coping skills also contribute significantly to the development of psychiatric illnesses. These emotional or psychological patterns and coping skills that predispose a person to develop a psychiatric illness depend upon certain factors the person is exposed to during childhood. These factors are mentioned below:

1. Exposure to physical, sexual, or emotional abuse during childhood
2. Significant life events during childhood such as the loss of a parent.
3. Neglect during childhood by parents

Social Factors

Various social factors such as family environment, support system, workplace environment, etc. also contribute significantly to the development of certain psychiatric illnesses. Some important social factors which predispose a person to develop a psychiatric illness are:

1. Marital disharmony or divorce
2. Dysfunctional family environment
3. Lack of support system (family and friends)
4. Loss of job or frequent changing of job and
5. Lack of job satisfaction

All these factors (biological, psychological, and social factors) interact in a complex way and contribute to the development of the disease. No single factor is solely responsible and cannot give rise to the illness in its own right. Therefore, all these factors should be taken into consideration while planning management protocols for any psychiatric illness. A wholesome treatment approach must involve all these components and their possible contribution to the development of the illness.

SUMMARY

1. Some of the biggest breakthroughs in psychiatry are introduction of ECT in 1938, discovery of the first antipsychotic chlorpromazine in 1952 and introduction of criteria based diagnostic systems in ICD and DSM.
2. The concept of neurosis and psychosis is very fundamental in psychiatry, although a bit controversial. Psychoses are differentiated from neuroses by presence of one of the three defining criteria of psychosis: insight, reality contact and ego boundary.
3. Currently the diagnostic criteria mentioned in DSM-5 (Diagnostic and Statistical Manual for mental disorders, 5th edition) and ICD-10 (International Classification of Diseases for Mental and Behavioural Disorders, 10th edition) are in widespread use for diagnosis of psychiatric illnesses worldwide.
4. Psychiatric interview involves psychiatry history taking and mental status examination known as MSE in short. Establishing rapport with the patient is the most important part of psychiatric interview.
5. Components of a good psychiatric history consist of patient's personal information, chief complaints, history of present illness, history of past illness, present medical history, family and birth history, personal and sexual history and history of substance abuse and premorbid personality.
6. MSE is considered as the jewel of psychiatric interview. It consists of observation of the general appearance of the patient, assessment of mood and affect, speech, thought disturbances, perceptual disturbances, assessment of cognitive functions and insight.
7. After a thorough history, mental status examination and physical examination, a diagnosis is established and further pragmatic management is planned.
8. Management in psychiatry can be diagnosis based (e.g. treatment of schizophrenia) or symptom based (treatment of troublesome symptoms, e.g. positive or negative symptoms in a case of schizophrenia) based on the preference of the concerned psychiatrist and prevalent practice of the institute.
9. Lastly, the concept of normality is very controversial in psychiatry. As per the DSM-5, nothing is considered abnormal in psychiatry unless it causes significant impairment in the socio-occupational functioning of an individual.

BIBLIOGRAPHY

1. Mental Health History and Timeline. Studymore.org.uk. Retrieved 15 April 2014
2. Heckers, S and Kendler, KS. The evolution of Kraepelin's Nosological principles. World psychiatry: official journal of the World Psychiatric Association (WPA), 2020. 19(3), 381–8.
3. Beer MD. The dichotomies: psychosis/neurosis and functional/organic: a historical perspective. Hist Psychiatry. 1996 Jun;7(26 Pt 2):231-55.
4. Wig NN, Singh G. A proposed classification of psychiatric disorders for use in India. Indian J Psychiatry. 1967;8:157–71
5. Fish, FJ (Frank James). Clinical Psychopathology: Signs and Symptoms in Psychiatry. Bristol: J. Wright, 1967.
6. Sadock, and Pedro Ruiz. Kaplan & Sadock's Synopsis of Psychiatry: Behavioral Sciences/clinical Psychiatry. Eleventh edition. Philadelphia: Wolters Kluwer, 2015.
7. Jaspers, K. General Psychopathology, 1997. (Vol. 2). JHU Press.
8. Stahl, SM, & amp; Grady, MM. Stahl. Essential Psychopharmacology: The prescriber guide, 2011. (4th ed.). Cambridge, UK; New York: Cambridge University Press.
9. Tripathi A, Das A, Kar SK. Biopsychosocial Model in Contemporary Psychiatry: Current Validity and Future Prospects. Indian J Psychol Med. 2019 Nov 11;41(6).

Chapter 4

Organic Psychiatric Disorders

Competency achievement: Students should be able to

1. **PS3.7** Enumerate and describe common organic psychiatric disorders and their magnitude, etiology, and clinical features
2. **PS3.8** Enumerate and describe the essential investigations in patients with organic psychiatric disorders
3. **PS3.9** Describe the steps and demonstrate in a simulated environment the importance of family education in patients with organic psychiatric disorders
4. **PS3.10** Enumerate and describe the pharmacologic basis and side effects of drugs used in organic psychiatric disorders
5. **PS3.11** Enumerate the appropriate conditions for specialist referral in patients with organic psychiatric disorders

DELIRIUM

Introduction

Consciousness is the ability to be **aware of the self and the surroundings** and the ability to react appropriately to external stimuli. Consciousness is a **basic function of the CNS** just like the maintenance of cardiovascular functions, respiration, reflexes, and maintenance of bodily homeostasis.

At the **brainstem level**, consciousness is maintained by a network of neurons spanning from the upper spinal cord to the midbrain, known as a **reticular activating system (RAS)**. Any condition causing injury to the RAS presents with a **lowering of consciousness**. On the other hand, consciousness at the **cortical level** is maintained by a set of neuronal activities known as **thalamocortical resonance**. Thalamocortical resonance is nothing but the synchronous oscillation of **neurons in the thalamus and layer V** of the cerebral cortex. Any disruption in this synchronous activity of the thalamocortical loop presents with **impairment in consciousness**. Impairment in consciousness is the **hallmark feature of delirium.**

Clinical Presentation

Delirium is a clinical condition presenting with **acute onset impairment in consciousness** along with **impairment in attention and cognition**. It is also known by various other names such as acute confusional state, acute organic psychosis, acute brain syndrome, etc.

Impairment in consciousness is the most important feature of delirium (a **hallmark sign of delirium**). Along with impairment in consciousness, the patient also presents with impairment in attention and cognition. Because of impaired attention, the person has difficulty sustaining attention (being focused on one topic) and shifting attention from one topic to another. Along with the above defining criteria, a case of delirium may present with other features like:

- Psychomotor agitation (hyperactive delirium) or retardation (hypoactive delirium)
- Impaired memory formation
- Sleep cycle reversal
- Disorganized speech and behavior
- Thought disturbances like delusions
- Perceptual disturbances like illusions and hallucinations

Depending upon the clinical presentation, **delirium is classified into:**

1. **Hyperactive delirium** presenting with agitation and restlessness
2. **Hypoactive delirium** presents with a lowering of activity and lethargy and
3. **Mixed state delirium** presenting with features of both hypoactive and hyperactive delirium.

Delirium is a **medical emergency** and a proper diagnosis should be made with a detailed history and clinical assessment. Delirium is frequently **confused with acute psychosis, severe depression, and dementia.** However, there is no impairment in consciousness in these cases. A case of delirium always has an underlying medical condition that affects the functioning of the CNS. Prompt diagnosis of the underlying condition and proper treatment proves life-saving in all cases of delirium. To identify the underlying cause we must keep in mind various medical conditions that can present with delirium as mentioned below:

1. *Conditions of the CNS*
   - **CNS infections** like meningitis, encephalitis, and meningoencephalitis
   - **Head trauma** causing raised ICT or diffuse axonal injury
   - **CVA** (ischemic or hemorrhagic)
2. Systemic conditions affecting CNS
   - Septicaemia
   - Brain hypoxia due to any cause
   - Dyselectrolytemia
   - Severe dehydration
   - Hypo- or hyperglycemia
   - Hypo- or hyperthermia
   - Hepatic or uremia encephalopathy
3. Substance intoxication or withdrawal
   - Alcohol intoxication
   - Alcohol withdrawal
   - Opioid intoxication

Pathophysiology

Delirium is the result of the widespread brain dysfunction arising from an inflammatory response or brain hypoxia caused by CNS or systemic infection or injury.

CNS or systemic inflammation results in increased levels of proinflammatory cytokines which can increase the permeability of the blood–brain barrier, exposing the neural tissue to endogenous toxins and inflammatory cytokines. Inflammation also results in the deposition of fibrin on the CNS microvascular causing neural tissue dysfunction. CNS or systemic infection or injury also results in subclinical hypoxia of the neural tissue leading to oxidative damage.

This widespread hypoxic damage causes global cortical dysfunction, especially impairment in the synchronous activity of the **thalamocortical loop** which results in impairment of consciousness. Brain hypoxia also causes **decreased synthesis of acetylcholine neurotransmitters**. As we know, acetylcholine is involved in the maintenance of attention and cognition, poor acetylcholine activity results in impairment in attention and cognition in cases of delirium. Furthermore, brain hypoxia also results in **increased dopaminergic activity** which explains agitation and psychosis in cases of delirium.

Diagnosis

Diagnosis of a case of delirium is made clinically with detailed history and proper clinical assessment. Level of consciousness is assessed using **Glasgow Coma Scale** and a score of less than 13 indicates impairment in consciousness. **The delirium assessment scale** can be applied to cases where there is doubt about the diagnosis. A differential diagnosis which includes acute psychosis, conversion reaction, severe depression, and dementia should be kept in mind while diagnosing a case of delirium.

Suggested Investigations

Delirium is a medical emergency; hence, all necessary investigations must be done to find out the underlying cause as treatment is dependent on the cause of delirium. Following investigations may be needed in a case of delirium (laboratory investigation depends upon the presenting condition in a case of delirium).

1. Complete blood count with differential counts
2. Blood electrolyte levels
3. Renal function test
4. Liver function test
5. Chest X-ray
6. CSF analysis
7. Urine analysis
8. Brain imaging studies such as CT scans and MRI scans
9. Electroencephalogram
10. Ultrasonography of abdomen

Treatment

Treatment of delirium consists of treatment of the **underlying medical condition**. Correction of electrolyte imbalance, hypoglycemia or dehydration, and parental antibiotics for systemic or cerebral infections, etc. are definite treatments for a case of delirium. Prompt identification and treatment can save the patient from dying. The **behavioral and psychiatric aspects** can be managed by low-dose **antipsychotic drugs** like haloperidol or risperidone whenever needed. An acutely agitated patient can be put under physical restraint to avoid harm to themself and others. Parenteral antipsychotics (haloperidol) also help calm the patient. Benzodiazepines should be avoided as they further add to the confusion, delay recovery, and can cause paradoxical effects in these patients leading to agitation and aggression. Oral melatonin can significantly improve sleep, and orientation and hasten recovery from delirium and should be considered in all cases of delirium to improve sleep and orientation.

DEMENTIA

Introduction

Cognitive functions are higher mental functions that fall under the purview of **cortical functions**. Different cerebral cortices are tasked with different cognitive functions. Memory, judgment and reasoning, mathematical abilities, language, etc are examples of cognitive functions. **Deterioration of already acquired cognitive functions is known as dementia**.

Memory is the most known cognitive function. Memory function has been described in detail in Chapter 2.

The language function is another important cognitive function. Language function involves two distinct domains: **comprehension domain and expression domain**. Language comprehension involves a perception of spoken language and its subsequent processing to make it understandable to the self and is the function of **Wernicke's area** in the parietal cortex. Language expression involves proper pronunciation with the use of syntax to make it understandable to others. Language expression is the function of **Broca's area** situated in the frontal cortex.

Executive functions are special types of cognitive functions that involve **proper planning and processing of information** and are functions of the **dorsolateral prefrontal cortex (dlPFC).** Judgment, reasoning, problem-solving, complex analysis, and developing abstract and innovative ideas are examples of executive functions. **Working memory** is also an executive function that involves holding and manipulating information at hand to perform a specific task (for example memorizing the number and name of a person to make an urgent phone call).

Praxis or the ability to carry out **purposeful motor actions** is another important cognitive function. Similarly, **gnosis** is the ability to **identify objects or faces**. Praxis and gnosis are functions of parietal-temporal cortices.

Orientation is also a cognitive function governed by the person's orientation. It is clinically assessed by checking his **orientation to person, place, and time in the same order**. The order should be maintained while checking orientation as it is quite easy to orient oneself to a person than to a place and orienting to time is the most difficult one.

Definition and Clinical Presentation

Dementia means the **deterioration of mental abilities**. It is defined as the **impairment of previously acquired global cognitive functions**. Cognitive functions include all the higher mental functions which fall within the domain of cortical functions such as memory, learning, concentration, judgment-reasoning, planning, mathematical ability, language functions, praxis, gnosis, etc. The term global signifies that cognitive impairment in dementia involves not only memory but an array of cognitive functions mentioned above. Therefore, a case of dementia generally presents with impairment in memory, judgment, reasoning, planning, purposeful motor activities (praxis), calculation, etc. However, clinical presentation depends largely on the type of dementia and the state of progression of the disease. Because of poor memory, dementia patients are frequently not oriented to time and place but they are **fully conscious** and normally responsive to external cues which are the primary differentiating points between dementia and delirium. Initially these cognitive deficits hamper **instrumental activities of daily living (IADLs)** like decision-making, marketing, calculation, managing finances, etc. Gradually, when cognitive impairment becomes more severe it starts hampering normal **activities of daily living (ADLs)** such as eating, dressing, going to the toilet, etc. Along with cognitive impairment, patients with dementia often show behavioral and psychiatric symptoms known as **BPSD** (behavioral and psychiatric symptoms of dementia).

Differential Diagnosis

Dementia is frequently confused with delirium, however, in dementia, the patient is fully conscious although he might not be oriented to time, place, or person (Table 4.1). Other conditions that are frequently confused with dementia are **severe depression, chronic schizophrenia,** and **mental retardation.** In mental retardation, higher mental functions are never achieved at their full potential while in dementia already acquired cognitive functions are gradually lost.

Causes

Dementias are primarily categorized into **idiopathic or irreversible dementias** and **reversible dementias. Idiopathic dementias**, also known as irreversible dementias, are a group of neurodegenerative conditions that affect the cerebral cortex and present with dementia and associated behavioral symptoms. These include:

- Alzheimer's disease
- Frontotemporal dementia
- Dementia with Lewi body or DLB
- Huntington's disease
- Parkinson's disease

Reversible dementias are the consequence of a known cause that leads to the atrophy of the cerebral cortex. Early detection and appropriate management of underlying causes can reverse the cognitive impairment or at least halt further progression of the condition. Various causes of reversible dementia include:

- Vascular dementia
- Vitamin B_{12} deficiency

Table 4.1: Differences between dementia and delirium

Clinical characteristics	*Delirium*	*Dementia*
Onset	Acute	Insidious
Course	Fluctuating	Gradually progressive
Consciousness	Always impaired	Always clear
Orientation	Impaired	May or may not be impaired
Recovery	Complete	Mostly irreversible
Causes	Acute medical conditions such as infection, injury, or toxicity of CNS	Degenerative diseases of the CNS such as Alzheimer's disease, FTD, DLB, etc.
Treatment	Treatment of the underlying medical condition	Treatment is mainly symptomatic

- Niacin deficiency (pellagra)
- Thyroid deficiency
- Alcohol-induced dementia
- Heavy metal poisoning (lead, mercury, etc.)
- Infection like HIV dementia, neurosyphilis (general paresis of insane)

(**Pseudodementia** is the term applied for patients with severe depression presenting with apparent cognitive decline. However, cognitive functions are regained with successful treatment of depression).

Behavioral and Psychiatric Symptoms of Dementia (BPSD)

Along with impairment of cognitive functions, dementia patients also present with **behavioral symptoms like irritability, restlessness, and aggression**. Frequent **mood swings** with anger outbursts are common. **Psychotic symptoms** such as delusions and hallucinations might also be present. Common delusions in patients of dementia are delusions of infidelity, the delusion of persecution, and the delusion of theft. Hallucinations can be auditory, visual, or tactile. One of the most common types of hallucination in patients of dementia is tactile hallucinations of bugs on the body also known as the **delusion of infestation or delusional parasitosis**. Many patients with dementia also develop **depression and anxiety disorders**. The presence of behavior or psychiatric symptoms further complicates the diagnosis and management of dementia.

ALZHEIMER'S DISEASE

As described for the first time by **Alois Alzheimer**, it is the **most common type of dementia** and accounts for almost 60–70% of all dementia cases. Alzheimer's disease involves **atrophy of parietal and temporal lobes** and presents with **memory impairment**, impairment in visuospatial functions, **apraxia** (inability to carry out purposeful motor activities), **acalculia,** receptive language impairment, etc. Memory impairment in Alzheimer's disease involves impairment in the formation of new autobiographical memories while long-term memories generally remain intact. With onset after 65 years of age, this disease is gradually progressive and ultimately leads to severe cognitive deterioration, vegetative state, and death.

Etiology

The exact cause of Alzheimer's disease is not known. Age is the most important risk factor and the incidence increases exponentially with an increase in age after 65 years. The second most common risk factor is genetic predisposition and the **ApoE4** gene is the most common candidate gene implicated. Apart from age and genetic risk, poor nutritional status, low level of education, poor intellectual capacity, mental idling, sedentary lifestyle, etc. are other important risk factors for Alzheimer's disease.

Pathology

Alzheimer's disease is the result of **neuronal loss (gray matter atrophy**) in the parietal and temporal lobes. It starts with the **deposition of amyloid beta (Aβ) plaques** outside the neurons. Amyloid beta is the end product of **amyloid precursor protein (APP),** a transmembrane protein when cleaved by beta or gamma-secretase instead of alpha-secretase. Stacks of amyloid beta are deposited outside the neurons and are known as **amyloid plaques**. In addition to this, the microtubules in the neural cell are coagulated and form deposits inside the neurons, known as **neurofibrillary tangles**. These depositions result in the excessive **excitation of NMDA** receptors and subsequent **calcium influx into the neurons**. Calcium ions trigger **apoplectic cell death** and subsequent neuronal cell loss. Initially, neural loss involves the **nucleus basalis of Meynert** causing depleted acetylcholine activity and leading to impairment in cognitive functions such as memory and executive functions. Subsequently, cell death involves the hippocampus and parahippocampal gyrus. As a result of **hippocampal atrophy**, there is an impairment in the formation of new long-term memory. Gradually, cell atrophy spreads to other parts of the cortex leading to diffuse cerebral atrophy, especially that of parietal and temporal cortices. Cerebral atrophy is evident in CT brain and MRI brain in the form of **prominent sulci and diminished gyri.**

Diagnosis

Diagnosis of a case of dementia is **made clinically** by proper history taking and examination. Mental status examinations involving assessment of short-term memory, orientation, attention concentration, judgment-reasoning, and tests for praxis are important points for evaluation. **Brain imaging studies** such as CT scans and MRI also add in diagnosis and are generally routinely done. In case of doubt, especially in the early stages, a **mini-mental state examination (MMSE)** can help in the screening of cases of dementia. A confirmed diagnosis can only be made by histopathological examination of brain tissue.

Comorbidity

Alzheimer's dementia is frequently complicated by **behavioral disturbances. Frank psychosis** with prominent delusions and hallucinations, **depression, anxiety,** and **sleep disturbance** are quite common in patients with dementia. These comorbidities can add to morbidity and mortality in demented individuals and add to the burden on caregivers.

Treatment

There is no specific treatment for Alzheimer's disease which can reverse the cognitive decline or halt the further progression of the disease. **Mild cases are managed with behavior modification**, diet, and mild exercise which improve day-to-day functioning. The behavioral modification involves good lighting of the bedroom, putting a clock and calendar in the room to help the patient in orientation, soothing music, and memory notes to help to remember. **Moderate-to-severe cases need treatment with cognitive enhancers** which improve cognition and general day-to-day functioning. **Acetylcholinesterase inhibitors** (donepezil, rivastigmine, tacrine) are the most commonly used cognitive enhancers. The **NMDA antagonist** memantine is also effective in cases with mild and moderate cognitive decline. Donepezil is frequently combined with memantine and is given twice daily.

Psychotic and behavioral symptoms are managed with the cautious use of **antipsychotics such as risperidone at low doses**. **Melatonin** is quite helpful in improving sleep and also in improving orientation. Sedatives like benzodiazepines should be avoided because of the fear of falls and further cognitive decline. In case of sleep disturbance not improving by melatonin, low-dose quetiapine or antihistamines are helpful.

FRONTOTEMPORAL DEMENTIAS

Frontotemporal dementias or FTDs are characterized by **atrophy of frontal and temporal lobes**. FTDs are the second most common cause of dementia after Alzheimer's disease and the most common cause of **early-onset dementia**. Onset is generally **before 65 years** of age and can affect persons as young as 45 years. FTDs are gradually progressive and the patient generally lives between 2 and 20 years after the onset of the disease. Frontotemporal dementias include the following three variants.

- Behavioral variant (bvFTD)
- Primary progressive aphasia (PPA)— Semantic variant
- Primary progressive aphasia (PPA)— Non-fluent aphasia

Behavioral Variant

The behavioral variant of frontotemporal dementia (bvFTD) is also **known as Pick's disease.** It is the most common variant and there is primary **involvement of the frontal lobe**. It presents with **drastic changes in personality** leading to impulsiveness, apathy, socially inappropriate behaviors, mood swings, poor self-care, and lack of insight. Along with personality changes, there is **cognitive decline** with impairment in judgment, reasoning, attention, concentration, and executive functions. Memory and spatial cognitions are generally intact due to the non-involvement of the parietal lobe.

PPA—Semantic Variant

It presents with **receptive language disturbance** with intact language fluency. **Atrophy of the temporal lobe** is the most conspicuous feature in this variant.

PPA—Non-fluent Aphasia

This variant of FTD presents with **non-fluent aphasia (motor aphasia)** and the patient has no difficulty in language comprehension but profound difficulty in language expression. It is due to atrophy of the ventrolateral **frontal cortex involving Broca's area**.

Treatment

Currently, there is neither any cure nor any effective pharmacological treatment for FTD. Cholinesterase inhibitors such as donepezil and NMDA antagonists such as memantine are not effective in FTD. **Behavioral modifications** may help in some cases. Mood swings and impulsivity generally respond to therapy with SSRIs. Antipsychotics and sedatives are also sometimes needed to control neuropsychiatric symptoms.

DEMENTIA WITH LEWY BODY

Dementia with Lewi body (DLB) presents with impairment in attention and concentration, fluctuating consciousness, delusions, visual hallucinations, and features of Parkinsonism (tremor, rigidity, and bradykinesia). Impairments in memory, language and praxis are late findings. Pathologically, there is **deposition of Alpha-synuclein (synucleinopathy)** in the neuron and these deposits are known as **Lewi bodies**. Neural atrophy starts primarily in the subcortical structures like **basal ganglia, limbic structures, and thalamus** leading to the development of Parkinsonian features and psychotic features early in the disease process. Gradually, neural atrophy progresses to involve cortical tissue, and impairment of cognitive functions becomes prominent. There is no treatment to reverse the disease or halt its progression. Donepezil and memantine may be effective in improving cognitive functions. Behavioral modification is particularly important in the cases of DLB. Antipsychotic drugs should be given cautiously as they can aggravate Parkinsonian features or may lead to the neuroleptic malignant syndrome.

VASCULAR DEMENTIA

Vascular dementia or **multi-infarct dementia** is the most **common cause of reversible dementia** and the second most common cause of dementia after Alzheimer's disease. Cardiovascular risk factors like diabetes, hypertension, dyslipidemia, and cigarette smoking are important risk factors for vascular dementia. Presenting features depend upon the cerebral lobe involved. Frontal lobe involvement presents with personality changes, disinhibition, socially inappropriate behaviors, mood swings, apathy, impairment in judgment reasoning, etc. Visuospatial impairment, apraxia, and acalculia are typical of parietal lobe involvement. The patient presents with memory impairment, receptive aphasia and visual or auditory hallucinations when the temporal lobe is involved.

Cortical atrophy is due to **microvascular changes and ischaemic damage** (infarction) of the neural tissue. The **step ladder pattern** presentation is typical in vascular dementia. Cognitive impairment remains non-progressive for some time then there is a sudden worsening of cognitive functions which is maintained for another few months to years till further sudden decline occurs. It is due to discrete cerebrovascular infarction events occurring from time to time causing mass neural tissue loss.

Good control of blood sugar level, blood pressure, lipid profile, abstinence from cigarette smoking, mild physical exercise, and high fiber diet can halt or slow down the progression of vascular dementia. **Cognitive enhancers** like donepezil and memantine are also effective in improving cognitive functions. **Antioxidants like ginkgo biloba** and other drugs promoting neural plasticity such as **cerebroprotein hydrolysate** are particularly important in this category of dementia. Behavioral symptoms and sleep disturbance can be taken care of by prescribing low doses of antipsychotics and melatonin respectively.

Binswanger's disease or subcortical leukoencephalopathy is a form of vascular dementia caused by vascular infarcts involving subcortical white matter tissue of the brain.

HIV DEMENTIA SYNDROME

HIV is the causative agent of AIDS. Persons with **long-standing HIV infection** can present with impaired attention concentration, forgetfulness, poor judgment-reasoning and personality changes with apathy and impulsiveness, motor impairment, etc. This category of dementia in a person with HIV infection is known as **HIV-associated dementia (HAD) or AIDS dementia complex (ADC).**

HIV are non-neural virus and doesn't attack the neural cells directly. Instead, they attack perivascular macrophages and astrocytes in the brain and trigger an immune response. Subsequent **release of inflammatory cytokines** can cause neural dysfunction or **apoptotic neuronal cell death**. Gradually neural loss leads to widespread grey matter atrophy involving the cerebral hemispheres, subcortical structures, and cerebellum.

Highly active antiretroviral therapy (HAART) is effective in decreasing viral load and delaying the onset of dementia. Earlier, around 30% of AIDS patients used to develop dementia complex, but with the advent of HAART, this has been reduced to less than 10%. Along with HAART therapy, cognitive enhancers can improve cognitive functions and antipsychotic drugs are frequently prescribed to control behavioral symptoms.

ORGANIC AMNESIC SYNDROME

Amnesic disorders present with **impairment of memory as the primary presenting symptom** caused by certain CNS conditions excluding delirium and dementia. Impairment of memory primarily involves declarative memory (especially episodic memory) and may be anterograde (inability to form new memories) or retrograde (inability to recall previously learned information). Some of the leading causes of the organic amnesic syndrome are:

1. **Korsakoff syndrome** occurs in chronic alcoholics due to thiamine deficiency. Korsakoff syndrome generally follows untreated cases of Wernicke's encephalopathy but not always. The primary CNS lesions are in the components of the Papez circuit such as mammillary bodies and the anterior nucleus of the thalamus. The primary presenting symptom is anterograde amnesia due to impairment in the formation of new memories. What is interesting is that patients of Korsakoff syndrome don't have insight, therefore they make-up stories to fill up the memory gaps, which is known as **confabulation**. Other symptoms of Korsakoff syndrome are apathy, personality change, and psychosis.
2. Head trauma causing injury to the hippocampus or other structures in the medial temporal cortex may present as an amnesic syndrome.
3. Transient global amnesia causing hypoxia of medial temporal cortical structures presents with loss of memory surrounding the event. However, this condition is transient in nature and improves by itself.
4. Complex partial seizure or CPS occurs due to injury and scarring of cortical matters in the medial temporal cortex (especially the CA3 region of the hippocampus). Mesial temporal gliosis is the prominent finding in cases of CPS. Many cases of CPS present with anterograde amnesia.
5. Herpes simplex encephalitis generally involves structures of the medial temporal cortex and can present as an amnesic syndrome.
6. Electroconvulsive therapy may lead to retrograde amnesia.

Organic Psychotic Disorders

Psychosis is a clinical state presenting with delusions, hallucinations, and disorganized behaviors. Psychosis generally occurs in the context of functional psychiatric illnesses such as schizophrenia and delusional disorder. However, some organic illnesses (involving CNS or systemic illnesses affecting CNS) may present with psychotic features. It is necessary to differentiate organic psychosis from that functional ones for proper treatment of the conditions. Following are a few characteristics features that point toward an organic cause for a case presenting with psychosis

1. Sudden onset of psychotic symptoms
2. The onset of psychotic symptoms in old age (after 60 years of age)
3. Associated soft or hard neurological features
4. Presence of confusion and disorientation
5. Presence of visual hallucinations

Once an organic cause for the presenting psychotic symptoms is suspected, confirmation may be done with requisite laboratory investigations and neuroimaging studies such as CT and MRI scanning of the brain. A few organic conditions which can present with psychosis are

1. CNS conditions such as CVA, traumatic brain injury, brain tumor, brain metastasis, etc.
2. CNS infections such as viral or bacterial meningitis or encephalitis, HIV encephalopathy, syphilis, prion disease, etc.
3. Neurodegenerative diseases such as Alzheimer's disease, Lewy body dementia, vascular dementia, etc.
4. Systemic illnesses such as hypo-/hypothyroidism, vitamin B_{12} deficiency, and paraneoplastic syndrome.
5. Autoimmune diseases such as SLE, autoimmune vasculitis, anti-NMDA encephalitis, etc.
6. Substance-induced psychosis is associated with alcohol, cannabis, cocaine, or phencyclidine abuse.

After confirmation, management involves the treatment of the underlying organic cause. However, antipsychotic medications are frequently needed to control psychotic symptoms. It should be kept in mind that these patients are very sensitive to antipsychotics and are prone to develop EPS. Second-generation antipsychotics such as olanzapine and risperidone are preferred over typical antipsychotics. Antipsychotic medications should be started at low doses and the dose is gradually increased to reach an optimum dose which is often less than that for functional psychoses.

Organic Mood Disorders

Several organic conditions may present with persistent alteration of mood and emotion. The presentation may be of a depressive or manic state depending upon the nature of the illness and the part of the CNS involved. Relevant laboratory investigations and imaging studies are needed to rule out possible organic causes for proper management of the condition for which probable causes should be kept in mind.

Organic causes of manic state:

1. CNS causes such as TBI, CVA, viral encephalitis, multiple sclerosis, etc.
2. Neurodegenerative conditions such as frontotemporal dementia, etc.
3. Complex partial seizure
4. Certain medications, especially steroids.
5. Hyperthyroidism
6. Amphetamine abuse

Organic causes of depressive mood state:

1. Hypothyroidism
2. Cushing syndrome
3. CNS causes such as CVA, CNS tumor, SLE, etc.
4. Neurodegenerative conditions such as Parkinson's disease, Huntington's disease, etc.
5. Medications-induced depression, e.g. beta blockers or digoxin-induced depression.

Once the underlying cause for the organic mood state is identified, management involves treatment of the underlying cause, if possible. If the condition is incurable then symptomatic management of the mood state is needed. Depressive mood states may be treated with SSRIs or TCAs. For example, SSRIs at low doses are the treatment of choice for post-stroke depression. Similarly, antiepileptic mood stabilizers, especially sodium valproate, may be used to control irritability, aggression, and grandiosity. Atypical antipsychotics, such as olanzapine, quetiapine, and aripiprazole may be indicated in some conditions but should be used with caution.

Organic Anxiety Disorder

Anxiety disorders are one of the most common psychiatric illnesses in the community. However, it is imperative to differentiate functional anxiety disorders from anxiety states arising from organic causes. Here are a few characteristic features that point toward an organic cause for presenting anxiety

1. Onset after 35 years of age
2. No history of anxiety neurosis in childhood
3. Lack of family history of anxiety disorders
4. Lack of stressful life events responsible for the onset of anxiety
5. Poor response to psychiatric treatment

Once an organic cause for the presenting anxiety symptoms is suspected then relevant investigations may be needed to confirm it. For this, we have to know some common organic causes presenting with significant anxiety symptoms such as:

1. Hyperthyroidism
2. Cardiac ailments leading to coronary insufficiency
3. COPD
4. Pheochromocytoma
5. Complex partial seizure
6. Diabetes mellitus presenting with frequent hypoglycemia
7. Substance withdrawal states e.g. alcohol or benzodiazepine withdrawal

Treatment involves the management of the underlying cause. Benzodiazepines and beta-blockers such as propranolol may be used for symptomatic control.

Organic Personality Disorder

Organic personality disorder presents with a change in premorbid personality due to CNS injury, infection, or toxicity. Common presenting symptoms are apathy, emotional incontinence, irritability and agitation, impulsivity, and disinhibited behaviors. Behavioral disinhibition may present with sexual disinhibition (hypersexuality or abnormal sexual approach) or social disinhibition (sudden aggression, impulsivity, lack of shame, disorganized behaviors, etc.). These patients generally do not have insight into their condition which contributes to difficulty in their behavioral management and treatment.

Personality changes occur following injury to the orbitofrontal cortex, anterior cingulate cortex, and dorsolateral prefrontal cortex due to head injury or any other CNS condition (CNS infection, tumor, CVA, etc.). This condition presenting with personality changes following injury to the prefrontal cortex is known as **frontal lobe syndrome**.

The most effective management approach for frontal lobe syndrome is behavioral therapy and family therapy (psychoeducation and behavioral modification approach). However, many patients need medications to manage disinhibited and problematic behaviors. Antiepileptic mood stabilizers such as sodium valproate and carbamazepine are effective in controlling mood swings, irritability, and aggression. Apathy, emotional outbursts, anxiety, and depression are better managed with SSRIs and TCAs. Antipsychotics may be prescribed at low doses to manage sexually and socially disinhibited behaviors.

Appropriate conditions for referral to a mental health specialist

1. All cases of delirium should be referred to a tertiary care hospital for proper evaluation and management
2. Advanced cases of dementia
3. Organic mental illnesses not responding to initial treatment
4. Cases requiring behavioral intervention
5. Patients with complicated medical conditions such as CVA, head injury, etc.
6. Patients presenting with poor nutritional status

SUMMARY

1. Delirium is a medical emergency characterized by impairment in consciousness, attention, and cognition associated with disorganized thoughts and behavior, fleeting delusions and hallucinations, and increased or decreased psychomotor activity.
2. Delirium is caused by CNS infection, injury, toxicity, space-occupying lesions, and systemic causes secondarily causing CNS hypoxia or inflammation.
3. Treatment of delirium involves the correction of underlying causes. Psychiatric intervention is needed to control agitation, aggression, and psychosis such as delusion and hallucinations.
4. Dementia is a clinical condition characterized by gradual impairment in global cognitive functions in clear consciousness. It presents with impairment in memory, language, intelligence, judgment-reasoning, and impairment in other cognitive functions.
5. Alzheimer's disease is by far the most common cause of dementia followed by vascular dementia, mixed dementia, frontotemporal dementia or FTD, Lewi body dementia, etc. In the majority of cases, dementia is irreversible; however, it is prudent to rule out any treatable cause for dementia such as vitamin deficiency dementia.
6. Alzheimer's disease is characterized by the presence of amyloid plaques in the extracellular space and neurofibrillary tangles inside the neurons. The hippocampal region is the first brain region to be involved followed by gradual onset atrophy of temporal and parietal cortices.
7. Many cases of dementia present with psychiatric symptoms such as irritability, mood swings, aggression, delusions and hallucinations collectively known as behavioral and psychiatric symptoms of dementia or BPSD.
8. Amnesic disorders present with impairment of memory as the primary presenting symptom caused by systemic illnesses or certain CNS conditions excluding delirium and dementia. Causes of amnesic syndrome are Korsakoff's syndrome, head trauma, transient global amnesia, HSV encephalitis, etc.
9. Organic causes such as hormonal imbalance, CNS injury or infections, intake of medications, etc can present with various psychiatric symptoms such as delusions, hallucinations, depression or mania, and anxiety. These cases are managed primarily by treatment of underlying causes. However, psychotropic medications are often prescribed to control symptoms.
10. Injury to the frontal lobe due to head injury, brain surgery, space-occupying lesion, or infection can present with a change in personality, aggression, loss of social inhibition, impaired executive functions, etc which is collectively known as frontal lobe syndrome.

BIBLIOGRAPHY

1. De Sousa A. Towards an integrative theory of consciousness: part 1 (neurobiological and cognitive models). Mens sana monographs, 2013;11(1):100–50.
2. Robyn P Thom et al. Delirium. Am J Psychiatry 2019Oct 1;176(10):785–93.

3. Grover, S, Avasthi, A. Clinical Practice Guidelines for Management of Delirium in Elderly. Indian journal of psychiatry, 2018. 60(Suppl 3).
4. McDougall GJ. A critical review of research on cognitive function/impairment in older adults. Archives of psychiatric nursing, 1995;9(1):22–33.
5. Cerejeira J, Lagarto L, Mukaetova-Ladinska EB. Behavioral and psychological symptoms of dementia. Frontiers in neurology, 2012;3:73.
6. Schachter AS, Davis KL. Alzheimer's disease. Dialogues in clinical neuroscience, 2000;2(2):91–100.
7. Young JJ, Lavakumar M, Tampi D, Balachandran, S, Tampi, RR. Frontotemporal dementia: latest evidence and clinical implications. Therapeutic advances in psychopharmacology, 2018;8(1):33–48.
8. Kopstein M, Mohlman DJ. HIV-1 Encephalopathy and Aids Dementia Complex. [Updated 2021 Jun 30]. In: StatPearls [Internet]. Treasure Island (FL): StatPearls Publishing; 2022 Jan.
9. Erickson KR: Amnestic disorders-Pathophysiology and 152:159–66 patterns of memory dysfunction. West J Med 1990 Feb.
10. Keshavan MS, Kaneko Y. Secondary psychoses: an update. World Psychiatry. 2013 Feb; 12(1):4–15.
11. Rundell JR, Wise MG. Causes of organic mood disorder. J Neuropsychiatry Clin Neurosci. 1989 Fall;1(4):398–400.
12. Chen JP, Reich L, Chung H. Anxiety disorders. West J Med. 2002 Sep;176(4):249–53.
13. Lang FU, Dudeck M, Becker T, Jäger M. Die organische Persönlichkeitsstörung: Konzeptuelle Grundlagen, Klinik und Therapie [Organic personality disorder: conceptual principles, clinical symptoms, and treatment]. Nervenarzt. 2015 Mar;86(3):332-4, 336-9.

Chapter 5

Substance Use Disorders

Competency achievement: Students should be able to
1. **PS4.1** Describe the magnitude and etiology of alcohol and substance use disorders
2. **PS4.2** Elicit, describe, and document clinical features of alcohol and substance use disorders
3. **PS4.3** Enumerate and describe the indications and interpret laboratory and other tests used in alcohol and substance abuse disorders
4. **PS4.4** Describe the treatment of alcohol and substance abuse disorders including behavioral and pharmacologic therapy
5. **PS4.5** Demonstrate family education in a patient with alcohol and substance abuse in a simulated environment
6. **PS4.6** Enumerate and describe the pharmacologic basis and side effects of drugs used in alcohol and substance abuse disorders
7. **PS4.7** Enumerate the appropriate conditions for specialist referral in patients with alcohol and substance abuse disorders

INTRODUCTION

Substance use disorders **are mental and behavioral disorders** characterized by engagement in the use of **addictive substances** despite known adverse consequences. The person spends a good amount of time procuring the substance, abusing it, and getting out of its intoxicating effects, leaving aside his obligations. Substance abuse behavior leads to physical and/or psychological harm, interpersonal conflict, and general impairment in day to day life of the person. Despite its known adverse consequences, the person cannot control this behavior. The **brain disease model** is the prevalent model to explain the characteristic pattern of behaviors seen in cases of substance use disorders.

EPIDEMIOLOGY

The Ministry of Social Justice and Empowerment, Government of India, has published a report titled, "Magnitude of Substance Use in India, 2019". The survey has found major variations in different states in the prevalence of overall substance abuse and also in the use of various substances. Alcohol is the most common psychoactive substance used in India followed by cannabis and opioids such as morphine and heroin. As per the data, the prevalence of alcohol use is 4.6%. The problem of alcohol abuse is significantly greater in males than in females with the ratio being 17:1. The prevalence of cannabis use is 2.8% and that of opioids is 2.1%.

ETIOLOGY

The exact cause of substance use disorder is not known. However, certain risk factors fall within the **biopsychosocial model** that can explain why some people engage in substance abuse while others don't.

1. ***Genetic risk:*** The genetic risk of substance abuse disorder has been supported by family studies. The presence of substance abuse in parents or a family member significantly increases the risk of substance abuse in a person. Identical twins who share 100% genetic components share a substance abuse risk of 50–70%. Therefore, it is quite evident that not all cases can be explained by genetic risk alone.

2. ***Peer pressure:*** Peer pressure is a known risk factor for substance abuse, especially in adolescents. Persons having friends abusing addictive substances are at greater risk of developing substance abuse disorder. The curiosity to explore new things (novelty seeking) with friends in the adolescent age group carries the greatest risk.

3. ***Socio-economic status:*** Persons from a lower socioeconomic background more often engage in substance abuse behavior. The financial burden and economic pressure, lack of personal identity are responsible for these behaviors in this group.

4. ***Adverse life events:*** A history of physical or sexual abuse in childhood is a known risk factor for substance addiction. Stressful life events in adolescence or adulthood also lead to substance abuse behavior. The euphoric and mood-altering effects of addictive substances are the reason people under stress abuse them.

5. ***Personality factors:*** Persons with a well-adjusted personality seldom engage in substance abuse behavior. Substance abuse risk is greatest in persons with disorganized and externalizing personality traits and persons with poor emotional regulation. Risk is highest in persons with cluster B personality traits such as antisocial, borderline, and narcissistic personality traits.

BIOLOGY OF SUBSTANCE ABUSE: THE BRAIN DISEASE MODEL

All of us have a brain circuit known as the **pleasure circuit**, which projects from the **ventral tegmental area (VTA)** in the midbrain to the **nucleus accumbens** (**NAc**) in the basal part of the brain (Fig. 5.1). Nucleus accumbens is also known as the pleasure center of the brain. It is activated by various stimuli such as eating good food, spending good time with friends, having fun trips, having sexual intercourse, and personal achievements. It is necessary for personal **motivation** and the survival of the species. Pleasure-producing stimuli activate this circuit leading to the secretion of **dopamine** neurotransmitter in the nucleus accumbens which is primarily involved in producing pleasure sensation. Addictive substances when used regularly **hijack this pleasure circuit** that makes the person dependent on the substance of abuse.

Regular use of addictive substances in significant amounts leads to changes at a genetic and neuronal level which are primarily responsible for the specific pattern of behaviors seen in substance abuse disorders.

Genetic Changes

Animal studies have shown that abusing addictive substances for a significant period leads to the **expression of ΔfosB** in the medium spiny neurons of the **nucleus accumbens. Overexpression** of this transcription factor is the necessary and sufficient event for

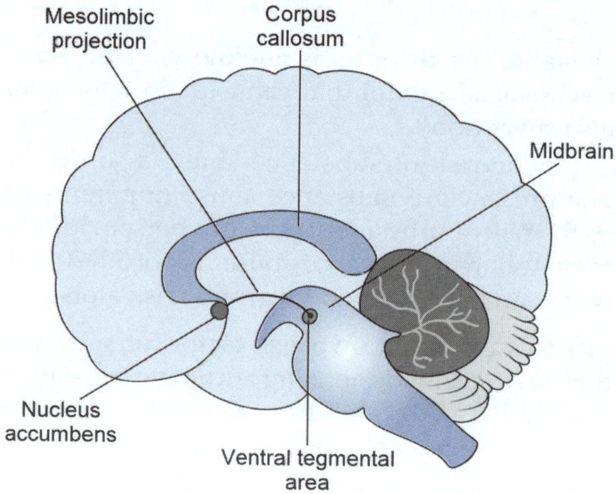

Fig. 5.1: Reward circuit in the brain responsible for substance addiction.

substance addiction which is achieved by inducing **neuroplasticity** in the pleasure circuit.

Changes at the Neural Level

Overexpression of **ΔfosB** brings certain neuroplastic changes in the neural pathway responsible for a pleasure sensation. These neuroplastic changes include decreased levels of dopamine secretion, a decrease in the activity of dopamine receptors in the medium spiny neurons of the nucleus accumbens, etc. Alteration in the pleasure circuit makes it **less sensitive** to natural pleasure-producing stimuli like food, sex, exercise, and achievements and makes it entirely dependent on the addictive substance for activation. Hence addictive substances hijack our pleasure center and make us dependent on them, which leads to substance-seeking behavior, craving, and lack of interest in other activities.

Learning Theory and Substance Abuse

Consumption of an addictive substance activates the pleasure circuit leading to a subjective sense of well-being known as euphoria. This euphoric effect of the addictive substance makes a person **compelled to take it again and again**. The self-reinforcing effect of an addictive substance is known as **positive reinforcement**. After consuming a substance impulsively or in a social gathering or under peer pressure, positive reinforcement sets in and compels the person to use the substance again and again. Regularly abusing the substance for a significant time may lead to the **development of addiction and dependence**. Once dependence has been established, stopping the substance will lead to **withdrawal symptoms** which **cause subjective distress**. Now, the person is compelled to take the substance to get rid of distressing withdrawal symptoms. These distressing withdrawal symptoms act as **negative reinforcement** and make the person compelled to take the substance even if there is the desire to cut down the substance intake.

DIAGNOSIS OF SUBSTANCE ABUSE DISORDER

The mere use of an addictive substance does not qualify for the diagnosis of substance abuse disorder. In ICD-10, certain criteria must be fulfilled to diagnose a case of substance addiction. Out of the 6 mentioned criteria, 3 or more criteria must be present at some point of time during the previous year to establish a diagnosis of substance dependence.

1. **Craving** or a strong urge to take the substance comes from time to time.
2. **Difficulty in controlling substance** abuse behavior in terms of its onset, termination or level of use.
3. **Physiological withdrawal reaction** which means suddenly stopping the intake of the substance leads to withdrawal symptoms. Withdrawal symptoms are specific to a substance of abuse and vary from substance to substance.
4. **Evidence of tolerance**, is more and more amounts of the substance are needed over the period to get the same intoxicating effects.
5. **Lack of interest** in other pleasurable activities apart from substance abuse behavior. The person **spends a significant amount of time** procuring the substance, abusing it, and getting rid of its intoxicating effects putting aside all his duties and obligations.
6. **Harmful use**, continuing abusing the substance despite known physical harm or psychosocial harm (**frequent conflict** in the family or society) due to substance abuse behavior.

GENERAL TERMINOLOGY

1. **Intoxication** is a state of altered mood, perception, cognition, and behavior due to the intake of a psychoactive substance in sufficient quantity.
2. **Addiction** is a state in which the person is engaged in compulsive abuse of an addictive substance despite its known adverse consequences.
3. **Dependence** is a state in which the continuous presence of the substance of abuse is needed in the body to function normally due to substance-induced physiological changes. Sudden stoppage of its use may result in withdrawal symptoms.
4. **Tolerance** is the phenomenon under which more and more amounts of the addictive substance are required to achieve the same mood-altering effects over some time.
5. **Withdrawal** is a state presenting with a consortium of symptoms as a result of sudden stoppage of the intake of an addictive substance in a dependent person. Withdrawal symptoms can be physical or psychological or both.
6. **Craving** is the urge to take an addictive substance coming from time to time.
7. **Adverse** use is abusing a substance despite knowing that it can cause harm.
8. **Harmful use** is abusing a substance despite knowing that it has already caused some physical or psychological harm.
9. **Abstinence** is a state in which an addicted person is no longer abusing the substance for a significant period.
10. **Relapse** is the term used to denote when the person starts abusing the substance after a period of abstinence.

ALCOHOL USE DISORDERS

Ethyl alcohol or ethanol is the active ingredient in all alcoholic beverages. In India, two types of alcoholic beverages are available such as **country-made liquor (CML)** and **Indian-made foreign liquor (IMFL).** Country-made liquors such as rice wine (*handia*), palm wine (*toddy*) and *mahuli* (from *Mahua* flower) generally contain around 30% of ethanol. Indian-made foreign liquors greatly vary from one another in terms of alcoholic content. Beer contains 5–8% of ethanol, wine contains 15–20% and ethanol content in whiskey is around 42%. They vary from one another in their taste not because of varying content of ethanol but because of the presence of other ingredients.

Calculation of Risk of Alcoholism

1 unit of alcohol means 10 mL of pure ethanol. For example, 100 mL of wine containing 20% of ethanol amounts to 2 units. It is considered safe to take up to 14 **units of alcohol per week** at intervals. Binge use of alcohol at once is harmful even if it is taken infrequently. More than **21 units of alcohol per week in females** and more than **35 units per week in males** pose the greatest risk of alcohol addiction and dependence.

Effects of Alcohol on the Brain

Ethanol is a **central nervous system depressant**. It mimics the activities of the inhibitory neurotransmitter **GABA** in the brain. It also activates the **pleasure circuit** via the activation of opioid receptors (alcohol induces secretion of endogenous opioids) leading to **euphoria and a general sense of well-being** which is primarily responsible for the addictive potential of alcohol (positive reinforcement). CNS depressant action is responsible for relieving anxiety, inducing sleep, and causing sedation and respiratory suppression. Regular intake of alcohol makes available an external source of CNS depressant hence the brain starts making less and less inhibitory neurotransmitter GABA. Gradually more and more amount is needed to get the same high which is known as **tolerance. Receptors desensitization** is the mechanism underlying the development of tolerance. Sudden stoppage of alcohol intake leads to over-excitation of the brain due to lack of inhibitory neurotransmitter GABA and excessive glutamate activity resulting in withdrawal symptoms like agitation, insomnia, sympathetic hyperactivity, and life-threatening conditions like withdrawal seizure and delirium tremens. Alcohol withdrawal symptoms are highly distressing which compels the person to take alcohol again and again (negative reinforcement).

Alcohol Intoxication

Alcohol intake leads to alteration in mood, perception, and cognition (thought process). Mild alcohol intake gives a general sense of well-being (euphoria), relaxation, increased confidence, and talkativeness. It is because this affects people who take alcohol while in stress to cope with anxiety. Consuming moderate amounts leads to sedation, psychomotor impairment, and clouding of thought processes. Slurred speech, gross motor disturbance, ataxia and staggering gait, and disorganized behaviors are symptoms of severe alcohol intoxication. Alcohol overdose leads to respiratory suppression, coma, and sometimes death from respiratory failure or aspiration.

Medical and Recreational Use of Alcohol

As such, there is no pharmacological use of ethanol except in the treatment of methanol poisoning. However, its **anxiolytic, hypnotic, and euphoric properties** are exploited by the general public. Stage performers frequently take alcohol before getting on the stage to get rid of **performance anxiety** and to increase confidence. Persons with social anxiety also abuse alcohol to get confidence and improve socialization. Persons having sleep difficulty abuse alcohol to get rid of insomnia.

Since antiquity, the recreational use of alcohol has been a favorite pastime for mankind. Alcohol is not an illicit drug and is frequently served at booze parties and social gatherings.

How our Body Handles Alcohol

Alcohol is **highly lipophilic** and immediately, after intake, is taken by the brain tissues. This leads to symptoms of intoxication. After some time, it is redistributed throughout the body and subsequently metabolized. The **enzyme alcohol dehydrogenase** converts ethanol into **acetaldehyde** which is a toxic by-product. Increased levels of acetaldehyde in the blood result in dysphoria, irritability, generalized weakness and muscle aches, headache, and hypotension. Increased level of acetaldehyde in the blood after a booze party is **responsible for an alcohol hangover** in the morning. Symptoms of a hangover can be alleviated by consuming sufficient amounts of water and oral rehydration solution which help dilute the level of acetaldehyde and its subsequent washout from the body. Acetaldehyde is metabolised by **alcohol dehydrogenase** into **acetone** which is excrete via kidneys and lungs and also by sweat glands albeit in small quantities.

Alcohol Dependence Syndrome

Regular intake of sufficient amounts of alcohol leads to a mental and behavioral disorder known as alcohol dependence syndrome characterized by the following features:

1. **Craving—strong** alcohol-seeking behavior leaving aside other important activities.
2. Using alcohol at an amount or for a period not intended at the start of using it and **inability to control or cut down** alcohol intake despite the strong will to do so.
3. **Withdrawal symptoms**—sudden stoppage of alcohol intakes leads to physical symptoms such as agitation, insomnia, autonomic hyperactivity or withdrawal seizure or delirium.
4. **Tolerance**—gradually increased amount of alcohol is needed to get the same mood-altering effects.
5. **Neglecting personal obligations** like family and social responsibilities, absenteeism from work.
6. **Harmful use**-taking alcohol despite its harmful effects on the body or **alcohol abuse behavior causing interpersonal conflict**.

Harmful Use of Alcohol

Regular use of alcohol can cause **physical damage** to various organs like the liver, heart, GI tract, pancreas, etc. Alcohol abuse is the single most important cause of liver cirrhosis and also for pancreatitis. Harmful use of alcohol is taking alcohol despite knowing that it has already caused damage to one or more organs and can further aggravate it.

Pathological Drunkenness

Pathological drunkenness is a state in which a seemingly normal person becomes **aggressive and violent after drinking alcohol**. The person becomes aggressive and violent, frequently indulging in a physical fight or verbal aggression, destroys property, and can harm himself and others. It is believed to be due to the paradoxical **action of alcohol** on the brain (also known as **idiosyncratic intoxication**). Persons with a history of seizures, head trauma, and cluster B personality disorders are at the highest risk. Complete abstinence is the only known treatment although prophylactic use of mood stabilizers like **lithium** and antiepileptics like carbamazepine and sodium valproate can decrease the frequency and severity of these episodes.

Alcohol Withdrawal Syndrome

Suddenly stopping alcohol intake in a dependent person results in physical and psychological symptoms collectively known as alcohol withdrawal syndrome. The severity of symptoms depends upon the degree of dependence and time elapsed since the last use. Depending upon the severity of symptoms withdrawal state can be categorized into the following stages (Fig. 5.2).

1. ***Stage I (stage of autonomic hyperactivity):*** It is characterized by irritability, agitation, tremor, insomnia, palpitation, etc. It starts 6–8 hours after the last intake. The absence of alcohol in the brain tissue leads to the activation of brainstem gray matters such as locus coeruleus which is responsible for autonomic hyperactivity.

2. ***Stage II (alcohol hallucinosis):*** It is characterized by the sudden onset of psychotic symptoms such as delusions and hallucinations in clear consciousness. It appears after 12–14 hours since the last intake. It is due to the activation of limbic system structures (Mesolimbic pathway) which is responsible for the development of psychosis.

3. ***Stage III (alcohol withdrawal seizure):*** If the withdrawal state is not treated for up to 20–24 hours the brainstem activation can spill over to the cerebral hemispheres resulting in generalized seizure. Alcohol withdrawal seizures are of GTCS type in presentation and the person seldom develops more than one episode of seizure. A history of epilepsy or withdrawal seizures increases the tendency to have further alcohol withdrawal seizures.

4. ***Stage IV (delirium tremens):*** If the withdrawal state remains untreated for more than 24 hours then the whole of the cerebral hemisphere gets activated leading to short-circuiting of information processing. The patient gradually develops confused behaviors, becomes agitated and disoriented, and actively hallucinates which mainly involves visual hallucination. Cognitive processes are deranged with inattention, impaired memory, disorganized thought, and disorganized behaviors. Sleep is frequently disturbed and the patient becomes very restless with the tremor of hands and body (tremens means tremor). A special type of hallucination known as Lilliputian hallucination is observed in delirium tremens in which the patient can see miniature humans and other creatures. Alcohol withdrawal delirium lasts for 1–3 days and seldom appears after 7 days since

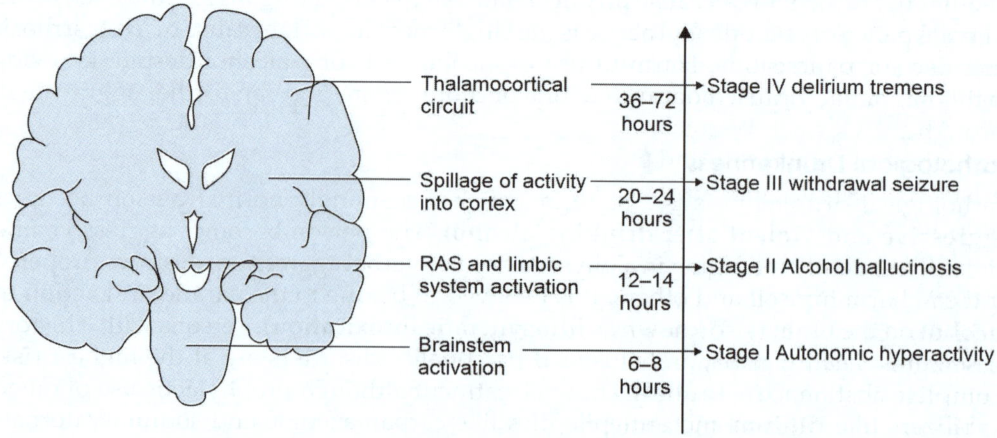

Fig. 5.2: Sequential activation of brain regions during various stages of alcohol withdrawal.

the last intake. Delirium tremens carry the greatest risk of dying from dehydration, aspiration, or accidents if left untreated. Old age, poor nutritional status, dehydration, organic brain diseases like dementia, and a history of delirium tremens are risk factors for the development of delirium tremens.

Treatment of Alcohol Withdrawal Syndrome

Alcohol withdrawal symptoms are managed with oral or parenteral **benzodiazepines** which enhance GABAergic activity and decrease neuronal hyperactivity. They help in calming down the patient, induce sleep and prevent further seizure episodes. In the past barbiturates were used for this purpose but benzodiazepines have replaced them for this use because of their better safety profile.

The first two stages of alcohol withdrawal (Stages of autonomic hyperactivity and alcoholic hallucinosis) are categorized as **uncomplicated withdrawal** and generally managed on an outpatient basis with **oral benzodiazepines**. Oral **chlordiazepoxide** given in tapering doses is the standard treatment option. However, it is contraindicated in patients with deranged liver functions in which case **oxazepam** or **lorazepam** are alternative medications available. Along with benzodiazepines, oral **vitamin B_1 supplementation** is necessary to prevent the development of Wernicke–Korsakoff syndrome.

Alcohol **withdrawal seizures and delirium** tremens are medical emergencies and warrant **hospitalization.** These two stages are also categorized as **complicated withdrawal** and managed with **parenteral benzodiazepines**, hydration with IV fluids, and **parenteral thiamine** (vitamin B_1) supplementation. Long-acting benzodiazepines like lorazepam and diazepam are given parenterally which helps in calming down the patient and prevents further seizure episodes. Vitamin B_1 should be administered before or along with intravenous fluid containing dextrose. Once dextrose is infused into the body it starts using thiamine via the G6PD pathway and further depletes thiamine level and makes it unavailable to the brain tissue which can precipitate Wernicke's encephalopathy, when given before thiamine administration.

NEUROLOGICAL CONSEQUENCES OF ALCOHOL USE

Wernicke's Encephalopathy

Wernicke's encephalopathy occurs due to **thiamine deficiency** in patients with chronic alcohol abuse. Persons with chronic alcohol abuse have generally low levels of thiamine due to their poor nutritional status and impaired absorption of thiamine through the GI tract. Wernicke's encephalo-pathy is a medical emergency because of the high level of mortality and morbidity associated with it. It presents with the characteristic triad: **confusion, ataxia, and ophthalmoplegia**. However, all these 3 signs are rarely found together. Ophthalmoplegia may present as lateral **rectus palsy** or commonly as **lateral nystagmus**.

1. *Mechanism:* Thiamine is an important cofactor in the **G6PD pathway** that generates **reducing agents (H•)**. These reducing agents are essential in activating **free radical scavengers** like glutathione. Lack of thiamine can render these free radical scavengers ineffective leading to **free radical damage** of cell membranes and intracellular organelles. As the brain is the most metabolically active organ, free radical damage is quite early and extensive in brain tissues. Damage to mitochondrial membranes leadsss to the

outpouring of **calcium ions** into the plasma which activates **cellular apoptosis**. Free radical damage of cell membranes leads to **water leakage** into the neural cells and subsequent **cellular swelling**. Cell damage due to apoptosis and cellular swelling results in **encephalopathy** clinically presenting with confusion or impaired consciousness. Brain tissue swelling increases the intracranial pressure with impingement on the fourth and sixth cranial nerves (they have the longest intracranial course) causing ophthalmoplegia. Similarly, cerebellar swelling presents with ataxia and movement incoordination.

2. *Treatment:* **Parenteral thiamine supplementation** at high doses is the standard of care. The patient should be hospitalized. It is also prudent to give thiamine before giving parenteral fluid containing dextrose to prevent further worsening of symptoms. Thiamine supplementation should be given at high doses till the patient becomes fully orientated and the cardinal signs of encephalopathy subside. Thereafter oral thiamine is generally given for a period of 3–6 months.

Korsakoff Syndrome

Korsakoff syndrome or Korsakoff psychosis is the usual **consequence of Wernicke's encephalopathy** if treatment is delayed. Korsakoff psychosis is almost always preceded by Wernicke's encephalopathy and collectively known as Wernicke–Korsakoff syndrome. Korsakoff psychosis is characterized by the following features:

1. **Amnesia-Anterograde amnesia** due to the inability to form new memories is the primary symptom of Korsakoff syndrome.
2. **Confabulation** is characterized by telling false stories unintentionally to fill up the memory gap (also known as honest lying). Confabulation can be provoked in response to a question or it can be spontaneous. Provoked confabulation lacks detailed explanation and the patient generally feels inhibited. In contrast, spontaneous confabulation is elaborative with fantastic details and is expressed with grandiosity.
3. **Cognitive** impairment such as lack of judgment, reasoning, and poor planning ability.
4. **Apathy** with lack of self-initiated actions accompanied by affective flatness and lack of emotional involvement.
5. **Psychosis** in the form of paranoia with a secretive, suspicious attitude.

Korsakoff psychosis is the consequence of **thiamine deficiency** in chronic alcoholics. Lack of thiamine can induce **free radical damage** to various diencephalic structures like the **anterior nucleus of the thalamus** and **mammillary bodies** which are involved in memory formation as a part of the **Papez circuit**. Along with diencephalic structural damage, there is also widespread cortical neuronal loss in patients of KS due to the toxic effects of alcohol on neurons which explains executive dysfunction and psychosis.

Marchiafava Bignami Disease

Chronic alcohol abuse for a long time can lead to a rare neurological condition known as Marchiafava Bignami disease. It occurs due to demyelination and subsequent necrosis of the corpus callosum in these individuals. It presents with fluctuating consciousness, disorientation, spasticity, dysarthria, ataxia, gait abnormalities, and occasional seizures.

Alcohol-induced Psychosis

This term is strictly applied to the development of psychotic features while a patient is chronically abusing alcohol and gradually develops features of psychosis. Alcohol-induced psychosis generally presents with **schizophrenia-like features** with prominent **auditory hallucinations, paranoia, and pan-anxiety**. Persons with a family or personal history of psychosis are at the greatest risk. **High dopamine activity** and a decrease in serotonin activity with chronic use of alcohol are possible causes. Alcohol-induced psychosis is difficult to differentiate from schizophrenia but the prominence of positive and affective symptoms (anxiety and depression), absence of negative and disorganized symptoms, and late age of onset give some clues. Persons who have developed psychosis are at greater risk of developing depression and suicidality.

Treatment involves abstinence from alcohol with tapering doses of benzodiazepines to cope with withdrawal symptoms. Alcohol-induced psychosis generally subsides by itself within 6 months of abstinence from alcohol. Psychosis can be managed with **antipsychotics** like olanzapine, risperidone, or haloperidol.

Suggested investigations in a case of alcohol use disorder

1. Complete blood count with differential count
2. Blood sugar level
3. Serum protein analysis, chronic alcoholism causes albumin depletion
4. Liver function test
5. Nerve conduction test in cases presenting with peripheral neuropathy
6. Brain imaging studies in cases of suspected Wernicke's encephalopathy, Korsakoff psychosis

Treatment of Alcohol Dependence

1. Detoxification phase: When a person with alcohol dependence comes for treatment he is advised to stop drinking alcohol. To get rid of withdrawal symptoms he has been prescribed medications such as **benzodiazepines**. Benzodiazepine **helps in overcoming withdrawal symptoms** by calming the patient, inducing sleep, and preventing withdrawal seizures and the emergence of delirium. Long-acting benzodiazepines such as c**hlordiazepoxide** are the first choice which is prescribed in tapering doses and stopped within 7–10 days. Chlordiazepoxide is contraindicated in patients with **deranged liver function** in which cases other long-acting BZD such as oxazepam and lorazepam are preferred. BZD should not be continued for more than 2 weeks and residual symptoms like sleep disturbance are taken care of with other medications like first-generation antihistamines.

2. *Deaddiction phase:* After detoxification, the primary goal of management is to keep the person abstinent from alcohol and **prevent relapse**. A combined pharmacological and psychotherapeutic approach is most effective in this regard. The pharmacological approach helps in decreasing craving for alcohol or inducing aversion toward alcohol use while psychotherapy is focused on relapse prevention by various means.

Pharmacological agents are grouped as **anti craving** drugs and **anti-abuse** drugs depending upon their mode of action.

A. Anticraving Agents

These drugs help reduce the urge to take alcohol in an addicted person. **Naltrexone** is an **opioid receptor antagonist** (μ antagonist) which suppresses the euphoric effect of alcohol by binding to opioid receptors in the pleasure center of the brain and makes alcohol no more effective in producing euphoria.

Another agent **acamprosate is an NMDA antagonist** and itself imparts some CNS effects of alcohol causing mild euphoria and relaxation. Therefore, it is also known as **artificial alcohol.** Mimicking the actions of alcohol makes alcohol no more desirable. Acamprosate is useful in patients with impulsivity and novelty-seeking behaviors. These patients have excessive glutamate activity leading to hyperactivity of the striatum. Acamprosate being an NMDA antagonist reduces striatal activity and subsequent impulsivity and novelty-seeking behaviors.

Baclofen is another anticraving agent which acts by enhancing GABAergic actions. Baclofen is mostly suitable for patients taking alcohol as self-medication to cope with anxiety, sleep problems, and low self-esteem. Baclofen being an anxiolytic with sedative properties helps maintain abstinence.

B. Anti-abuse Drug

Disulfiram is the only anti-abuse drug approved for alcohol de-addiction. It acts by inhibiting the enzyme **aldehyde dehydrogenase** and blocking the conversion of acetaldehyde to acetic acid leading to the accumulation of acetaldehyde in the body. As we know, acetaldehyde is a toxic by-product and causes dysphoria, irritability, generalized weakness, headache, vomiting, etc. (**disulfiram reaction**). When a person on disulfiram takes alcohol there is an accumulation of acetaldehyde in the body with above mentioned problematic symptoms which produces an aversion to alcohol intake. A person on disulfiram can also develop a similar reaction when he uses other alcohol-containing products such as body deodorant, after shaving lotion, etc., and must be alerted about their use.

Psychotherapy and Family Intervention

Psychotherapy is principally focused on **relapse prevention**. The first task is to identify the factors that can cause relapse such as stressful situations, interpersonal conflict, loneliness, etc. The patient is taught to cope with the stressful situation without returning to drinking alcohol. He is advised to spend more time with family and friends and in productive work. One of the important aspects of psychotherapy is to avoid cues that can induce craving such as wine shops, friends, parties, etc. Many patients benefit from joining self-help groups like **alcoholics anonymous**.

Family therapy involves psychoeducation regarding the nature of the illness. Family members should understand that alcohol abuse is a brain disorder and not due to moral failure on the part of the patient. Emotional, social, and financial support by the family members is the most important factor in achieving and maintaining abstinence in cases of substance abuse disorders. They should also be vigilant regarding the risk of relapse and seek help from a psychiatrist in cases of relapse.

CANNABIS USE DISORDERS

Canna**bis or marijuana** is obtained from the female flowering stalk **(female inflorescence)** of the cannabis plant, ***Cannabis sativa***. Cannabis is known by various **street names** such as **ganja, weed, grass, mary jane,** etc. Cannabis is the **most widely used** illicit psychoactive substance in the world. Various parts of the cannabis plant contain **psychoactive alkaloids,** but female flowering stalks contain them in the highest quantities. Important components found in cannabis that has psychoactive properties are

tetrahydrocannabinol (THC), cannabidiol (CBD), and cannabinol (CBN). Marijuana is cultivated worldwide, especially in Afghanistan and South-East Asia. **Myanmar–Laos–Thailand** together forms a geographical boundary known as the **golden triangle** which is notorious for marijuana cultivation.

Recreational Use of Cannabis

Cannabis use is one of the favorite pastimes of adolescents and **college-going students** in many countries. It is frequently smoked in cigarettes, **joints, *chillum*, and *hookah*.** Cannabis can also be taken orally in the form of **cakes and beverages** known as ***bhang*.** ***Bhang*,** a milk-based beverage containing cannabis is frequently consumed in India during various religious festivals.

Cannabis Intoxication

When smoked, the effects of cannabis can be felt within minutes; however, it takes 1–2 hours to exert its effect when taken orally. However, the bioavailability of orally taken cannabis is considerably high. The primary effect is a **sense of well-being** known as a **stoned feeling or high feeling**. Along with euphoria, it can also produce a sense of relaxation, elevated self-confidence, talkativeness, increase appetite and increase libido. At a slightly higher dose, it causes a heightened perception of the surroundings with an altered perception of the flow of time (time slows down) and can cause delusions and hallucinations. These effects last for 1–2 hours and gradually wean out.

Sometimes cannabis can also produce nervousness with **panicky feelings**, restlessness, **palpitations, paranoia**, the delusion of persecution, and **scary visual and auditory hallucinations**. This effect of cannabis is known as a **'bad trip'** and frequently occurs after oral intake of cannabis because of higher bioavailability in this route. However, cannabis has minimal or **no effects on the vital functions** of the brain due to the lack of its action on the brain stem region and not a single case of death due to cannabis overdose has been reported so far from any part of the world.

Effects of Cannabis on CNS

Various psychoactive effects of cannabis are mediated via **cannabinoid receptors CB1 and CB2**. We have **endogenous cannabinoids such as anandamide** (the name has been derived from the Sanskrit word '*ananda*' meaning pleasure) which act on these receptors. Activation of the CB1 receptor in the pleasure circuit potentiates the action of endogenous morphine (endorphins) causing euphoria and a sensation of high. Cannabis receptors are also present in large quantities in the cerebral cortex which mediates their mood and perception-altering effects. Cannabis receptors are conspicuously absent in the brain stem which explains little or no effect of cannabis on vital functions of the brain.

Cannabis Addiction

Because of instant euphoric and mood-altering effects, cannabis has **high addiction potential**. Cannabis addiction is characterized by the following features:

1. Craving or drug-seeking behavior
2. Tolerance
3. Inability to cut down cannabis abuse
4. Lack of interest in other activities other than taking cannabis

5. Lack of responsibilities toward personal obligations
6. Interpersonal conflict due to cannabis abuse and indulgence in dangerous activities like rash driving and physical fight in an intoxicated state.

Although cannabis has high addiction potential it **does not cause physical dependence**. Stopping cannabis after a period of regular intake has no effects on bodily functions. Withdrawal symptoms are mainly psychological like drug craving, irritability, dysphoria, agitation, and insomnia.

Cannabis-induced Psychosis

Long-term use of cannabis can result in **psychosis**. However, there is debate whether the psychosis is caused by cannabis itself or whether the person is prone to develop psychosis while cannabis use acts as an aggravating factor. The risk of developing cannabis-induced psychosis is highest in persons with a **family history of psychotic disorders** such as schizophrenia or BPAD.

The presentation of cannabis-induced psychosis can vary from person to person. **Affective psychosis** with euphoric or irritable mood, aggressive behavior, and ideas of grandiosity is the most common presentation. Some also present with schizophrenia-like symptoms with prominent delusions, hallucinations, poor self-care, and wandering behavior. Persecutory delusions and auditory hallucinations of a threatening type are the most common symptoms. It is quite difficult to differentiate cannabis-induced psychosis from true cases of psychosis and both these disorders can overlap in many cases. However, the symptoms of cannabis-induced psychosis (or any psychoactive substance-induced psychosis in general) should subside within 6 months of stopping the substance use.

It should be noted that psychotic features with delusions and hallucinations can also appear during **cannabis intoxication**. However, these symptoms are less severe and insight into the symptoms is generally intact. Psychotic features appearing during intoxication generally resolve within 24 hours.

Cannabis-induced Amotivational Syndrome

Regular intake of cannabis for a prolonged period results in **amotivational syndrome**. It is characterized by idleness, loss of interest in pursuing life goals, and aversion toward pleasurable activities (anhedonia). The patient is mostly confined to a home environment with poor socialization. There is no specific treatment for amotivational syndrome and abstinence from cannabis also does not reverse the condition.

Treatment of Cannabis Addiction

Because of the lack of physical withdrawal symptoms in the case of cannabis withdrawal, **detoxification is not needed in a person** with cannabis addiction. Psychological withdrawal symptoms can be controlled with mild anxiolytics like low-dose clonazepam given for a short period (5–7 days). **Deaddiction** phase mainly involves psychotherapeutic approaches such as **motivational enhancement therapy (MET)** and **cognitive behavioral therapy (CBT).** MET focuses on relapse prevention by avoiding cues and developing coping strategies to cope with stress and boredom. CBT focuses on deranged thought processes regarding life, interpersonal relations, and drug use.

There is **no specific pharmacological agent** for the treatment of cannabis addiction. However, recent evidence is piling up for high doses of **acetylcysteine** in decreasing cannabis cravings and preventing relapse.

OPIOID USE DISORDERS

Opium is a psychoactive substance obtained from the opium **poppy plant (*Papaver somniferum*).** It is obtained by drying the **latex** oozing out from the outer fleshy part of poppy fruits. Dried latex contains many psychoactive substances such as morphine, thebaine, codeine, etc. Opium is a controlled substance and both cultivation and distribution of opium products are illegal in many countries. Afghanistan produces and exports the largest amount of opium in the world. The mountainous regions spanning **Pakistan, Afghanistan, and Iran** harbor the highest numbers of poppy fields and are notoriously known as the **'golden crescent'**.

What are opioids?

Opioids are substances that have similar psychoactive properties as opium under their **action on opioid receptors**. Opioids can be **natural, semisynthetic, or synthetic** as shown in Table 5.1.

Recreational Use of Opioids

Opioids are illicit substances with **high addiction and dependence potential**. Crude opium has been abused as a recreational drug since antiquity. Currently, because of the ban on the cultivation of opium and the difficulty in procuring crude opium, many are turning toward medically prescribed opioids. Those who have been prescribed opioids for pain relief are at the highest risk of developing opioid addiction and dependence. Opioids are generally taken orally or intravenously. Other modes of abuse are inhalation by heating heroin in a container and by sniffing.

Action of Opioids on CNS

The pleasure center in the brain has various opioid receptors which modulate the activities of the pleasure circuit. There are **3 principal opioid receptors; μ, δ, and κ receptors,** which mediate various actions of endogenous opioids. **Endogenous opioids** such as **beta-endorphin** (endogenous morphine), **dynorphin, and enkephalins** act on these receptors to exert their actions. Activation of the mu receptor leads to the release of dopamine in the pleasure center (nucleus accumbens) which gives the sensation of being high. μ receptor is also coupled with inhibitory G-protein and causes neuronal inhibition which explains the CNS suppressing, analgesic and anesthetic actions of opioids. μ receptor mediates strong euphoric, analgesic, reduces GI motility, and pupillary constricting actions, and is principally responsible for physical dependence, δ receptor mediates euphoric, analgesic, and antidepressant actions while activation

Table 5.1: Different categories of opioids

Opioid category	*Natural opioids*	*Semisynthetic opioids*	*Synthetic opioids*
Source	The poppy plant	Produced by processing opium products in the laboratory	Purely synthesized in the laboratory
Examples	Morphine, codeine and thebaine.	Heroin*, hydrocodone, hydromorphone, oxymorphone, etc.	Tramadol, methadone, fentanil, sufentanil, alfentanil etc.

*Heroin is chemically diacetyl-morphine obtained by attaching two acetyl groups to the naturally obtained morphine which makes it highly lipophilic and more potent.

of κ receptor in contrast causes dysphoria and analgesia. Actions of exogenous opioids taken for medical or recreational purposes are mediated via these receptors to exert their euphoric, analgesic, and sedative actions.

Opioid Intoxication

Intravenous injection of heroin gives intense pleasure akin to orgasm. Along with euphoria, it also produces a general sense of relaxation, increased confidence, lack of inhibition, and increased libido. They also produce cognitive impairment (impairment in judgment-reasoning, memory, attention concentration, etc.) and psychomotor retardations. Opioid intoxication also causes appetite suppression, nausea or vomiting, and constipation. A slightly increased amount can lead to sedation, profound analgesia, and sleepiness.

Opioid overdose results in a constricted pinpoint pupil, respiratory suppression, coma, and ultimately death. Opioid overdose is a medical emergency and the patient is managed with securing of the airway and stabilization of cardiovascular functions. The effects of opioids can be effectively reversed with opioid antagonist **naloxone given intramuscularly or intravenously**. Naloxone injection should be repeated at frequent intervals till the patient gains consciousness and respiration becomes normal.

Opioid Addiction

Opioids have high addictive potential mediated by their intense **pleasure-**producing actions which act as **positive reinforcement** for their repetitive use. **Tolerance develops rapidly** because of receptors desensitization and decreased levels of endogenous opioids. **Unpleasant withdrawal symptoms** act as **negative reinforcement** which further enhances their addictive effects. Regular intake of opioids causes permanent changes in the pleasure circuit and other parts of the brain (prefrontal cortex, insular cortex, and striatum). Changes in the pleasure circuit include receptors desensitization and decreased effects of other endogenous chemicals (e.g. endorphins) on them, leading to a lack of motivation and interest in other activities apart from taking opioids.

Opioid Withdrawal Syndrome

In cases of opioid withdrawal, the **hyperactive prefrontal cortex** results in subjective symptoms of withdrawal such as dysphoria, irritability, and intense craving while **hyperactivity of noradrenergic neurons** in locus coeruleus is responsible for much of the objective feature. A case of opioid withdrawal presents with the following features

1. Dysphoria and irritability
2. Excessive lacrimation and rhinorrhea
3. Stomach ache and myalgia
4. Nausea, vomiting, and diarrhea
5. Hyperarousal symptoms like palpitation, tachypnoea, high blood pressure and tremor and
6. Sleep disturbance

Treatment of Opioid Withdrawal

Definitive treatment of opioid withdrawal is done with prescription opioids such **as tramadol and methadone**. Prescription opioids effectively control both subjective and somatic symptoms of opioid withdrawal. In cases of severe withdrawal symptoms tramadol injection is given in twice daily or thrice daily doses and gradually tapered and stopped within 5–7 days. Cases with less severe withdrawal symptoms can be managed with oral tramadol or methadone. The dose of these medications should be gradually tapered and stopped within 7 days. **Symptomatic management** can also be done by following medications.

1. **Clonidine** is indicated to control hyperarousal symptoms
2. **Loperamide** effectively controls diarrhea
3. **Promethazine** can be used to control rhinorrhea and lacrimation
4. **NSAIDs** such as aceclofenac and ibuprofen are used for controlling pain
5. **Cyclobenzaprine** has good efficacy in controlling musculoskeletal pain
6. **Sedatives such as lorazepam** may be used to calm down the patient and induce sleep

Treatment of Opioid Addiction

Proper management of opioid dependence is necessary for reducing dependence on opium, reducing the financial burden, and living a meaningful and productive life. Treatment of opioid addiction can be done in two phases as described below.

1. *Detoxification phase:* It involves washing out the opioid from the body and making the body get rid of opioid dependence to function normally. It starts with abstinence from opioids and effectively controlling withdrawal symptoms. It generally takes 5–7 days to clear the body off the opioid. After the detoxification phase, the patient is put on either the deaddiction phase or oral replacement therapy (ORT) as per the patient's preference.

2. *Deaddiction phase:* The goal of the deaddiction phase is to maintain abstinence from opioid use and to prevent relapse. The pharmacological approach involves treatment with opioid antagonists such as naltrexone. **Naltrexone is a μ receptor antagonist** which effectively suppresses any euphoric or reinforcing effects of an opioid in case of relapse. Naltrexone should be continued for a period of 6–12 months and then gradually stopped. Administration of naltrexone to a still dependent person (in the detoxification stage) can induce severe withdrawal symptoms; hence it should be started only after opioid washout from the body which takes 5–7 days of abstinence.

3. *Risk reduction approach with oral replacement therapy:* In patients who are unwilling to stay abstinent from opioids or where treatment adherence with anti-craving drugs is questionable, the patient can be put on oral opioid replacement therapy. Oral opioid replacement therapy minimizes the risks associated with abusing opioid injections such as
   - Contraction of viral infections (HIV, HBV, and HCV infections) via needle sharing
   - Endocarditis
   - Venous thrombosis
   - Septicemia
   - Scarring of the skin

   Methadone and buprenorphine are used for oral replacement therapy. These drugs are opioids themselves but are far less potent than heroin. They prevent withdrawal symptoms and produce euphoria and relaxation. Sudden stoppage of methadone can also precipitate withdrawal symptoms which are less with buprenorphine.

   Psychotherapy such as motivational enhancement therapy or MET can motivate a person to stay abstinent and increase treatment adherence. Group therapy is also highly effective in this regard. Family therapy has some role in understanding the illness, reducing stress and miscommunication among the family members, and increasing familial support for the patient's cause.

STIMULANT USE DISORDERS

Stimulants are substances that **increase the activity of the CNS** by increasing the levels of excitatory chemicals. They make the person **alert, confident, and energetic** with a subjective sense of **well-being**. Many stimulants such as **cocaine and nicotine** are **naturally obtained** from plants while others such as amphetamine and its derivatives are **synthesized in illicit laboratories**. Most of these substances are illicit substances (except nicotine) and some are used as prescription drugs for various psychiatric conditions.

COCAINE

Cocaine is a **naturally obtained** psychoactive substance derived from the leaves of the plant ***Erythroxylon coca***. Coca plant is widely cultivated in northern **South American countries** such as Bolivia, Columbia, and Ecuador. Cocaine consumption is highest in North American and European countries and least in Asian countries because of its cost and availability.

Recreational use of Cocaine

Cocaine is a **white crystalline substance** available in freebase form (known as **crack**) and also in an adulterated form mixed with chalk, sugar, and other white substances. The most common method of consumption is via **nasal inhalation** also known as **snorting**. Other methods are intravenous or subcutaneous **injection** and via **smoking** of freebase cocaine.

Cocaine is a highly addictive substance and produces **immense pleasure and excitement**. Even a single use of cocaine can produce psychological dependence with extreme craving and drug-seeking behavior. Physical dependence can occur; however, it is not as pronounced as heroin abuse.

Effects of Cocaine on CNS

Cocaine acts as an **inhibitor of dopamine reuptake** (by blocking dopamine transporter or **DAT**) causing increased activity of dopamine in the synaptic cleft. **Increased dopamine activity** in the pleasure circuit (projecting from the VTA to the nucleus accumbens) causes immense pleasure akin to orgasm. Increased dopamine level in other parts of the brain such as in the **frontal cortex** increases attention, confidence, and clarity of thinking and in the brainstem causes increased sympathetic activity (due to increased level of noradrenaline) leading to increased blood pressure, heart rate, and psychomotor activity. Cocaine also causes inhibition of the reuptake of serotonin and noradrenaline.

Health Hazards of Cocaine Abuse

1. The snorting of finely chopped cocaine crystals can cause **nasal inflammation, nasal ulcer,** and bleeding and on long-term use, it can cause **perforation of the nasal septum**.
2. Smoking crack cocaine can cause bronchospasm, aggravation of bronchial asthma, and **COPD** on long-term use.

3. Intravenous use can cause **vasculitis, cellulitis, endocarditis,** and transmission of viral infections such as HIV and hepatitis viruses.
4. Long-term use of cocaine can cause adverse cardiovascular events such as **myocardial infarction, cerebrovascular infarction,** and **hemorrhage**.
5. **Seizure** is most commonly associated with cocaine among all the substances of abuse. A seizure is generally a single episode of GTCS but recurrent episodes of seizure and status epilepticus can also happen.

Psychiatric Complications

Cocaine use can lead to the development of **paranoia with delusions and hallucinations**. Delusions of persecution, reference and infidelity, and auditory hallucinations are common with cocaine abuse. Delusion of **insects crawling under the skin** is typically seen in cocaine abusers and known as **formication or 'cocaine bug'**.

AMPHETAMINES

Amphetamines are widely used psychoactive substances which are synthesized in illicit laboratories across the world, especially in the US and Europe. The forms of amphetamines used for this purpose are:

1. **Dextroamphetamine**
2. **Methamphetamine** and
3. A **mixture** of dextroamphetamine and amphetamine

Effects of Amphetamine on CNS

Amphetamines are **CNS stimulants** that increase the activities of the neurons and sharing of information between them. This is achieved by **inhibiting the reuptake of dopamine** by blocking the dopamine transporter or DAT in the presynaptic terminal thereby increasing the availability of dopamine in the synaptic cleft and subsequent increase in its activity on dopamine **D_1 and D_2 receptors**. Increased dopamine activity in the **reward circuit** causes euphoria and a subjective feeling of well-being which acts as the major reinforcer of amphetamine abuse. Increased dopamine activity in other parts of the CNS leads to increased confidence, enhanced interest, alertness, and increased clarity of thinking. Higher doses may cause restlessness, insomnia, aggression, paranoia, delusions, and hallucinations.

Recreational Use of Amphetamines

Amphetamines are one of the most **commonly abused illicit drugs** second only to cannabis. Because of their potent psychoactive effects, they are highly addictive substances of abuse. Amphetamines are available by various **street names such as ice, crystal, crystal meth, speed,** etc. These drugs can be taken by inhalation, smoking, and as intravenous injections. Intravenous injection of methamphetamine causes intense euphoria.

Amphetamines on long-term use can cause chronic insomnia, weight loss, and **features of paranoid schizophrenia**. These patients present with paranoia and delusions of persecution, reference, and infidelity. Auditory hallucinations of a threatening type are also common in chronic amphetamine abusers. However, negative and deficit symptoms are conspicuously absent. This observation of the appearance of features of paranoid schizophrenia with amphetamine use led to the development of the dopamine **hypothesis of schizophrenia**.

MDMA

3,4-methylenedioxymethamphetamine or MDMA is a methamphetamine derivative available by the street names **ecstasy, E, X, and Molly**. What is peculiar about MDMA is; it produces effects that resemble that of stimulants amphetamines and psychedelics LSD. This is because; it **increases the activities of both dopamine and serotonin in the CNS**.

Club Drugs

These are illicit drugs frequently **consumed in dance parties** and especially in all-night dance parties **known as raves** and hence are named club drugs. Club drugs mostly include stimulants such as

1. Gamma hydrobutyrate
2. Methamphetamine
3. MDMA also known as ecstasy and
4. Ketamine

NICOTINE

Nicotine is the **active ingredient of all tobacco products** which is obtained from the leaves of the plant *Nicotiana tabacum*. Tobacco products can be consumed by smoking in beedis and cigarettes and also orally as chewable products. Because of legality, easy availability, and low cost, tobacco products are the most common addictive substance used by the general public. Tobacco use is a major health concern in every country because of associated morbidity and mortality due to its health effects such as the risk of cancer, cardiovascular risks, GI problems, etc.

CNS Effects of Nicotine

Nicotine exerts its effects by acting as an **agonist at nicotinic acetylcholine receptors (NAChRs).** Increased activity of these receptors leads to **increased levels of monoamine neurotransmitters** such as dopamine, serotonin, and noradrenaline which produce the peculiar stimulating effects associated with nicotine use. Nicotine use leads to a sense of well-being, elevated mood and interest, increased cognitive performance, and enhanced motor performance.

Treatment of Nicotine Addiction

Nicotine is a **highly addictive substance** and addiction to nicotine is established quickly and is difficult to get rid of. Both pharmacological and psychological management approaches are available which help a person to quit tobacco use if motivation is there.

1. ***Pharmacological approach:*** **Nicotine replacement therapy or NRT** is available for those who are finding it difficult to quit nicotine even if with the presence of motivation. This approach uses **nicotine patches, gums, and lozenges** to be used by the person in place of tobacco. This **eliminated the health hazard** associated with tobacco use.

   Other medications such as **bupropion and varenicline** can be used to **get rid of cravings** and other psychological withdrawal symptoms such as dysphoria, irritability, and lethargy occurring after stopping tobacco use.

2. ***Psychological approach:*** **Brief intervention psychotherapy techniques** based on motivational enhancement therapy such as the **5 As (ask, assess, advise, assist,**

and arrange) and **5 Rs (relevance, risk, reward, roadblock, and repeat)** approaches (formulated by WHO) are highly effective in motivating a person to quit tobacco use and maintaining abstinence.

HALLUCINOGEN USE DISORDERS

Hallucinogens are psychoactive substances that cause alteration in perception (causing illusions and hallucinations) and alteration in mood, thought process, and consciousness. Hallucinogens, obtained from plant sources are in use for thousands of years especially as recreational drugs and in religious festivals. **Albert Hoffman**, in 1938, produced the first synthetic hallucinogen, **LSD** or **lysergic acid diethylamide**, which is far more potent than its botanical counterparts.

Effects of Hallucinogens on CNS: Deactivating the Default Mode Network

There is a **network of interconnected neurons** involving various cortical regions known as the default **mode network or DMN**. It includes such cortical areas as **the** medial prefrontal cortex, posterior cingulate cortex, and angular gyrus. DMN is primarily involved in **subjective awareness of self and surrounding**, awareness of perception of time and external reality, self-thoughts and actions, etc. DMN determines what we are, and makes us aware of our thoughts and behaviors and our **ego boundaries**. It is revealed that hallucinogens, especially **psychedelics, deactivate this default mode network** by acting on serotonin receptors (and NMDA and ACh receptors) resulting in alteration in the subjective sense of self, mood, and thinking. Many people describe this state as **'out of the body ' experience (due to the dissolution of ego boundary)** or a sense of unison with divinity or the supreme being. Because of these effects, psychedelics are also considered substances that reveal the unconscious mind and can help in 'out of the box' thinking.

Classification of Hallucinogens

Hallucinogens are typically grouped into the following three classes:

1. ***Psychedelics or classical hallucinogens:*** They primarily produce vivid hallucinations along with alterations in mood and thinking. **LSD** is a classical example of psychedelics. These drugs act as **partial agonists at the serotonin 5HT receptors** in the cerebral cortex to produce alteration in thinking, perceptions, and emotions. LSD can produce a special type of hallucination known as **reflex hallucination** or **synesthesia**, in which stimuli in one sensory modality are perceived in another sensory modality such as hearing colors and seeing music! It is hypothesized to be due to its effect on the **angular gyrus** (a part of the **default mode network**) which is tasked with converting stimuli in one sensory modality to perception in another modality (when we look at the written words in book we feel as if someone is reading them aloud inside our mind, this conversion of visual stimuli into auditory sensation is the function of angular gyrus). **Psilocybin,** obtained from the fungus ***Psilocybe mexicana,*** and **mescaline,** obtained from **peyote cactus** plants are famous examples of naturally available psychedelics. Both psilocybin and mescaline are used in religious rituals as god-revealing substances.

2. ***Dissociatives:*** **Dissociatives** are drugs that **induce dissociation, a trance-like state** in which the person is conscious but is unresponsive to external stimuli with minimal perception of the somatic sensations (e.g. pain) with a feeling of detachment from self and the surrounding (**depersonalization and derealization**). Phencyclidine

(PCP) also known as **angel dust** and its derivative **ketamine** are the most commonly used dissociative drugs. Ketamine is an anesthetic agent categorized as a **dissociative anesthetic**. Phencyclidine is available as a crystalline substance and is frequently abused alone or in combination with cannabis to enhance its effects. These drugs act **as NMDA antagonists,** blocking the actions of glutaminergic neurons in the cerebral cortex to produce their effects.

3. ***Deliriants:*** Deliriants, as the name indicates, are substances that **induce a confused delirium-like state** with impairment in consciousness and alteration of mood and perception. Deliriants act as **anticholinergic agents** in the cerebral cortex to impart their mood-altering effects. **Atropine**, obtained from Atropa plants frequently causes delirium at higher doses. Other well-known deliriants are **scopolamine and hyoscyamine obtained from the Datura plant**. Deliriants are seldom used for recreational purposes as they cause dysphoria and unpleasant effects.

Hallucinogen Use Disorder

Along with inducing altered states of perception, mood, and cognition, hallucinogens also **activate the pleasure center of the brain** to produce a sense of well-being, the basis of their abuse potential. **Tolerance** with these agents develops very rapidly within 4–5 days; however, they do not cause physical dependence and withdrawal reactions.

Hallucinogen Intoxication

Ingestion of hallucinogens causes a euphoric mood, heightened sense of self with clarity of thinking, and diminished perception of pain. Higher doses result in vivid visual and auditory hallucinations, altered perception of time, cognitive impairment with confusion and sometimes **the person can hear colors and see music!** (Also known as **synesthesia or reflex hallucination**). Apart from these subjective feelings, hallucinogen intoxication results in increased heart rate with palpitation, facial flushing, excessive sweating, etc.

Some persons, who take an excess dose of hallucinogen, experience a panicky **feeling** with extreme fearfulness, palpitation, shortness of breath, and scary visual and auditory hallucination, known as **'BAD TRIP'**. Bad trips are common **with LSD and phencyclidine**. Hallucinogen intoxication state can be treated by putting the patient in a quiet environment, giving verbal reassurance, and oral or parenteral benzodiazepines such as clonazepam and lorazepam. Neuroleptics should be avoided as they can cause worsening symptoms.

Hallucinogen-induced Persisting Perception Disorder

It is characterized by **re-experiencing** the mood-altering effects of hallucinogens in the form of **flashbacks l**ong after the subsiding of their effects. Flashbacks are spontaneous dissociative episodes in which there is a feeling that the person is re-experiencing the events once again. Flashbacks are common after the experience of bad trips with LSD and phencyclidine. Flashbacks can be long-lasting and can be treated with long-acting benzodiazepines such as **clonazepam** and mood stabilizers such as **sodium valproate** and **carbamazepine.**

Hallucinogen-induced Psychosis

Persistent use of hallucinogens, especially phencyclidine, can induce a state akin to schizophrenia with the delusion of persecution, referential ideas, auditory hallucinations, etc. This state is known as hallucinogen-induced psychosis. Positive symptoms are prominent with minimal negative symptoms and the person's functionality is more or less preserved. Hallucinogen-induced psychosis can be effectively treated by **abstinence from the drug** combined with **antipsychotic medications** such as olanzapine and risperidone given for a short-term duration (6–9 months).

Conditions for specialist referral in substance use disorders

1. Cases presenting with substance overdose, e.g. coma due to opioid overdose
2. Cases presenting with severe withdrawal state, e.g. delirium tremens
3. Cases presenting with substance-induced complications such as Wernicke's encephalopathy, Korsakoff psychosis, etc.
4. Poor response to initial deaddiction therapy
5. Patients requiring psychotherapeutic intervention
6. When substance abuse is secondary to a psychiatric illness
7. Patients with underlying personality disorder

SUMMARY

1. Substance addiction is characterized by repetitive indulgence in the abuse of a substance despite known harmful consequences leaving aside other important aspects of life. Dependence is different from addiction and is characterized by a state in which the continuous presence of a substance of abuse is needed for the maintenance of bodily homeostasis.
2. Alcohol is the most important substance of abuse with high addiction and dependence potential. Chronic use of alcohol is associated with liver cirrhosis, neuropathy, dementia, psychosis, and Korsakoff's syndrome.
3. Alcohol withdrawal presents with sympathetic hyperactivity, seizure, or delirium. Alcohol withdrawal is treated with intravenous fluid therapy, benzodiazepines, and thiamine supplementation.
4. Cannabis or marijuana can cause addiction and psychological dependence via the action of its active ingredient tetrahydrocannabinol (THC) on cannabinoid CB1 receptors in the CNS. Chronic use of cannabis can lead to psychosis and amotivational syndrome.
5. Opioids are natural or synthetic substances that act on opioid receptors in the CNS similar to opium products such as morphine. Opioids are associated with significant abuse potential and addiction and dependence is quickly established with them.
6. Stimulants such as cocaine, MDMA, and amphetamine derivatives act on the CNS by inhibiting the reuptake of dopamine from the synaptic cleft causing extreme euphoria and well-being.
7. Hallucinogens such as LSD are substances that cause alteration in consciousness, mood, perceptions, and subjective experience of self and surrounding. Chronic use of hallucinogens is associated with the development of psychosis akin to schizophrenia.

BIBLIOGRAPHY

1. Ambekar A, Agrawal A, Rao R, Mishra AK, Khandelwal SK. The magnitude of Substance Use in India. New Delhi: Ministry of Social Justice and Empowerment, Government of India; 2019. On behalf of the Group of Investigators for the National Survey on Extent and Pattern of Substance Use in India.
2. Jadidi N, Nakhaee N. Etiology of drug abuse: a narrative analysis. Journal of Addiction, *2014*, 352835.
3. World Health Organization. (1992). The ICD-10 classification of mental and behavioral disorders: Clinical descriptions and diagnostic guidelines. Geneva: World Health Organization.
4. Koob, George F, and Nora D Volkow. "Neurobiology of addiction: a neurocircuitry analysis." The Lancet. Psychiatry 2016; vol. 3,8:760–73.
5. Sadock, and Pedro Ruiz. Kaplan and Sadock's Synopsis of Psychiatry: Behavioral Sciences/clinical Psychiatry. Eleventh edition. Philadelphia: Wolters Kluwer, 2015.
6. Taylor DM, Barnes TRE, Young AH. The Maudsley prescribing guidelines in psychiatry (13th ed.). 2018. John Wiley and Sons.

7. Pervin, Z, Stephen JM. Effect of alcohol on the central nervous system to develop neurological disorder: pathophysiological and lifestyle modulation can be potential therapeutic options for alcohol-induced neurotoxic action. AIMS Neuroscience 2021;8(3):390–413.
8. Archie, SR, and amp; Cucullo L. Harmful Effects of Smoking Cannabis: A Cerebrovascular and Neurological Perspective. Frontiers in Pharmacology 2019;10:1481.
9. Pearson, NT, and amp; Berry JH. Cannabis and Psychosis Through the Lens of DSM-International Journal of Environmental Research and Public Health 2019;16(21):4149.
10. lum K, Khalsa J, Cadet JL, Baron D, Bowirrat A, Boyett B, Lott L, Brewer R, Gondré-Lewis M, Bunt G, Kazmi S and Gold MS. Cannabis-Induced Hypodopaminergic Anhedonia and Cognitive Decline in Humans: Embracing Putative Induction of Dopamine Homeostasis. Front. Psychiatry 2021;12:623403.
11. Weinstein AM, and amp; Gorelick, DA. Pharmacological treatment of cannabis dependence. Current Pharmaceutical Design, 2011;17(14):1351–8.
12. Rosenblum A, Marsch LA, Joseph H, and Portenoy RK. Opioids and the treatment of chronic pain: controversies, current status, and future directions. Experimental and Clinical Psychopharmacology, 2008;16(5):405–16.
13. Pathan H and Williams J. Basic opioid pharmacology: an update. British Journal of Pain, 2012;6(1):11–16.
14. NIDA. 2016, November 1. Effective Treatments for Opioid Addiction. Retrieved from https://nida.nih.gov/publications/effective-treatments-opioid-addiction on 2022, May 22.
15. Stotts AL, Dodrill CL, and Kosten TR. Opioid dependence treatment: options in pharmacotherapy. Expert Opinion on Pharmacotherapy, 2009;10(11):1727–40.
16. Farzam K, Faizy RM, Saadabadi A. Stimulants. [Updated 2022 May 2]. In: StatPearls [Internet]. Treasure Island (FL): Stat Pearls Publishing; 2022 Jan.
17. Chan, B, Kondo, K, Freeman, M et al. Pharmacotherapy for Cocaine Use Disorder—a Systematic Review and Meta-analysis. J Gen Intern Med 2019;34:2858–73.
18. Heal, DJ, Smith, SL, Gosden, J, & Nutt, DJ. Amphetamine, past and present—a pharmacological and clinical perspective. Journal of Psychopharmacology (Oxford, England), 2013;27(6):479–496.
19. Widysanto A, Combest FE, Dhakal A, et al. Nicotine Addiction. [Updated 2022 May 2]. In: StatPearls [Internet]. Treasure Island (FL): StatPearls Publishing; 2022 Jan.
20. World Health Organization. Toolkit for delivering the 5A's and 5R's brief tobacco interventions in primary care; 2014.
21. Müller F, Dolder PC, Schmidt A, Liechti ME and amp; Borgwardt S. Altered network hub connectivity after acute LSD administration. NeuroImage Clinical. 2018;18:694–701.
22. Garcia-Romeu A, Kersgaard B, and amp; Addy PH. Clinical applications of hallucinogens: A review. Experimental and Clinical Psychopharmacology, 2016;24(4):229–68.

Chapter 6

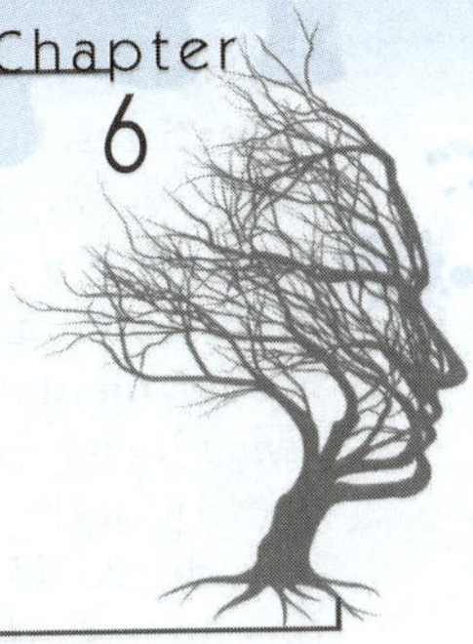

Psychotic Disorders

Competency achievement: Students should be able to
1. **PS5.1** Classify and describe the magnitude and etiology of schizophrenia and other psychotic disorders
2. **PS5.2** Enumerate, elicit, describe, and document clinical features, and positive and negative symptoms of schizophrenia
3. **PS5.3** Describe the treatment of schizophrenia including behavioral and pharmacologic therapy
4. **PS5.4** Demonstrate family education in a patient with schizophrenia in a simulated environment
5. **PS5.5** Enumerate and describe the pharmacologic basis and side effects of drugs used in schizophrenia
6. **PS5.6** Enumerate the appropriate conditions for specialist referral in patients with psychotic disorders

SCHIZOPHRENIA

Introduction

Schizophrenia is the most interesting of all psychiatric illnesses. It is also the most known one among the general population because of its commonality and frequent portrayal in media and television. Schizophrenia is considered a highly debilitating psychiatric illness associated with significant morbidity and mortality. A diagnosis of schizophrenia has a tremendous impact on the life of a person with significant ramifications on the socio-occupational well-being of the patient himself and of his family members at large. Although effective treatment for schizophrenia is widely available, there is general hesitation in seeking psychiatric care for these patients because of a lack of awareness and the high level of stigma associated with it.

History

Over a century ago, **Emil Kraepelin**, a German psychiatrist, was the first to suggest that not all psychotic illnesses are the same in presentation and were also the first to propose a system of classification for psychotic illnesses. As per his observations, some psychotic illnesses have had a gradually deteriorating course after the onset of the illness in the late teenage period while others have had an episodic course. Based on this observation, in 1893 he classified psychotic illnesses into two categories.

1. ***Dementia praecox,*** which means early onset deterioration of the mind. This illness arises in late adolescence or early adulthood, follows a gradually deteriorating course and the patient never reaches his premorbid level of functioning once the disease starts.
2. ***Manic depressive psychosis*** follows an episodic course with the patient achieving complete remission (reaching his premorbid level functioning) in between the

episodes. As an episode in this illness can present with either depressive or manic features, hence the name *manic depressive psychosis*.

However, **Eugene Bleuler**, another German psychiatrist, argued that the term ***'dementia praecox'* is a misnomer** as there is no deterioration of memory or other higher mental functions in these patients (dementia technically means deterioration of higher mental functions including memory). He proposed that in this illness (named *dementia praecox* by Kraepelin) the basic problem is that the behavior is not under the control of the mind of the patient. To signify this **splitting of mind and behavior** he introduced the term **schizophrenia** (***schizein*** means splitting and ***phren*** means mind) for this illness. After meticulous observation and investigation, he identified the following 4 core symptoms of schizophrenia, famously known as **Bleuler's 4 As** which are:

1. **Autism**
2. **Ambivalence**
3. **Affective blunting and**
4. **Association loosening** (or loosening of association)

(Schizophrenic patients are mostly confined to themselves and do not interact much with others which are denoted by the term **autism. Ambivalence** is the inability to decide for or against a confusing situation. They show minimum or no emotional reaction in response to emotion-laden stimuli such as a funny joke or the loss of a family member, which is signified by the term **affective blunting**. Schizophrenia is characterized by disorganized speech due to a lack of connection between spoken words or logical association between sentences (**association loosening**).

According to **Kurt Schneider**, although **Bleuler's 4 As are core features of schizophrenia**, they are less significant in bringing the patient to the clinical realm as they lack dramatic presentation (a patient comes to notice only when he becomes delusional or becomes aggressive). He identified **11 symptoms of schizophrenia** which are dramatic in presentation and bring the patient to the clinician. These symptoms are known as **Schneiderian first-rank symptoms (FRS)** which are as mentioned in the box below.

A. Thought alienation phenomena:
   1. **Thought insertion**, the patient claims that the thoughts in his mind are not his thoughts and are being inserted by some outside agent.
   2. **Through withdrawal**, the patient claims that people are being aware of his thoughts by some means.
   3. **Through broadcasting**, the patient claims that whatever he is thinking, everyone is being aware of it and it is also coming in television and newspapers.

B. Three auditory hallucinatory phenomena:
   4. **Thought echo** means the patient can hear his thoughts being spoken aloud from outside. When the thought comes first in mind and then is heard from outside, it is known as ***echo de la pensee***. When the thought is simultaneously heard at the same time when it comes into the mind, it is known as ***gedankenlautwerden***.
   5. **Voices commenting or commanding**, the patient hears the voices of a single person giving a running commentary on his activities or commanding him to do certain activities.
   6. **Voices discussing**, the patient hears the voices of two or more persons discussing the patient among themselves.

C. Three made phenomena:
   7. **Made impulse**, sudden impulsive actions (such as fire setting) are claimed to be forced by some outside agent.

8. Made affect, sudden bursts of affective expressions (sudden smiling or crying) are claimed to be induced by some outside agent.

9. Made volition, whatever the patient is doing is claimed to be under the control of some outside agent.

D. Rest two are:

10. Somatic passivity, bodily functions such as sensation, thought and emotion are claimed to be under the control of an outside force.

11. Delusional perception, normal occurrences in day-to-day life are perceived in a delusional way and are given special meaning with self-respect. (Flickering of light may be perceived as some special message from god!)

Symptom Domains

In the late 1980s, **Nancy Andreasen** introduced the concept of **positive and negative symptoms in schizophrenia**. Apart from positive and negative symptom domains, patients with schizophrenia also present with affective symptoms and subtle cognitive impairment. All these symptoms in schizophrenia can be grouped under the following 4 symptom domains.

1. ***Positive symptoms:*** These are the features that are generally not present in a normally functioning individual and are added when a person develops schizophrenia (positive means an **addition of symptoms**). This includes:

- Delusions,
- Hallucinations,
- Disorganized speech or behavior,
- Catatonic behavior and
- Aggressive behavior

Delusion, which is defined as a **false and unshakeable belief** that remains even after there is evidence to the contrary, is the most common symptom in a case of schizophrenia. Delusions of persecution and reference are the most common types of delusions in these patients. **Bizarre delusions** (beliefs that are not logically possible, e.g. patient claiming that he can control the movement of clouds) when present are characteristics of schizophrenia.

Hallucinations in the auditory modality are also seen in most patients with schizophrenia. Auditory hallucinations of a **commanding type** or **giving a running commentary** or **voices discussing** among themselves about the patient are characteristics of schizophrenia.

Disorganized speech, which is either **incoherent (not understandable)** or **irrelevant** to the point is also found in schizophrenia. This occurs due to the **loosening of association** between trains of thought. **Disorganized behaviors** are socially awkward behaviors (undressing in front of people, passing urine and stool in inappropriate places, etc.) that are also seen in schizophrenia which are considered regressive behavior.

2. ***Negative symptoms*:** These symptoms appear due to the subtraction of functions from the normal functioning of an individual when the illness is developed. Negative symptoms of schizophrenia include:

- **Alogia** (poor verbal communication),
- **Anhedonia (**loss of interest in pleasurable activities),
- **Asociality** (lack of socialization),

- **Avolition** (loss of goal in life and the will to do work) and
- **Affective blunting** (lack of facial expression).

Negative symptoms arising due to schizophrenia itself are considered primary **negative symptoms.** However, negative symptoms can also appear as a result of antipsychotic treatment or out of positive symptoms or due to the development of depression (post schizophrenic depression) in which cases they are considered as **secondary negative symptoms**. For example, a paranoid schizophrenic patient may avoid socialization out of fear of persecution (asociality secondary to paranoia). Similarly, a patient may develop anhedonia if he develops post-schizophrenic depression. Furthermore, treatment with typical antipsychotics can lead to masked facies (Parkinsonian features) which may be confused with affective blunting.

3. *Affective symptoms* include anxiety, perplexity, depression, elation, etc.

4. *Cognitive symptoms* are impairment in higher mental functions such as attention-concentration, planning, decision making, abstract ability, etc. Cognitive impairment is the root cause of poor functionality in a case of schizophrenia.

Diagnosis

Diagnostic criteria for diagnosis of schizophrenia have been mentioned in **ICD-10 and DSM-5**. ICD diagnostic criteria are based on **Schneiderian first-rank symptoms** and are a bit elaborative. DSM diagnostic criteria are more comprehensive and clinically useful. DSM-5 criteria necessitate the presence of 2 of the following 5 symptoms for **a period of 6 months** (with symptoms actively present for at least 1 month) for a diagnosis of schizophrenia.

1. **Delusions**
2. **Hallucinations**
3. **Disorganized speech**
4. **Disorganized or catatonic behavior**
5. **Negative symptoms**

One out of the first 3 symptoms must be present for a diagnosis of schizophrenia. The presence of these symptoms should cause **significant impairment** in the socio-occupational well-being of the individual. These symptoms cannot be better explained by another psychiatric or medical illness and must not be due to the intake of a substance.

Types

Depending upon the most prominent symptoms in a case of schizophrenia, it can be categorized into one of the following types.

1. *Paranoid schizophrenia:* It is the most common type and presents with prominent delusions and hallucinations (**paranoid symptoms**). Delusional themes mostly involve persecutory, referential, grandiose, religious, or bizarre content. Persecutory delusions (the patient believes that he is being spied on, conspired against, being followed, etc.) are by far the most common type of paranoid delusion in schizophrenia. Hallucinations are mostly present in the auditory modality and involve **voices commenting** (giving a running commentary on the patient's actions), **voices commanding** or **voices discussing**. Somatic hallucinations (e.g. a hand protruding from the back of the body) can also be present. Visual hallucinations are rare. The personality of the patient with paranoid

schizophrenia is more or less preserved with little impact on hygiene and self-care although impairment in occupational functioning can be marked. Paranoid schizophrenia has a late age of onset with a female predisposition. Paranoid schizophrenia has a better prognosis (best among all the categories) as it is more responsive to treatment with antipsychotics, both typical and atypical.

2. *Disorganized schizophrenia or hebephrenia:* It is characterized by the prominence of **disorganized speech and behavior**. These patients are aloof and self-absorbed with giggling, self-smiling, and muttering. Mirror gazing may be noted in some patients. Self-care is neglected, the goal in life is lost and many patients become vagrants. Disorganized behaviors such as spitting here and there, and loss of shame with getting naked in front of others (non-purposive) are common. Delusions and hallucinations are seldom present in cases of hebephrenia. This category carries the worst prognosis among all and death from starvation, suicide, accidents or infections is common.

3. *Catatonic schizophrenia:* A case of **catatonic schizophrenia** presents with at least 2 weeks of catatonic features such as **catatonic stupor** characterized **by mutism** (lack of verbal communication), **rigidity** (muscle rigidity), **waxy flexibility** (patient maintains an externally imposed posture even if it is discomforting), **posturing** (maintaining an odd posture for a prolonged period) **or catatonic excitement** characterized by over-excitation, involuntary movements, and aggression. Catatonic features were common in cases of chronic untreated schizophrenia; however, are becoming less and less common due to early interventions. Catatonic features respond readily to benzodiazepines and ECT and this category carries a good prognosis (**antipsychotics should be avoided** in acute cases of catatonic).

4. *Undifferentiated schizophrenia:* When symptoms are mixed and the patient cannot be confidently put in any of the 3 categories then the diagnosis of undifferentiated schizophrenia is made.

Deficit Schizophrenia

It is a type of schizophrenia presenting with poor functioning, loss of volition, negative symptoms, disorganized symptoms, and progressive impairment in cognitive functions. The most striking feature is **atrophic or degenerative changes** in the brain imaging studies such as enlarged ventricles or prominent sulci and gyri. The prognosis is very poor in this type of schizophrenia.

Simple Schizophrenia

It is a controversial and debated subtype of schizophrenia. Characterized by **gradually evolving negative symptoms** such as odd and eccentric behaviors, diminished socialization, poor communication, anhedonia, and loss of goal in life, simple schizophrenia causes significant impairment to the general functioning of the individual. ICD-10 requires at least 1 year of slowly developing negative symptoms to be present for the diagnosis. Positive symptoms such as delusions and hallucinations are conspicuously absent.

Egocentric thoughts are common in some cases of schizophrenia. The patient thinks that he is at the center of the universe and every event occurring in his surroundings carries a special meaning for him. He may believe that the chirping of the birds, the blowing of winds, and the sound of flowing rivers have some hidden meaning for him.

Some patients may develop odd thought patterns involving **pseudophilosophical, pseudoscientific, and pseudo-religious contents.**

Epidemiology

The prevalence of schizophrenia in the general population is about **1%**. The onset of this debilitating illness is in the late adolescent or early adulthood period. Incidence is slightly more in males than females, the basis of which is still not understood properly. It might be due to more incidence of substance abuse (such as cannabis) in males and female hormones such as estrogen might have some neuroprotective properties. The onset of the illness is earlier in males and the prognosis is also poorer in males than females. About 20% of schizophrenic patients attempt suicide at some point in time. Schizophrenic patients are also victims of violence, homelessness, and chronic infections.

Etiology

The exact etiology of schizophrenia is poorly understood. The **biopsychosocial approach** emphasizes the complex interplay between genetic predisposition and environmental risk factors in the development of schizophrenia.

1. ***Genetic risk:*** The genetic risk of schizophrenia has been established by family studies, twin studies, and adoption studies. The heritability is determined to be around 60–70%. A few findings from these studies have been presented below as risk of developing schizophrenia

- When one parent is affected is 12%
- When both parents are affected is 40%
- When one sibling is affected is 14% and
- When one of the identical twins is affected is 50%

Linkage studies and association studies have identified the location of risk genes on chromosomal segments: 1q, 5q, 6p, 8p, 10p, 13q, 17q and 22q. Search for candidate genes have implicated **DISC1 and DISC2** (disrupted in schizophrenia genes), **reelin gene, neuregulin gene, dysbindin gene**, the gene for D_2 dopamine receptors, etc. Protein products of these genes are involved in neural migration and synaptic orientation (e.g. axon guidance) during the process of brain development (see neurodevelopment in Chapter 22).

2. ***Environmental factors:*** Any environmental factor which hampers the normal development of the brain can be a risk factor for the development of schizophrenia. Prenatal factors such as **maternal malnutrition, maternal infections** (e.g. TORCH infection), and chronic medical conditions (e.g. maternal diabetes mellitus, COPD, etc.) can disrupt normal neurodevelopment *in utero.* Similarly, birth trauma and **hypoxia** and childhood infections such as meningitis or encephalitis, childhood head trauma, etc. also pose a significant risk of developing schizophrenia. Long-standing childhood abuse and neglect can also contribute to the development of this disease to some extent.

Neurobiology

A few prevalent hypotheses to explain the peculiar signs and symptoms of schizophrenia have been discussed below.

1. ***Dopamine hypothesis:*** As per the dopamine hypothesis, **dopaminergic hyperactivity** in the **mesolimbic pathway** which projects from VTA (ventral tegmental area) to NAc (nucleus accumbens) is responsible for psychosis (Fig. 6.1). Increased dopamine activity on the D_2 receptor in NAc causes **delusions and hallucinations**. This hypothesis is supported by the efficacy of D_2 antagonists in alleviating symptoms of psychosis (delusions and hallucinations). Psychiatrist **Shijit Kapur** argues that dopamine activity in the mesolimbic pathway is responsible for giving personal meanings to external events but in a controlled manner. Excessive dopamine activity in this pathway results in attaching a **personal meaning** to almost all events occurring out there no matter how trivial it is. This leads to the formation of delusions.

However, symptoms of psychosis are just a part of the whole story of schizophrenia. Negative symptoms and cognitive deficits in schizophrenia are in fact due to decreased levels of dopamine in the **mesocortical pathway,** projecting from VTA to the prefrontal cortex **(Fig. 6.1)**. Therefore, it is dopamine imbalance (and not just dopamine hyperactivity) that is responsible for the different symptoms of schizophrenia.

2. ***Serotonin imbalance is schizophrenia:*** Dopamine imbalance is hypothesized to be due to an imbalance **in serotonergic activity** in the brain. Excessive serotonin activity is thought to mediate both positive and negative symptoms of schizophrenia. Evidence in favor of serotonin dysfunction is from the fact that serotonin antagonists such as clozapine and olanzapine are effective in controlling both positive and negative symptoms. However, the root cause of schizophrenia is glutamate hypoactivity rather than serotonin hyperactivity as described below.

3. ***Glutamate hypothesis:*** Recently, hypoactivity of the glutamate system in the cerebral cortex has been implicated in schizophrenia. This stems from the observation that certain antiglutaminergic drugs (**phencyclidine and ketamine**) can induce both negative and positive symptoms of schizophrenia. As per this hypothesis what is happening in schizophrenic patients is, the parvalbumin-containing **GABAergic interneurons** fail to inhibit the glutaminergic pyramidal cells in the cerebral cortex leading to their hyperactivity. These cells are, in turn, directly wired to dopaminergic neurons in the mesolimbic pathway and inversely (via an inhibitory interneuron) to the mesocortical pathway. The hypoactive glutamate system in the cortex leads to increased dopamine levels in the mesolimbic and decreased dopamine level in the mesocortical pathway accounting for positive and negative symptoms of schizophrenia, respectively (Fig. 6.2).

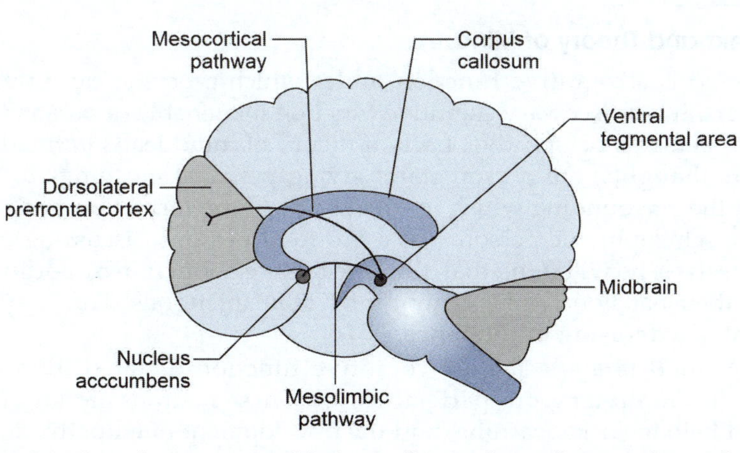

Fig. 6.1: Dopaminergic pathways responsible for positive and negative symptoms of schizophrenia.

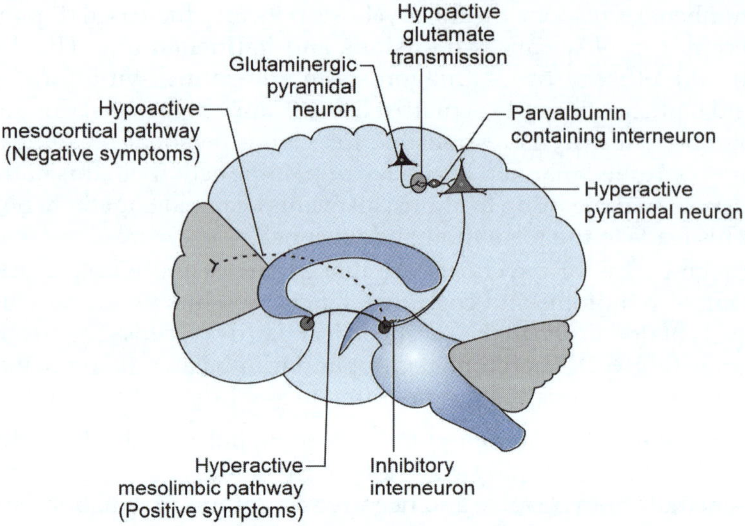

Fig. 6.2: Glutamate hypoactivity in schizophrenia.

4. ***The neurodevelopmental hypothesis:*** According to the neurodevelopmental hypothesis, **abnormal neurodevelopment in-utero** and during childhood can lead to the development of schizophrenic symptoms in the late adolescent or early adulthood period. The risk factors for schizophrenia (both genetic and environmental risk factors) have a tremendous impact on the normal process of neurodevelopment which ultimately leads to **abnormal wiring of neurons** in the cerebral cortex. These risk factors generally hamper the normal process of **neural migration** and formation of neural connections such as dendritic sprouting and axon guidance during brain development (*see* Chapter 22). **Abnormal information processing** due to abnormal wiring of neurons is the fundamental defect that leads to various symptoms of schizophrenia. The abnormal distribution of parvalbumin-containing GABAergic Interneurons due to abnormal neural migration leads to the failure of these cells to inhibit the glutaminergic pyramidal cells which explain the glutamate hypothesis.

Schizophrenia and Theory of Mind

Theory of mind is **a cognitive function** under which a person can **infer the intentions of others.** It is a necessary cognitive function that enables a person to see things from another person's perspective. Lack of theory of mind leads to the development of **egocentric thoughts;** the person starts giving personal meanings to every event occurring in the surrounding which in turn leads to the formation of **delusions.** For example, if a schizophrenic person sees a group of persons discussing their matters among themselves, he will think that they are talking about him by adding a personal meaning to their behavior, as he cannot infer their intentions. This may lead to the development of a **delusion of reference**.

Theory of mind is a specialized cognitive function dictated by a **network of neurons in the fronto-temporo-parietal cortex**. These neurons are known as **mirror neurons** and help in social learning, and the development of **empathy** and judgment skills.

Course and Prognosis

Schizophrenia is a lifelong illness but in the majority of cases, symptoms can be controlled with treatment. With treatment, about 40% of cases become symptoms free, another 40% respond somewhat moderately while the remaining 20% respond poorly to treatment. Factors that are associated with a good prognosis in a case of schizophrenia are:

1. Late age of onset
2. Female gender
3. Good premorbid functioning
4. Absence of negative symptoms
5. Paranoid and catatonic subtypes
6. Lack of other comorbidities like substance abuse

Complications

A case of schizophrenia, if left untreated, may develop following complications:

1. ***Post schizophrenic depression:*** Depressive symptoms can arise as the aftermath of schizophrenia especially when psychotic symptoms are resolving and the condition is known as post-schizophrenic depression. The patient presents with sadness, lack of interest in activities, hopelessness, and helplessness along with some residual symptoms of psychosis. Post-schizophrenic depression is associated with poor functional improvement, high morbidity, and mortality from suicide. It must be differentiated from **residual schizophrenia** which is characterized by the persistence of negative symptoms after the resolution of positive symptoms with treatment.

2. ***Suicide:*** Suicide is fairly common in schizophrenia with a lifetime risk of 10%. Suicidal risk is highest within 10 years of the onset of illness. Risk factors of suicide include male gender, early age of onset, presence of commanding hallucinations, good premorbid functioning with high expectations in life, history of suicidal attempts, etc. The presence of insight into the illness also substantially increases suicidal risk. Many patients also yield to commanding hallucinations and commit suicide. The post-schizophrenic depressive episode carries the highest risk of suicide. Proper adherence to medication is the best strategy to prevent death from suicide in schizophrenia.

3. ***Aggression and violence:*** It is a widely held myth that schizophrenic patients are always aggressive and dangerous; however, these patients are more commonly **victims of violence** rather than the perpetrators. Only a few patients with schizophrenia sometimes get aggressive and violent. Violence can be in reaction to **delusions of persecution, infidelity,** etc. or response to **commanding hallucinations**. Nonetheless, proper control of these symptoms (delusions and hallucinations) with antipsychotics effectively controls aggression and violence in these patients.

4. ***Medical complications:*** Schizophrenic patients are at increased risk of contracting infectious diseases such as **tuberculosis, leprosy, HIV infection,** etc. due to poor self-care, poor nutrition, and vagrancy. Furthermore, treatment with antipsychotics (especially second-generation antipsychotics) makes them prone to develop metabolic syndrome which increases the risk of cardiovascular adverse events.

Suggested Investigations in a Case of Psychosis

Diagnosis of schizophrenia is mainly clinical, although certain laboratory investigations are needed to rule out organic causes presenting with psychosis and for planning proper management strategies as described below.

1. **Blood sugar level** and **lipid profile** as many antipsychotics are contraindicated in persons with diabetes and/or dyslipidemia.
2. **Complete blood count** with differential counts.
3. **The absolute neutrophil** count is mandatory before the start of therapy with clozapine.
4. **Brain imaging studies** such as CT and MRI scans are done when underlying organic causes are suspected. CT scanning of the brain is often indicated in cases presenting with acute psychosis.

Treatment

1. ***Hospitalization:*** A patient with schizophrenia may be managed on an OPD basis or may be admitted to a hospital with a psychiatric inpatient facility. Hospitalization is necessary for the following conditions.

1. Violent and aggressive patient
2. Patients refusing medications
3. Patients with poor nutritional status causing emaciation or electrolyte imbalance
4. Actively suicidal or homicidal patient
5. Patients presenting with stupor.

After hospitalization, violence and aggression can be controlled with parenteral antipsychotics such as haloperidol injection. It is mandatory to give promethazine with haloperidol to prevent the development of acute EPS such as dystonia or Parkinsonian features. Sedation with lorazepam or diazepam also helps in controlling aggression. Homeostasis is maintained with intravenous fluid therapy and nutrition can be maintained via nasogastric tube wherever needed. The stupor can be broken with parenteral lorazepam given for a few days. ECT has a special role in rapidly controlling suicidal and homicidal behaviors because of the rapid onset of actions and also in breaking stupors not responding to lorazepam or diazepam.

2. ***Pharmacotherapy:*** **Antipsychotic medications** are the mainstay of treatment for schizophrenia. Antipsychotics are very much effective in controlling positive symptoms such as delusions, hallucinations, and aggression and somewhat effective in improving negative symptoms. Antipsychotics used in the treatment of psychosis are generally categorized into two groups.

a. **Typical or first-generation antipsychotics** are chlorpromazine, haloperidol, flupentixol, trifluoperazine, pimozide, etc. Being dopamine D2 blockers **(DRA or dopamine receptor antagonists)**, they act by decreasing dopamine activity in the mesolimbic pathway. They are very much effective in controlling positive symptoms but are not effective in improving negative symptoms. They are also notorious for causing EPS like Parkinsonism and tardive dyskinesia.

b. **Atypical or second-generation antipsychotics (SGA)** also known as **serotonin dopamine antagonists (SDA)** which include clozapine, risperidone, olanzapine, quetiapine, aripiprazole, amisulpride, lurasidone, etc. They are effective in improving positive symptoms and also negative symptoms to some extent. Long-term treatment with some SGAs can cause metabolic syndrome.

When a patient is diagnosed with schizophrenia, treatment should be started with an SGA and should be awaited for 4–6 weeks. If no improvement occurs within this period then another SGA or DRA can be started after tapering and stopping the initial drug. **Clozapine is reserved** for cases not responding to at least two antipsychotics given for an adequate period (**resistant schizophrenia**).

Benzodiazepines such as lorazepam and clonazepam can be given for a short duration (2–4 weeks) along with antipsychotics. They help in improving sleep, controlling aggression, and speedy improvement in symptoms. However, it should be tapered and stopped within 2 weeks and in no cases should be given for more than 4 weeks for fear of dependence.

Treatment with antipsychotics after the **first episode** is generally **continued for one year** and then medication doses are gradually tapered down and stopped. After one year of treatment, if **symptoms reappear (relapse)** then treatment with antipsychotics should be **continued for life**.

3. *Brain stimulation methods* such as ECT are reserved for actively suicidal or homicidal patients and patients presenting with stupor. ECT can also be considered in treatment-resistant cases.

4. *Psychosocial approach:* Psychosocial approaches in schizophrenia are aimed at following aspects of the life of the patient

1. Social skills
2. Interpersonal skills
3. Practical skills and
4. Self-sufficiency

Social Skills Training

Many patients with schizophrenia have poor social skills due to poor eye contact, odd facial expressions, inadequate perception of emotions, and lack of spontaneity in social situations. Social skills tainting aims to improve social interaction and **integration of the patient back into society**. It is achieved via videotapes of other schizophrenic patients and of the patient, role-playing therapy, and homework assignment for the specific skills to be practiced.

Cognitive Remediation

It is a fairly recent approach that aims at improving the cognitive skills of the patients to make them self-sufficient in life. It employs computational approaches such as computer-generated exercises, neural networks, virtual reality, etc. to improve cognition, working memory, spontaneity, and working capacity.

Family Education in Schizophrenia

Family members play an important role in the treatment and care of patients suffering from schizophrenia. Psychoeducation regarding the nature of the illness and the importance of treatment and regular follow-up is given to family members. Caregivers are also made aware of how to recognize signs of relapse and deterioration of the condition or the emergence of complications such as depression and suicidal tendencies. Counseling regarding the marriage of the patient and the risk of children developing the disease is also explained.

OTHER COMMON PSYCHOTIC DISORDERS

BRIEF PSYCHOTIC DISORDER

A case of brief psychotic disorder (BPD) presents with **sudden onset** of schizophrenia-like psychotic symptoms lasting for no more than a month. The patient reaches his premorbid level of functioning after the episode. However, **relapse may occur** in which case it is known as **recurrent BPD**. Symptoms in most cases are polymorphic in nature presenting with a combination of symptoms of schizophrenia and affective psychosis with disorganized speech and behavior. **Acute and transient psychotic disorder** (**ATPD**) in **ICD-10** is equivalent to BPD in DSM-5.

Clinical Presentation

A case of BPD presents with acute onset of psychosis characterized by the following symptoms.

1. **Delusions** (delusion of persecution, reference, possession by spirits, etc.)
2. **Hallucinations** (mostly auditory but transient visual hallucinations may occur).
3. **Affective symptoms** like pan anxiety, perplexity, depression, crying spells, a burst of euphoria or elation, and giggling may present.
4. **Disorganized speech** which presents as irrelevant or incoherent speech.
5. **Disorganized or catatonic behavior** such as poor self-care, spitting behavior, undressing in front of others, stupor, sudden aggression with excitement, etc.

These symptoms should be present **for 1 day to 1 month. The resolution is complete** and the person reaches his premorbid level of functioning after the episode. Relapse may occur or the patient may progress to develop other psychotic disorders like schizophrenia, BPAD, and schizophreniform disorders.

Depending upon the presence of **preceding stress,** BPD has been categorized into the following 3 types.

1. ***BPD with significant stress*** also known as **acute reactive psychosis:** Acute reactive psychosis generally occurs following a major stressful event which should cause distress in almost all individuals exposed to such stress. These types of stress include the loss of a spouse or a close relative, the loss of a job, and exposure to major life-threatening events like war, motor vehicle accidents, natural disasters, etc. Acute reactive psychosis is thought to develop due to poor resilience to stress and coping skills. Reactive psychosis is more common in females and persons with personality disorders.
2. ***BPD without significant stress:*** It develops in a person without exposure to any major stressful event.
3. ***BPD with postpartum onset:*** Presentation is within 4 weeks of delivery.

Treatment

Hospitalization is needed if the patient is grossly disorganized or aggressive or in case of poor oral intake or cases presenting with a stupor. The patient is put on parenteral antipsychotics such as haloperidol with promethazine and sedatives like lorazepam or diazepam for adequate sedation. The patient should be put on oral medications as early as possible when aggression or disorganized behaviors subside and he starts taking them orally.

Second-generation antipsychotics such as **olanzapine, risperidone, and quetiapine** are the mainstay of treatment for BPD. **Short courses of benzodiazepines** may be added in agitated and aggressive patients. However, benzodiazepines should be tapered **and stopped within 2–3 weeks**. The symptoms should subside within one month as per definition but antipsychotic medications should be continued for a period of one year. Periodic evaluation for relapse and residual symptoms is necessary for adequate management. In case of frequent relapse, reviewing the diagnosis is necessary to rule out BPAD and schizoaffective disorder. **In the case of recurrent BPD, long-term treatment** with second-generation antipsychotics (olanzapine or risperidone) in low doses is necessary.

Psychotherapy has a special role in reactive psychosis. Supportive psychotherapy teaches the patient how to cope with extreme stress. Insight-oriented psychotherapy helps the patient and family members to understand the disease and the importance of treatment adherence.

DELUSIONAL DISORDERS

Delusional disorders are characterized by **prominent well systematized delusions** without much deterioration in personality and socio-occupational functioning. These delusions must not conform to the cultural and religious background of the patient and **must be non-bizarre**, which means they can occur in real-life settings. Apart from delusions, **other psychotic symptoms are conspicuously absent** and even if present are secondary to the delusional theme (persons with delusion of persecution may become aggressive or might experience auditory hallucinations). Apart from delusions and associated behavioral problems, the patient's socio-occupational functioning is generally not impaired. **Insight is always absent** and hence it might be challenging to bring the patient to a psychiatrist and put on treatment.

Delusional disorders are **rare psychiatric disorders** with a prevalence of 0.02% in the general population as per DSM5. Onset is generally in late age (after 35 years and both males and females are equally prone to develop delusional disorders, although the theme of delusion can vary in both genders. A patient's socio-cultural background has a great influence on the type of delusion the patient develops.

Common Types

1. **Persecutory type:** The patient is convinced that he is being conspired against, harassed, or being tried to be harmed. This is the most common theme of delusion in patients with delusional disorder. The patient may become aggressive, irritable, and litigious.
2. **Jealous type:** The patient is convinced that one's spouse is being unfaithful even if there is substantial evidence to the contrary. It is more commonly seen in males than in females and the patient may become aggressive and develop suicidal or homicidal ideas. It is also known by other names such as **morbid jealousy** or **Othello syndrome**.
3. **Erotomanic type:** The patient claims that someone of higher status is in love with her or him. Mostly these patients are socially withdrawn with poor functionality and are sexually inhibited. It is associated with **'paradoxical conduct'** which means that any attempt to deny or avoid advances by the patient is perceived as an affirmation of love. **De Clerambault syndrome** presents solely with erotomanic delusion.
4. **Somatic type:** The patient claims with conviction that he has been suffering from some bodily illness or deformity. The most common presentations are delusion of

infestation, bad body odor or halitosis, and body dysmorphic delusions. The belief is held with conviction even if there is sufficient evidence to the contrary.

5. **Grandiose type:** A false belief that one is superior to others in some aspects. It is also known as **megalomaniac delusion** and the common themes are delusion of position, power, possession, and relation.
6. **Mixed type:** The patient presents with two or more delusional themes.
7. **Unspecified type:** Include Capgras syndrome, Fregoli's delusion, and Cotard's delusion.

Capgras syndrome is a special type of delusional disorder characterized by the **misidentification of family members or friends**. In this disorder, the patient thinks that a family member or close relative has been **replaced by an imposter**. Studies by **VS Ramachandran** and colleagues have revealed a **break in the emotional processing** of the perceived image in cases of **Capgras delusion**. When we perceive an image a signal is sent to the emotional circuit for **emotional appraisal** of the object we see. Lack of emotional appraisal results in the only physical perception of the image without the required emotion attached to it. It means if the patient sees his mother he will perceive the physical image only without the emotional component of a mother. This forces the individual to infer that his mother is not the real one and has been replaced by an imposter.

Fregoli's delusion is another special type of delusion characterized by the **delusion of identity swapping**. The patient believes that someone (the persecutor) is changing appearances and identity in disguise to pursue him by masking himself as a close relative or family member.

Cotard's syndrome is characterized by nihilistic delusion or delusion of nihilism. The person is convinced that he is dying or the world has come to an end. Some people also believe that their body parts are dying or rotting and that a foul smell is emanating from them. Cotard's delusion is most commonly seen in **organic brain cases such as dementia**.

Theories of Delusion

Delusion is thought to arise from a combination of neurobiological, cognitive, and psychological dysfunctions. Neurobiology researchers have pointed out dysfunctions in the prefrontal cortex, limbic system, and other subcortical regions. The cognitive hypothesis suggests a **mismatch between the patient's expectations and current inputs from reality** leading to the formation of the delusion. In these patients, there is a **lack of cognitive flexibility** to ascertain this mismatch because of cognitive bias and impaired social learning. At a neurological level, this cognitive inflexibility arises due to impaired information processing in the reward circuit due to the **increased firing of dopaminergic neurons in the mesolimbic pathway**.

Treatment

Antipsychotic medications are the mainstay of treatment. Antipsychotics with strong D2 blocking activities such **as risperidone, amisulpride, haloperidol, and pimozide** are primarily selected as first-line medications. Pimozide is specially indicated for patients with somatic delusions. The most problematic aspect of the treatment is putting the patient on medications and subsequent treatment adherence due to a lack of insight into such patients. In case of poor compliance long acting antipsychotic injections may be considered and has better outcomes than oral medications.

SHARED PSYCHOTIC DISORDERS

Shared psychotic disorder (***folie e Deux***) is a rare but interesting psychiatric condition characterized by sharing of delusions between two or more individuals. The term ***Folie a Deux*** was coined by **Lasegue and Falret** in 1877. The delusions can be shared by two or more individuals or with a group, e.g. between family members (***folie en famille***), between the individuals of a mass (***folie en mass***), etc., *folie e Deux* being the most common type. ***Folie e Deux*** involves sharing of delusion between the primary or inducer and the secondary or induced. The primary or inducer influences the thought process of the secondary in the following ways.

1. ***Folie imposee*** (imposed psychosis)—the primary is far dominant and both are in an intimate relationship. The condition resolves once both are separated from one another. Common between married couples.
2. ***Folie simultanee*** (simultaneous psychosis)—both primary and secondary share same genetic predisposition and develop the delusion almost simultaneously. Common between sisters or siblings.
3. ***Folie communiquée*** (communicated psychosis)—similar to *Folie impose,* but the secondary is far more convinced and it does not resolve even after separation.
4. ***Folie induite*** (induced psychosis)—in this type new kinds of delusions are induced by the primary in the secondary.

Psychopathology

Shared psychosis is generally found in individuals who are in an **intimate relationship** for a prolonged period. These individuals are generally **socially isolated** and the primary has a dominant role over and in many cases secondary is submissive or of subnormal intelligence. The primary might have a long-standing untreated psychotic illness such as schizophrenia. They may share genetic predispositions or have personality disorders.

The theme of delusion shared depends upon the sociocultural context. By far **persecutory and grandiose delusions** are the most common type in shared psychoses. However, in the Indian context, persecutory and religious delusions are common.

REFERRAL CRITERIA IN CASES OF PSYCHOSIS

General practitioners should be aware of the conditions when referring a case of psychosis to a mental health facility is required. Conditions for referral are as follows:

1. When the patient is a risk to the safety of others due to aggression and violence.
2. The patient is a risk to self due to the emergence of suicidal tendency.
3. Poor response to initial treatment or poor adherence to treatment.
4. The emergence of intolerable side effects due to antipsychotic treatment.
5. The emergence of secondary substance abuse behavior.
6. Patients presenting with catatonic symptoms.

SUMMARY

1. Schizophrenia is the most well-known and notorious psychiatric illness associated with significant morbidity, and morality and also carries a significant stigma in society.
2. The word schizophrenia was coined by Eugene Blueler who also described some core features of schizophrenia famously known as Blueler's 4 As which include autism, ambivalence, affective blunting, and association loosening in speech.

3. Currently, the clinical aspects of schizophrenia are described in terms of symptom domains such as positive (delusion, hallucination, disorganized speech and behavior, aggression, and catatonic features) and negative symptoms (alogia, asociality, avolition, anhedonia, and affective blunting).
4. Depending upon the predominant presenting symptoms, schizophrenia can be categorized as paranoid, disorganized, catatonic, or undifferentiated schizophrenia.
5. Both genetic predisposition and environmental factors interact in a complex way to develop schizophrenia.
6. Although dopamine is the main neurotransmitter implicated in schizophrenia, serotonin, and glutamate abnormality are at the core pathophysiology of schizophrenia which stems from abnormal neural development.
7. A case of schizophrenia must be differentiated from other psychotic illnesses such as acute psychosis (ATPD), BPAD, schizoaffective disorder, delusional disorders, and substance-induced psychosis.
8. Untreated schizophrenia can lead to suicide, homicide, violence, and vagrancy.
9. Treatment of schizophrenia mainly includes the use of medications such as antipsychotics to control symptoms. Treatment improves symptoms and the general well-being of the patient.
10. Rehabilitation programs are directed at re-integrating the patient into society to live a meaningful and productive life.

BIBLIOGRAPHY

1. Ebert A, Bär KJ. Emil Kraepelin: A pioneer of scientific understanding of psychiatry and psychopharmacology. Indian Journal of Psychiatry, 2010;52(2):191–2.
2. Ashok AH, Baugh J, Yeragani VK. Paul Eugen Bleuler and the origin of the term schizophrenia (SCHIZOPRENIEGRUPPE). Indian Journal of Psychiatry, 2012;54(1):95–6.
3. KMR Prasad. Current Status of First Rank Symptoms. NIMHANS Journal, Volume: 09 Issue: 02 July 1991. pp 59–69
4. Hany M, Rehman B, Azhar Y, et al. Schizophrenia. [Updated 2021 Nov 27]. In: StatPearls [Internet]. Treasure Island (FL): StatPearls Publishing; 2022 Jan. Available from:
5. Patel KR, Cherian J, Gohil K, Atkinson D. Schizophrenia: overview and treatment options. PT. 2014;39(9):638–45.
6. Stephen A, Lui F. Brief Psychotic Disorder. [Updated 2021 Oct 10]. In: StatPearls [Internet]. Treasure Island (FL): StatPearls Publishing; 2022 Jan.
7. Joseph SM, Siddiqui W. Delusional Disorder. [Updated 2021 Jul 13]. In: StatPearls [Internet]. Treasure Island (FL): StatPearls Publishing; 2022 Jan.
8. Hirstein W, Ramachandran VS. Capgras syndrome: a novel probe for understanding the neural representation of the identity and familiarity of persons. Proc Biol Sci. 1997 Mar 22;264(1380): 437–44.
9. Al Saif F, Al Khalili Y. Shared Psychotic Disorder. [Updated 2022 Jan 20]. In: StatPearls [Internet]. Treasure Island (FL): StatPearls Publishing; 2022 Jan.

Chapter 7

Depression

Competency achievement: Students should be able to

1. **PS6.1** Classify and describe the magnitude and etiology of depression
2. **PS6.2** Enumerate, elicit, describe, and document clinical features in patients with depression
3. **PS6.3** Enumerate and describe the indications and interpret laboratory and other tests used in depression
4. **PS6.5** Demonstrate family education in a patient with depression in a simulated environment
5. **PS6.6** Enumerate and describe the pharmacologic basis and side effects of drugs used in depression
6. **PS6.7** Enumerate the appropriate conditions for specialist referral in patients with depression

INTRODUCTION

Depression is a mood state characterized by persistent low mood associated with low self-esteem and loss of interest in pleasurable activities. Depression as the dominant presenting symptom can be found in several psychiatric conditions collectively known as depressive disorders. Major depressive disorder (MDD) is the most common clinical condition associated with depression and is considered a prototype of depressive disorders. Because of its severe impact on productivity and associated life risk, depression has gained considerable attention and coverage in recent times. Suicide is a major mortality factor associated with depression and around 80% of patients who attempt or commit suicide have had depression. A comprehensive understanding of the clinical presentation, etiology, pathophysiology, and treatment of depression is necessary for every medical professional.

DEPRESSIVE DISORDERS

Major Depressive Disorder (MDD)

It is the most common type of depressive disorder. Because of its clinical importance, it is described in detail in this chapter.

Endogenous Depression or Melancholia

Endogenous depression is a clinical condition **occurring due to some inner factors** (biological or cognitive) without any external stressor to trigger depression (in contrast to MDD). It presents with a severe low mood with a complete loss of energy and interest (hence the name melancholia). **Psychomotor abnormalities** (agitation or retardation) are present in almost all cases of melancholia and are one of the defining features. **Atypical features** such as increased appetite, excessive sleeping, and weight gain are also frequently present in melancholia.

Bipolar Depression

Depressive episodes in the context of BPAD are known as bipolar depression and are more common than manic episodes in patients with BPAD. Anxiety symptoms, restlessness and irritability, psychotic features, and atypical features are more common in bipolar depression. It is imperative to differentiate a case of bipolar depression from that of unipolar depression (MDD) for accurate treatment of the condition. History of an episode of mania or hypomania in the past firmly establishes this diagnosis.

Persistent Depressive Disorder or Dysthymia

PDD is a distinct mood disorder characterized by **less severe depressive features lasting for years**. Depressed mood, low self-esteem, and loss of interest in pleasurable activities are predominant presenting symptoms in a case of dysthymia. Dysthymia follows a **relapsing-remitting course,** and is highly heritable which suggests a link between dysthymia and autoimmune disorders. The autoimmune hypothesis of dysthymia is supported by the onset of symptoms after immune activation by stress or viral infection and cytokine flare in these patients.

Seasonal Affective Disorder (SAD)

Patients with seasonal affective disorder develop depressive symptoms **only in winter**, almost every year. It is hypothesized to be due to **decreased light intensity in winter** and people with SAD have **low sensitivity to light** as compared to normal people and develop lethargy, sleepiness, low mood, and loss of energy and interest in pleasurable activities during winter.

Mixed Anxiety Depression

Mixed anxiety depression or anxious depression has been categorized as a distinct diagnosable condition in ICD-10. It presents with simultaneous symptoms of depression and anxiety, although, neither of which is sufficient enough to independently diagnose the case as depression or anxiety disorder. Treatment of mixed anxiety depression may slightly vary from a major depressive disorder.

Postpartum Depression

Postpartum is a period of tremendous physical and psychological stress. Many women develop low mood, tearfulness, and hopelessness in the postpartum period which is known as '**baby blues**' and lasts for 1–2 weeks and resolves by itself. Only a few women in the postpartum period develop depressive symptoms severe enough to **cause impairment in the general functioning of the patient and her relation with the child**, in which case it is diagnosed as postpartum depression and treatment is required.

Premenstrual Dysphoric Disorder (PMDD)

A case of PMDD presents with **mood swings, irritability, loss of interest, and hopelessness**, a few days before the onset of menstruation and resolves with the onset of menstruation. Although slight mood symptoms are common in many women before menstruation, PMDD is diagnosed only when symptoms are severe enough to impair the socio-occupational or scholastic life of the patient.

Secondary Depression

Depression occurring secondary to other neurotic illnesses or long-standing physical illnesses (long-standing anxiety disorders, OCD, personality disorder, diabetes mellitus, COPD, etc.) is known as secondary depression. Depression can also occur in schizophrenic patients after the successful resolution of psychotic symptoms and is known as **post-schizophrenic depression**.

Certain medications like steroids, beta-blockers, antiretroviral drugs, and chemotherapy can induce depression. **Antitubercular drugs** are also prone to induce depressive symptoms. Furthermore, features of depression are frequently associated with **hypothyroidism. Long-standing chronic illnesses** can also induce depression.

MAJOR DEPRESSIVE DISORDER (MDD)

It is the most common type of depressive disorder in the community setting. Major depressive disorder is generally associated with significant and/or long-lasting stress in life. Even if MDD can occur in any person, it is more commonly seen in persons with poor coping skills and those having significant stress in day-to-day life. Because of its commonality and clinical importance, MDD has been described in detail in this chapter.

Epidemiology

The point prevalence of MDD in India is 2–3% while lifetime prevalence is as high as 15%. MDD is more common in older age groups (after 40 years of age) and in females than in males (it is 2 times more common in females than in males). It is also more common in individuals with comorbid long-standing illnesses like diabetes mellitus, hypertension, connective tissue disorders, etc. MDD is also the leading cause of disability worldwide and is associated with high morbidity and mortality.

Clinical Presentation

A case of major depressive disorder, being a mood disorder, presents with **abnormal mood states with other associated features**. Clinical features of major depressive disorder can be grouped into:

1. Mood and associated symptoms
2. Impairment in biological functions
3. Psychotic symptoms
4. Cognitive symptoms and
5. Other associated features

Mood and Associated Symptoms

Persistent and pervasive depressed mood or sadness is the **hallmark feature** of **MDD**. However, mere sadness, as all of us feel sometimes, is not sufficient for the diagnosis of depression. Low mood or sadness must be persistent and pervasive, must be present throughout the day and almost every day for a **period of at least 2 weeks**, and is expressed in all situations. Low mood is almost always accompanied by a **loss of interest** in pleasurable activities **(anhedonia)**. The patient shows little or no interest in any kind of pleasurable activities and is mostly confined to himself. The patient also **feels drained of energy** with weakness, lethargy, and easy fatigability. Most patients start **ruminating** about past mistakes and failures and feel extremely guilty about their past activities.

One of the important features of major depression is what is known as **Beck's triad** (Beck's cognitive triad proposed by Aron T Beck). Beck's triad consists of **hopelessness, helplessness, and worthlessness.** The patient's perception of the surroundings is altered and he thinks that no one can help him out of his misery leading to helplessness. Similarly, the patient perceives his future as dark and unsuccessful, feeling hopeless. He also perceives himself as a failure, lacking self-confidence, and feeling worthless. These distorted perceptions about self and the future make the patient think that their life is not worth living. Many think of committing suicide to end their misery and suffering.

Impairment in Biological Functions

Biological functions are also impaired in the case of depression. Many complain about **early morning awakening** and find it difficult to go to sleep again. They experience a **lack of freshness after sleep** and feel drowsy and lethargic throughout the day. **Loss of appetite** and constipation is frequently associated with depression. The depressed patient also **loses interest in sexual activities** and also suffers from erectile dysfunction (psychological).

> **Atypical depression**
>
> In general, depression is associated with loss of appetite, weight loss, and insomnia (these symptoms are typical of depression). However, few patients with depression complain of **excessive sleep, increased appetite, and weight gain**. These features are considered atypical in the context of clinical depression. Atypical features are more common in depression in old age, melancholia, and in bipolar depression.

Psychotic Symptoms

Few patients with MDD who are severely depressed present with psychotic symptoms such as delusions and hallucinations. Mood-congruent delusions such as **delusion of guilt** (thinks that he has committed an unpardonable sin) and **nihilism** (thinks that they are dead, the world has ended or their body is rotting) are prominent in severe cases of MDD. Similarly, hallucinations are also mood congruent, and depressed patients may hear hallucinatory voices telling them that they are worthless, a sinner, and should commit suicide. Depression presenting with psychotic features is known as **psychotic depression**.

Cognitive Symptoms

Patients with severe depression often complain of **poor memory, lack of clarity of thinking, slowing of thoughts, and impaired judgment and reasoning**. These impairments in higher mental functions are known as cognitive symptoms of depression. Because of cognitive impairment, a severely depressed patient may be confused with a case of dementia. However, this impairment in cognitive symptoms is due to the slowing down of information processing in the cortex and improves automatically once the depression is treated. Hence, the term **pseudodementia** is often applied for impaired cognitive functions in cases of severe MDD.

Other Symptoms

Somatic symptoms such as burning sensation and pain over various parts of the body, tingling, numbness, fullness of stomach, etc. are also present in patients with MDD, especially in older individuals. **Anxiety symptoms** such as restlessness, agitation, apprehension, and palpitation are present in many cases. Older patients with depression also frequently present with irritable mood, restlessness, and prominent psychotic features. Irritable mood and restlessness are also defining features of childhood depression.

Etiology of Depression

1. Psychodynamic theory: As per **object relation theory** persons have special feelings for the objects they love (love objects may be persons they love or material objects they own). Loss of these love objects (death of family members or loss of a material object) leads to extreme guilt feeling and they start blaming themselves for their inability to protect their love objects. The **aggression** due to the loss is **turned inward** leading to self-blaming and self-harm behavior.

2. Behavioral model: **Learned helplessness** is the behavioral model which explains the occurrence of depression in individuals undergoing significant stress in life. According to this model when a person is exposed to a significant adverse live situation over which he has no control, the person gradually develops hopelessness, frustration, pervasive sadness, suicidal ideas, and other features of MDD. Learned helplessness was experimentally demonstrated in a controlled environment by behavioral psychologist **Martin Seligman** in 1967.

3. The cognitive model of depression: Aron Beck pioneered the cognitive model of depression. As per this model, it is the perception of the patient about self, the environment, and his future that leads to depression. Some persons have altered perceptions of self, their future, and of their surroundings. These faulty thoughts lead to feelings of worthlessness, hopelessness, and helplessness (also known as **cognitive triads of depression**). This cognitive model has paved the way for **cognitive behavioral therapy (Chapter 20)**.

4. The diathesis-stress model: Diathesis means an individual's inbuilt factors that make the individual vulnerable to certain illnesses. These factors can be the **genetic makeup of an individual, his psychological mindset and/or coping skills, etc.** These **inbuilt factors (diathesis)** interact in a complex way with external stress and ultimately lead to the development of depression.

A. **Genetic risk:** MDD tends to run in families signifying genetic underpinnings. Family studies have found that the risk of developing depression is highest when a first-degree relative has had depression. Similarly, twin studies have revealed that the contribution from genetic risk is around 40–50%. Genome-wide association studies have identified single nucleotide polymorphism in genes encoding CRH (corticotropin-releasing hormone), BDNF (brain-derived neurotrophic factor), SERT (serotonin transporter), etc. However, no single gene defect has been identified that is solely responsible for depression indicating a contribution of multiple susceptible genes toward the development of depression.

B. **Psychological risk:** Abnormal psychological development in childhood leads to poor **coping skills** and **poor emotional regulation**. **Childhood abuse** (sexual or physical) contributes to abnormal psychological development and poor emotional regulation. Similarly, broken families, insensitive parents, and troubled parental relationships also contribute to this. Poor coping skills and poor regulation of emotions lead to abnormal handling of life stress and disturbed attitude toward self and others which make the person more vulnerable to depression.

Pathophysiology

The neurobiology of different types of depression (endogenous depression, major depression, bipolar depression, or SAD) differs from one another. However, all of them ultimately arise due to the **depletion of monoamines** (serotonin, dopamine, noradrenaline) levels in the brain which results in mood and associated features characteristic of depression.

The major depressive disorder involves a **slew of neurochemical changes** following a stressful event or due to some ongoing significant stress. Any kind of stress induces hormonal and biochemical changes collectively known as **stress reactions (Chapter 2)**. Stress reaction can be divided into 3 phases:

1. Alarm phage (hyperarousal state)
2. A phase of resistance and
3. Phase of exhaustion

Stress is immediately followed by an alarm phase characterized by **hyperarousal symptoms** such as hypervigilance, autonomic hyperactivity, and sleep disturbance due to sympathetic hyperactivity and subsequent secretion of noradrenaline. It helps the individual in being attentive toward the stressful event and in finding out possible solutions. **The alarm phase** is followed by a phase **of resistance** characterized by increased secretion of corticosteroids due to activation of the HPA axis. Steroids soothe the mind with a general sense of well-being and help the patient cope with stress. However, **long-standing stress** can prolong the increased secretion of steroids which leads to a phase of exhaustion. The phase of exhaustion is characterized by poor immunity, impaired insulin resistance, increased vulnerability to infection and cardiovascular complications, and other bodily changes.

Sustained increased levels of **steroids** have a significant impact on brain functions and neural tissue. Sustained steroid action can lead to neural tissue loss in the form of **loss of dendrites or axons** or other neural substances, although neuronal cell loss doesn't occur. **Neural tissue loss** is especially prominent in the hippocampal **region** followed by the prefrontal **cortex**. Loss of connection between neurons due to loss of axons and dendrites and **neurochemical** changes like decreased levels of serotonin and other monoamines results in clinical symptoms characteristic of MDD. Low mood, decreased interest in pleasurable activities and decreased energy level are due to depletion in the levels of monoamines such as serotonin and dopamine. **Low level of dopamine** activity in the reward circuit results in **anhedonia and poor motivation**. On the other hand, poor memory, impaired concentration, poor judgment, and reasoning arise due to impaired information processing in the brain as a result of a loss of connection between neurons, especially in the prefrontal cortex. When depression is treated all these structural and chemical changes are gradually reversed.

Diagnosis

Diagnosis is made based on clinical presentation but laboratory tests are needed to rule out possible medical causes for depression. All cases of depression should be evaluated for thyroid function abnormality to rule out **hypothyroidism.**

Diagnostic guidelines such as ICD-10 and DSM-5 require the symptoms to be present for at least **2 weeks**. Symptoms should be pervasive and should present most of the time throughout the day and almost every day. ICD-10 also has categorized depression into mild, moderate, and severe depression depending upon the severity of symptoms and also has mentioned a special category known as depression with psychotic symptoms.

The differential diagnosis for major depressive disorder includes **bipolar depression, seasonal affective disorder, post-schizophrenic depression,** etc. Medical conditions that might present with depressive symptoms include hypothyroidism, steroid therapy, antitubercular drug therapy, HAART therapy for HIV-AIDS, etc. Clear differentiation of major depression from other illnesses (mentioned above) is necessary for the proper treatment of the condition.

Suggested Investigations

Depression is diagnosed based on clinical presentation. However, the following investigations may be needed.

1. Complete blood count with differential counts
2. Thyroid function tests to rule out hypothyroidism
3. Serum vitamin D level
4. Brain imaging studies to rule out organic pathology such as dementia, stroke, etc.

Comorbidity

A case of MDD frequently presents with other psychiatric comorbidities. By far, **anxiety disorders** (especially GAD) are the most common comorbid conditions. **Personality disorders** (borderline, histrionic, and cluster C personality disorders) are common comorbid conditions. Patients suffering from other neurotic illnesses such as **OCD, somatoform disorder, and sleep disorders** frequently develop secondary depression. Patients recovering from psychotic illnesses (schizophrenia or ATPD) are also prone to develop depression known as post-psychotic depression.

Complications

1. Loss of productivity: MDD is the leading cause of disability worldwide. The loss in disability-adjusted life years due to recurrent depressive episodes is around 10 years per individual with a diagnosis of depression.

2. Substance abuse: A depressive episode carries a significant risk for the emergence of substance abuse behavior such as alcohol, nicotine, and cannabis. Many patients use substances to get relief from their perceived misery in a depressive state. Others also get indulged in alcohol abuse for the sake of self-medication to improve sleep and anxiety.

3. Medical complications: Long-standing depression can lead to insulin resistance and type II diabetes mellitus, hypertension, etc. Poor immunity and poor self-care also make the patient prone to infections such as tuberculosis, pneumonia, and UTI.

4. Suicide: Depression is by far the most important risk factor for suicide. It is estimated that around 80% of patients who attempt suicide have underlying depression. Bipolar depression and geriatric depression which present with agitation are at the highest risk of suicide. It has been observed that suicide attempts are more common during the recovery phase as the patient becomes more active and can carry out suicidal activities.

Treatment

Prompt diagnosis and treatment are imperative to make the patient productive and to prevent mortality from suicide. Hospitalization is needed in the following cases:

- Actively suicidal patients.

- Patient with severe psychotic depression (e.g. presenting with a stupor or lack of insight).
- Patients with poor nutritional status due to poor oral intake.

Once a patient is admitted, homeostasis is maintained with IV fluid, and nutrition is maintained with NG tube feeding if needed. Actively suicidal patients should be kept under constant supervision and harmful objects (knives, blades, any poisonous products, etc.) should be kept out of the patient's reach. Antidepressant medications are started immediately. SSRIs are first-line medications but for actively suicidal patients mirtazapine (15–30 mg) given at bedtime have better effectiveness because of its sedative property. Other sedatives such as benzodiazepines are needed for a short duration to improve sleep, relieve anxiety, and also help in speedy recovery. Antipsychotic medications may be needed in cases with psychotic features. ECT may be considered in patients presenting with high suicidal risk or in a case of depressive stupor.

Pharmacotherapy

Medications are the mainstay of treatment in **moderate to severe cases** of depression. SSRIs are first-line drugs for any case of depression needing medications because of good efficacy and better safety profile. Out of six SSRIs**, one single drug is selected** based on the patient profile and presenting symptoms. TCAs are also equally efficacious but are falling out of favor because of troublesome side effects (anticholinergic and antihistamine side effects). **Newer antidepressants** such as **SNRIs** (duloxetine, venlafaxine, desvenlafaxine), and **multimodal agents** (vilazodone and vortioxetine) are reserved for patients not responding to first-line medications. Mirtazapine has a special role in patients with suicidal behavior or cases of mixed anxiety-depression.

Cases of MDD not responding to the above medications might need **augmentation therapy** to enhance the efficacy of first-line drugs. **Lithium, low-dose antipsychotics** (risperidone), **triiodothyronine (T_3), stimulants** (modafinil and armodafinil), etc. are generally used as augmentation agents in cases with poor response to antidepressants.

Psychotherapy

Psychotherapy is the treatment of choice for **mild to moderate depression** where medications are not considered good choices. **Cognitive behavioral therapy** which tries to improve a patient's thinking and perception about himself, his surroundings, and his future is the psychotherapy technique specifically developed for depression. Psychotherapy is quite efficacious for mild to moderate cases and also helps in a speedy recovery, augmenting treatment response to drugs and preventing relapse in moderate to severe cases.

Brain stimulation methods such as ECT, are preserved for treatment-resistant depression, depression with **active suicidal tendencies,** and those cases presenting with severe psychotic symptoms or **stupor**. Apart from ECT, other brain stimulation methods such as **vagus nerve stimulation**, **transcranial magnetic stimulation,** and **deep brain stimulation** also impart similar results as ECT.

Importance of Family Education

Depression **is** a highly debilitating illness associated with significant morbidity and mortality due to suicide. It is imperative to involve family members in the management of depression. Family members must understand the nature of the illness and the mortality factor associated with it due to the risk of suicide. Along with medical treatment (medication or psychotherapy), family support is of tremendous importance in recovery from acute depressive episodes and in preventing relapse. Family members are also taught about the warning signs of relapse and emerging signs of suicidal risk and should seek immediate psychiatric help in such cases.

Need for Referral to a Psychiatric Specialist

A case of depression should be referred to a psychiatrist under the following conditions:
1. Depression with risk of suicide
2. Psychotic depression with poor insight
3. When the case is suspected to be a case of bipolar depression
4. Poor response to initial antidepressant medications
5. When psychotherapy or counseling is needed
6. Cases of depression presenting with stupor

SUMMARY

1. Depressive disorders are a group of psychiatric illnesses sharing depressed mood, low self-esteem, and decreased interest in pleasurable activities as principal presenting symptoms.
2. Major depressive disorder or MDD is the most common of all depressive disorders with a prevalence of 5–17% in the general population. It presents with a depressed mood, decreased interest in pleasurable activities, and persistent guilt feeling, hopelessness, helplessness, and worthlessness. Many patients with MDD also harbor suicidal ideas or commit suicide out of misery.
3. The diathesis-stress model of depression emphasizes the complex interplay of genetic makeup, psychological predisposition (diathesis), and environmental factors in the causation of MDD.
4. Pathophysiology of MDD stems from abnormal activation of the HPA axis due to stress response which ultimately leads to a decreased level of serotonin in the brain leading to symptoms of depression.
5. Differential diagnosis of MDD includes other depressive disorders such as dysthymia, seasonal affective disorder, bipolar depression, post schizophrenic depression, depression associated with medical illnesses, etc.
6. MDD is associated with significant morbidity and mortality if left untreated. Suicide is the most common mortality factor associated with MDD.
7. Depression is treated by both psychotherapy and pharmacological means. Psychotherapy such as CBT is mainly indicated in mild to moderate depression while pharmacotherapy is well suited for moderate-severe cases.
8. SSRIs such as fluoxetine, sertraline, etc. are the mainstay of treatment for MDD. Other medications such as SNRIs, mirtazapine, bupropion, etc. are prescribed on a case-to-case basis.
9. Family education and coping skill training have special importance in preventing relapse and recurrence of symptoms.

BIBLIOGRAPHY

1. Benazzi F. Various forms of depression. Dialogues in clinical neuroscience, 2006;8(2):151–61.
2. Bains N, Abdijadid S. Major Depressive Disorder. [Updated 2022 Apr 14]. In: StatPearls [Internet]. Treasure Island (FL): StatPearls Publishing; 2022 Jan.
3. Jacob K. Major depression: Revisiting the concept and diagnosis. Advances in Psychiatric Treatment, 2009;15(4):279–85.
4. Hasler G. Pathophysiology of depression: do we have any solid evidence of interest to clinicians? World psychiatry: official journal of the World Psychiatric Association (WPA), 2010; 9(3):155–61.
5. Duval F, Lebowitz B, Macher JP. Treatments in depression. Dialogues in clinical neuroscience, 2006; 8(2):191–206.

Chapter 8

Bipolar Disorders

Competency achievement: Students should be able to
1. **PS7.1** Classify and describe the magnitude and etiology of bipolar disorders
2. **PS7.2** Enumerate, elicit, describe, and document clinical features in patients with bipolar disorders
3. **PS7.3** Enumerate and describe the indications and interpret laboratory and other tests used in bipolar disorder
4. **PS7.4** Describe the treatment of bipolar disorders including behavioral and pharmacologic therapy
5. **PS7.5** Demonstrate family education in a patient with bipolar disorders in a simulated environment
6. **PS7.6** Enumerate and describe the pharmacologic basis and side effects of drugs used in bipolar disorders
7. **PS7.7** Enumerate the appropriate conditions for specialist referral in patients with bipolar disorders.

INTRODUCTION: A COMPARISON BETWEEN EPILEPSY AND BIPOLAR AFFECTIVE DISORDER

Many authorities have conceptualized bipolar affective disorder (BPAD) in the line of epilepsy. This conceptualization has stemmed from the following characteristic features shared by both epilepsy and bipolar affective disorder.

1. Both of them are **lifelong illnesses with an episodic course** and the patient is completely normal in between the episodes.
2. Basic pathology in both of these disorders is thought to be **abnormal activation** of cortical tissue arising from a focus and gradually spreading to involve either one hemisphere or both the hemispheres (respectively known as partial or generalized activation).
3. Channelopathies (Na^+, K^+, Ca^{2+} channelopathy) or abnormality in intracellular activation cascade are the possible mechanisms underlying the abnormal cortical activation in these disorders.
4. A phenomenon known as **kindling**, which means each episode increases the propensity of further episodes, is seen both in epilepsy and bipolar disorder.
5. Management in both epilepsy and bipolar disorder involves **abortive treatment** for acute episodes and **prophylactic treatment** to prevent further episodes in both of these illnesses. Prophylactic treatment should be continued for at least 2–3 years and if further episodes occur then treatment is for life.
6. Certain factors such as stress, dehydration, and sleep deprivation can **trigger** an acute episode in both of these disorders.

Therefore, to understand bipolar disorder, it is a prerequisite to understanding seizure and epilepsy and to have a clear understanding of the presentation, neurobiology, and treatment of both these illnesses, it is necessary to know about the basic mechanism of neural activation.

Mechanism of Neural Activation

Neural activation starts with the generation of **action potential** via an opening of **Na^+ or Ca^{2+} channels** on its membrane. Subsequent entry of Na^+ or Ca^{2+} into the cell leads to the **activation of intracellular activation cascade** and other activities. Neurons can be activated either automatically or the activation can be induced by another neuron via the release of neurotransmitters. **Automatic activation** involves leaky sodium channels while **induced activation** involves **neurotransmitter-mediated** (mainly glutamate) opening of calcium channels (Fig. 8.1).

Similarly, **inhibition** of an activated neuron involves the opening of **K^+ or Cl^- channels**. Neural inhibition can also be **auto-inhibition** (mediated by opening of K^+ channels) or neurotransmitter-mediated **induced inhibition**. The principal inhibitory neurotransmitters **GABA and glycine** act on the GABA receptors and lead to the opening of Cl^- channels and subsequent inhibition of the neuron (Fig. 8.1).

SEIZURE AND EPILEPSY

Seizure is abnormal **and synchronized electrical hyperactivity of neurons in the cerebral cortex.** Seizure activity starts at a point known as **seizure focus** and subsequently spreads to other areas of the cortex. This activity may be limited to either one cerebral

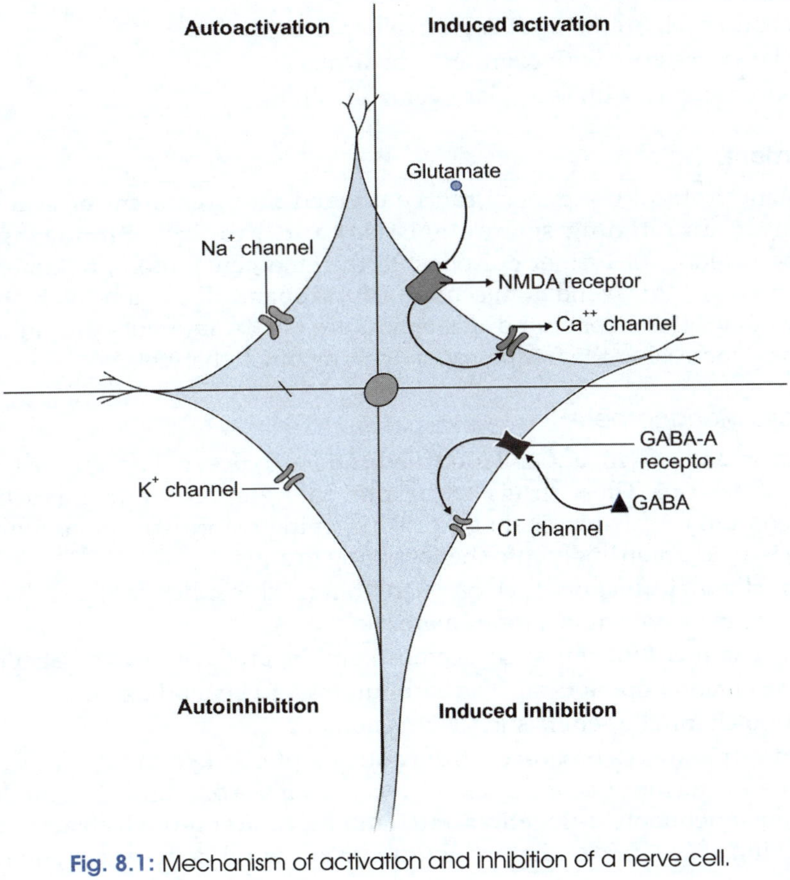

Fig. 8.1: Mechanism of activation and inhibition of a nerve cell.

hemisphere (known as a **partial seizure**) or may involve both cerebral hemispheres (known as a **generalized seizure**). **Convulsion** is the external motor manifestation of seizure activity in the brain. Convulsion can present as muscle contractions as in GTCS or loss of muscle tone as in absence seizure.

A seizure can be **provoked,** i.e. triggered by some **brain pathology** (infection, injury, toxicity, or mass occupying lesions) or **unprovoked in which** no brain pathology is detected. **Epilepsy is the occurrence of two or more unprovoked seizures occurring at least 24 hours apart**. Epilepsy is a **disorder of the brain** presenting with recurrent episodes of seizure and other associated features.

Classification

International League against Epilepsy (ILAE) has classified epilepsy into the following types.

1. Generalized onset seizure
   - Generalised tonic–clonic seizure
   - Tonic seizure
   - Atonic seizure
   - Absence seizure
   - Myoclonic seizure
2. Focal onset seizure
   - Focal onset seizure without cognitive impairment
   - Focal onset seizure with cognitive impairment
3. Focal onset seizure with secondary generalization

Management

Management protocol of epilepsy can be divided into **treatment of acute episodes** (treatment of an ongoing seizure episode) **and prophylactic management** to prevent occurrences of further episodes. In the emergency room, treatment of acute episodes involves intravenous injection of **lorazepam,** diazepam, or **fosphenytoin.** Benzodiazepines (lorazepam and diazepam) are GABA mimetics and inhibit neural activation by increasing the frequency of opening of Cl^- channels.

Prophylactic Management

It involves treatment with antiepileptic medications to **prevent occurrences of further episodes of seizure**. These drugs act by preventing excessive neural activation by blocking sodium or calcium channels or by opening chloride or potassium channels and are classified accordingly into the following groups

1. **Sodium channel blockers** such as phenytoin (and fosphenytoin), carbamazepine, oxcarbazepine, lamotrigine, topiramate etc
2. **Calcium channel blockers** such as ethosuximide, pregabalin, and gabapentin.
3. **Chloride channel openers** such as barbiturates and benzodiazepines
4. **Potassium channel openers** such as retigabine.
5. **Sodium valproate** is a broad-spectrum antiepileptic drug that acts by blocking both sodium and calcium channels and also acts as a GABA mimetic. Another broad-spectrum antiepileptic is **levetiracetam (and brivaracetam)** which acts by blocking the docking of synaptic excitatory neurotransmitter (glutamate) containing vesicles

by binding with synaptic vesicles glycoprotein 2A (SV2A). Currently, broad-spectrum antiepileptics are the drugs of choice for several epileptic conditions.

Prophylactic therapy should be **continued for a period of 2–3 years**. If no seizure episode occurs during this period then there is a good chance that the seizure focus has healed (due to the absence of kindling) and the seizure will not occur any further. However, even after 2–3 years of prophylactic treatment if any further seizure episode occurs, then there is less possibility that the focus will heal anymore and treatment should be for life.

BIPOLAR AFFECTIVE DISORDER

Introduction

Bipolar affective disorder is a complex **mood disorder** presenting with episodes of **mania, hypomania, depression, or episodes with mixed symptoms of mania and depression (mixed episodes).** BPAD is a fairly common and highly debilitating psychotic illness with a tremendous impact on the socio-occupational functioning of a patient. In between the episodes, the patient is completely symptom-free and generally **reaches the premorbid level of functioning**. It is a lifelong illness with an episodic course and treatment is necessary to preserve the general well-being of the patient. BPAD is also associated with significant aggression, violence, and suicidality.

BPAD is a common psychiatric illness with a prevalence of **1% in the general population**. Onset is generally in the third decade of life (**20–30 years of age**). Its incidence is almost the same in both males and females, but what is intriguing is that manic episodes are more common in males while depressive episodes are more common in females. Furthermore, Depressive episodes also become more frequent as the patient grows old.

Clinical Presentation

As already mentioned, bipolar disorder is an episodic illness characterized by episodes of mania, hypomania, depression, or mixed state (Fig. 8.2). In between these episodes, the patient is completely normal (asymptomatic) returning to his premorbid level of functioning. For easy memorizing and clarity, clinical features of an episode of BPAD can be grouped into the following headings.

1. Mood and associated features
2. **Impairment in biological functions** and
3. **Psychotic features**

Manic Episode

Being a mood disorder, **mood symptoms** are the primary and necessary features of BPAD. Patients in manic episodes present with **elevated or expansive moods** or sometimes mood can be irritable. Along with elevated mood, they have **increased energy levels** as evidenced by increased goal-directed activity (a student may read excessively), increased talkativeness and it seems thoughts are rushing into the patient's mind (known as the flight of ideas), overfamiliarity and at times restlessness and aggression. These patients have tremendous self-confidence with **expansive ideas and activities.** Many engage in risk-taking behaviors with harmful consequences such as increased and reckless spending, rash driving, substance abuse, and engagement in indiscriminate sexual behavior.

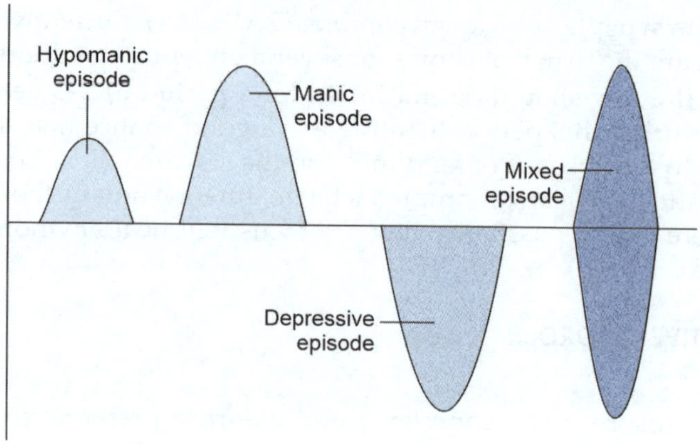

Fig. 8.2: Various mood episodes in a case of BPAD.

Apart from mood symptoms, these patients also present with **impairment in biological functions** such as a **decreased need for sleep** and **increased appetite**. Despite eating a lot, they might lose weight because of increased BMR due to increased activity. **Self-care and grooming** are markedly increased as evidenced by their stylish attire and excessive makeup. Increased engagement in **sexual activities** such as teasing, commenting, pursuing, and increased need for sexual intercourse is often present.

Many patients with mania show overt **psychotic symptoms** such as delusions and hallucinations. **Delusion of grandiosity** is most common, but some may develop persecutory delusions secondary to grandiosity. Grandiose delusion may involve following themes.

1. **Delusion of power:** Patient claims that he has special powers bestowed upon him by god.
2. **Delusion of possession or value:** Patient claims that he has a lot of money, several vehicles, or real estate properties.
3. **Delusion of position or identity:** Patient claims that he holds a special position in some authority or the government establishment, and
4. **Delusion of relation:** Patient claims that he has a special relationship with people in power such as CM, PM, or president.

Unlike delusions, hallucinations are seldom present in mania and if present are mood-congruent (hearing voices which give positive and encouraging comments about their appearance, abilities, and behavior).

Diagnosis

For a diagnosis of **manic episodes,** these symptoms should be present for a period of **7 days** with complete impairment in the socio-occupational functioning of the individual. **The presence of psychotic symptoms** or aggression which necessitates **hospitalization** also invites a diagnosis of **manic episodes** irrespective of the duration of the episode. The presence of the above symptoms for a period of **4–7 days** mandates a diagnosis of **hypomania.** In hypomania functional impairment is present but it is not complete. There should not be any psychotic features such as delusions or hallucinations although expansive ideas are commonly present in hypomania but not up to the level of delusion.

Depressive Episode

Depressive episodes in BPAD (commonly called **bipolar depression)** are characterized by **low mood** or sad feeling which is pervasive and present for the entire day and almost every day. Along with low mood, the person also complains of **decreased energy** level as evident by generalized weakness, decreased communication, and socialization, **decreased activity,** etc. There is a **loss of interest in pleasurable activities** such as going out with friends, watching television, hearing music, etc. And the patient becomes confined to themself with a loss of productivity.

Patients in depressive episodes also complain of **helplessness, hopelessness, and worthlessness.** These features of a negative attitude toward self, others, and one's future are known as **Beck's cognitive triad of depression**. These negative attitudes often lead to suicidal ideas and activities.

Marked **impairments in biological functions** are often present. These patients complain of **early morning awakening with the inability to go to sleep again**, lack of freshness after sleep with excessive daytime sleepiness. They also complain of **poor appetite** and constipated bowel. Self-care and personal hygiene have also decreased. There is a **lack of interest in any type of sexual activity** and the patient may complain of erectile dysfunction. Some patients present with atypical features such as excessive sleep and appetite with weight gain.

Few patients with severe depression also present with **psychotic symptoms such as delusion of guilt** (the patient is convinced that he has done an unpardonable sin) or **nihilism** (the patient believes that he is dead or dying or a part of his body is rotting etc.) or **auditory hallucination**. Auditory hallucinations in bipolar depression are mood congruent and the patient may hear derogatory voices (telling the patient that he is a sinner, a failure, and should commit suicide, etc.).

(It is difficult to differentiate an episode of bipolar depression from unipolar depression. A history of a clear-cut manic or hypomanic episode always establishes a diagnosis of bipolarity. Certain features are indications of bipolar depression such as the presence of agitation or restlessness, somatic features, atypical features, and psychotic features. Suicidal ideas and activities are also more common in bipolar depression than unipolar depression.)

Diagnosis

For a diagnosis of a depressive episode, depressive symptoms should be present for a period of at **least 2 weeks.** There must be marked impairment in the socio-occupational functioning of the individual. These symptoms must not be due to any other psychiatric disorder, medical illness, or substance abuse.

Mixed Episode

Mixed episodes in the context of BPAD are characterized by features of **both depression and mania or hypomania at the same time.** The patient may be expressing a sad mood but talking excessively or have hopelessness and expansive ideas at the same time. Generally, the patient has had either a clear depressive or manic episode for a few days and then develops mixed features. Agitation, restlessness, somatic symptoms, and suicidal ideas or activities are common in mixed episodes.

Types

Bipolar Type I

It is characterized by at least one episode of mania with episodes of depression, hypomania, or mixed state. This type is more common in men.

Bipolar Type II

It is characterized by the absence of any clear-cut manic episode. It is characterized by episodes of depression with few episodes of hypomania but manic episodes are never present. There is a female predisposition for this type of BPAD.

Rapid Cycling Bipolar Disorder

When a patient of BPAD presents with **at least 4 mood episodes** (either depression, mania, hypomania, mixed state, or their combinations) **within a period of one year**, then the condition is known as rapid cycling bipolarity. In the case of rapid cycling bipolarity, symptom-free periods are of short duration and difficult to discern and the patient is almost always having a mood episode. Rapid cycling bipolarity is associated with marked functional impairment and morbidity and high mortality from suicide and response to medications is also poor.

Cyclothymia

It is characterized by alternating episodes of hypomania and depressive episodes with less severe symptoms (not amounting to full-blown depression). Cyclothymia is a lifelong illness associated with significant functional impairment.

Etiology

The exact etiology of bipolar disorder is not known. The **biopsychosocial model** emphasizes genetic and environmental factors and the complex interplay between them.

1. Genetic Factors

The prevalence of BPAD in the general population is roughly 1%. Bipolar disorder tends to run in families. In fact, among all the psychotic illnesses, the heritability of BPAD is the highest, i.e. 80–85%. Twin studies have revealed a **genetic contribution of 70–90%.** However, no single gene is solely responsible and the inheritance pattern is polygenic. Genetic linkage studies have located the **risk genes on 18q and 22q.** Search for candidate genes that have implicated genes involved in neural activations (genes coding for **K^+ or Ca^{2+} channels** or proteins involved in **intracellular activation cascade**) or in the modulation of **monoamine neurotransmitter systems (e.g. COMT gene).**

2. Environmental Factors

Childhood risk factors include a history of abuse, troubled childhood development, or exposure to intrauterine or childhood infections. These factors (especially infections) can produce abnormally irritable tissue in the cortex ultimately leading to abnormal activation which may lead to the development of BPAD.

Environmental factors in a genetically predisposed individual can trigger an episode. These triggering factors include sleep deprivation, significant stress, substance abuse, physical illness, etc.

Neurobiology

Mood symptoms occur due to abnormal reciprocal activation of brain areas involved in regulation of mood and emotions such as **orbitofrontal cortex (OFC) and associated contralateral limbic structures**. This abnormal activation may arise due to defective ion channels **(K^+ or Ca^{2+} channelopathy)**, subtle structures defects (gliosis) or abnormality in regulation of intracellular activation cascade. This abnormal activation in BPAD is of low level but persists for weeks to months. As in case of seizure, abnormal activation can be limited to one hemisphere (right or left) or may involve both the hemispheres and accordingly presentation can be manic, depressive or that of mixed features as explained below.

Orbitofrontal cortex and its connection with structures of the limbic system regulate mood, emotions, impulsivity and aggression. OFC acts as the suppressing centre inhibiting activities of the limbic structures. Studies have revealed that **left OFC** is associated with **positive mood and emotions** while **right OFC** regulates **negative mood and emotions. Manic episodes** are associated with **hypoactivity of right OFC** (suppressing negative emotions) with consequent hyperactivity of contra-lateral (left sided) limbic structure resulting in increased levels of **dopamine** in sub-cortical structures (Fig. 8.3). **Elevated dopamine level** is associated with impulsivity, aggression and psychotic features (delusions and hallucinations).

Similarly, **hypoactivity of left OFC** and consequent activation of right sided limbic structures lead to **suppression of positive emotion** resulting in feeling of sadness, anhedonia and hopelessness which are characteristic features of depressive episode. If this abnormal activation involves **both hemispheres** then the patient presents with a mixture of symptoms of mania and depression **(mixed episode)**. This abnormal activation usually starts in one hemisphere (left or right) and then subsequently involves both the hemispheres (analogues to partial seizure with secondary generalisation). Hence, in most cases, mixed episodes are preceded by 2–3 days of either depressive or manic features.

Differential Diagnoses

BPAD is frequently confused with other psychiatric illnesses. Clear identification and diagnosis of the condition are imperative for proper management of the condition. The possible differential diagnoses are

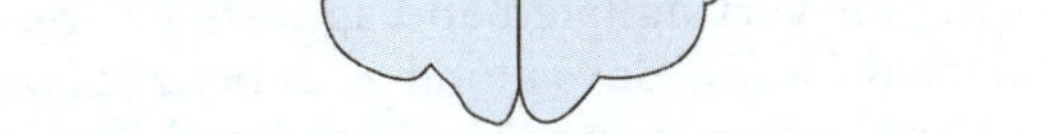

Fig. 8.3: Cerebral activation in manic episode

1. **A borderline personality disorder** is frequently confused with bipolar disorder because of frequent mood swings, self-harm behavior, and episodes of psychotic features. However, BPD, being a personality disorder is continuous in course and there is no clear-cut recognizable episodic pattern.
2. **Schizophrenia with affective symptoms**, however, affective symptoms in schizophrenia are mood incongruent.
3. **Schizoaffective disorder**
4. **Substance-induced psychosis** and
5. **Recurrent brief psychotic disorder**

Suggested Investigations

A case of BPAD is usually diagnosed clinically, although following investigations are often required for management purposes and to rule out any organic cause.

1. Complete blood count with differential counts
2. Thyroid function test to rule out hyperthyroidism
3. Liver function tests before starting sodium valproate
4. Renal function test and ECG before starting lithium
5. Blood sugar and lipid profile before starting second-generation antipsychotics
6. Imaging studies of the brain to rule out organic causes

Course and Prognosis

BPAD is a lifelong illness with an **episodic course**. The patient becomes completely symptom-free between the episodes and reaches his premorbid level of functioning. However, one mood episode in BPAD increases the probability of having further episodes, a phenomenon known as **kindling**. Depressive episodes are associated with more impairment in day-to-day functioning than manic episodes. Depressive episodes are also more common in females and older individuals with BPAD. BPAD, if not treated early in the course, can lead to the following complications.

1. Suicidality
2. Secondary substance abuse behavior
3. Aggression and violence
4. Impairment in the long-term functioning of the individual

MANAGEMENT

Management of BPAD involves treatment of **acute episodes** (manic or depressive) and **prophylactic management** to prevent further episodes.

1. Treatment of Manic Episodes

In some cases of acute mania, **hospitalization** is necessary and the circumstances include

A. Aggressive and violent patients

B. Manic episodes with excessive restlessness and agitation leading to dehydration (manic delirium)

C. Patients refusing medications

Currently, second generation antipsychotics are mainstay of treatment of acute manic episodes either alone or in combination with mood stabilisers. SGAs commonly used for this indication are olanzapine, quetiapine, risperidone and aripiprazole. In case the patient is very agitated and aggressive, injectable haloperidol with promethazine can be used for few days along with benzodiazepines. A short course of benzodiazepines such as lorazepam and clonazepam along with SGAs controls agitation and aggression, improve sleep and hasten symptoms remission.

Prophylactic Treatment

Prophylactic treatment should be started once acute symptoms subside or as early as considered necessary. **Mood stabilizers** such as **lithium, sodium valproate, and carbamazepine** are first-line drugs for the prophylactic treatment of manic episodes. Lithium is indicated in euphoric mania with clear-cut bipolarity while sodium valproate is specially indicated for irritable mania and in case of rapid cycling bipolar disorder. Sodium valproate is not preferred in young women of fertile age groups because of possible side effects like PCOS and neural tube defects if given during the first trimester of pregnancy. In these cases, either lithium or carbamazepine (or oxcarbazepine) is preferred.

2. Treatment of Bipolar Depression

Clear-cut diagnosis of a case of bipolar depression is necessary for proper treatment as bipolar depressive episodes are non-responsive to antidepressants such as SSRIs or the patient may switch to manic episodes if treated with these drugs. There is also fear of the development of rapid cycling bipolarity on treatment with conventional antidepressant medications. **First-line medications** for the treatment of bipolar depression are:

A. Olanzapine and fluoxetine combination
B. Quetiapine
C. Aripiprazole and
D. Lurasidone

There is the greatest evidence in support of the olanzapine and fluoxetine combination followed by quetiapine and lurasidone. Other second-generation antipsychotics such as risperidone and amisulpride have very poor evidence in support of them for use in bipolar depression. These medications should be continued **for a period of 6–9 months** after the resolution of acute symptoms. **ECT is reserved for non-responsive and resistant cases of bipolar depression**.

Prophylactic Treatment

Lamotrigine is the most preferred drug for prophylactic treatment in patients presenting with bipolar depression. Lamotrigine is an antiepileptic which acts by blocking sodium channels and possibly calcium channels and has better efficacy in preventing depressive episodes than manic episodes**. Lithium** has also some efficacy in preventing depressive episodes but is less effective than lamotrigine. Sodium valproate and carbamazepine are not effective in preventing depressive episodes in cases of BPAD.

Prophylactic treatment for BPAD should be continued for a period of 2–3 **years**. If any further episodes of mania, hypomania, or depression occur then treatment with prophylactic drugs should be **continued for life**.

3. Family Education

Being the primary support system, family members need to be educated about the nature of the disease, possible complications, and the need for treatment. Generally, it is seen that after recovering from acute episodes, many patients refuse to take medications as they feel completely normal and free from any symptoms. Family members should encourage the patient to adhere to the prescribed medications as they are mainly prophylactic in nature and are meant for the prevention of further episodes. Furthermore, family members should also be taught about the warning signs of relapse (emergence of any mood episode) and to seek psychiatric treatment as soon as relapse is suspected.

Conditions for Referral to a Psychiatric Specialist

1. Manic cases presenting with aggression and violence
2. Poor treatment adherence
3. Poor response to initial therapy
4. The emergence of intolerable side effects to medications

5. All cases of bipolar depression should be referred to, especially cases with psychotic features or suicidal risk
6. The emergence of secondary substance abuse.

SUMMARY

1. There is a significant overlap between seizure disorder and BPAD in terms of neurobiology and treatment response and both are thought to be due to abnormal activation of cortical tissue.
2. BPAD is a common psychiatric illness with a prevalence of 1% in the community associated with significant morbidity, mortality, and loss of productivity.
3. It is a lifelong illness with an episodic course presenting with episodes of mania, hypomania, depression, or mixed features.
4. Manic episodes are characterized by euphoric or irritable mood, increased goal-directed activities with expansile ideas, and increased energy levels. Hypomania is a less severe form of mania.
5. The bipolar depressive episode presents with a sad mood, decreased interest in pleasurable activities, and decreased energy level.
6. BPAD is mostly genetically determined by polygenic inheritance with some environmental factors leading to the precipitation of an episode in a patient with BPAD.
7. Episodes of BPAD occur due to abnormal over-activation of the frontal cortex leading to neurotransmitter imbalance. Differential activation of the left and right frontal cortex determines the presenting episode (either mania or depression).
8. A case of BPAD must be differentiated from schizophrenia, schizoaffective disorder, cannabis-induced psychosis, and organic mood disorder (e.g. hyper/hypothyroidism)
9. Manic episodes of BPAD are associated with significant aggression, violence, and socio-occupational impairment. Similarly, depressive episodes are associated with suicide and loss of productivity.
10. Treatment of acute episodes of BPAD is with antipsychotics (haloperidol, olanzapine) with benzodiazepines. Hospitalization may be required in some cases.
11. Prophylactic management is to prevent further episodes and is done with mood stabilizers such as lithium, sodium valproate, lamotrigine, etc.
12. Family therapy and psychoeducation are necessary for proper treatment adherence and understanding of the disease.

BIBLIOGRAPHY

1. Epilepsy and bipolar disorders. Marco Mula, et al. Expert Rev Neurother. 2010 Jan.
2. Stafstrom CE, Carmant L. Seizures and epilepsy: an overview for neuroscientists. Cold Spring Harb Perspect Med. 2015 Jun 1;5(6):a022426.
3. Jain A, Mitra P. Bipolar Affective Disorder. [Updated 2022 May 1]. In: StatPearls [Internet]. Treasure Island (FL): StatPearls Publishing; 2022.
4. Cerimele JM, Chwastiak LA, Chan YF, Harrison DA, Unützer J. The presentation, recognition, and management of bipolar depression in primary care. Journal of general internal medicine, 2013; 28(12):1648–56.
5. Ross ED. Differential Hemispheric Lateralization of Emotions and Related Display Behaviors: Emotion-Type Hypothesis. Brain Sci. 2021 Aug 3;11(8):1034.
6. Cerullo MA, Adler CM, Delbello MP, Strakowski SM. The functional neuroanatomy of bipolar disorder. Int Rev Psychiatry. 2009;21(4):314–22.
7. Cotovio G, Oliveira-Maia AJ. Functional neuroanatomy of mania. Transl Psychiatry. 2022 Jan 24;12(1):29.
8. Phillips ML, Kupfer DJ. Bipolar disorder diagnosis: challenges and future directions. Lancet (London, England), 2013;381(9878):1663–71.
9. Geddes JR, Miklowitz DJ. Treatment of bipolar disorder. Lancet (London, England), 2013; 381(9878): 1672–82.

Chapter 9

Anxiety Disorders

Competency achievement: Students should be able to
1. **PS8.1** Enumerate and describe the magnitude and etiology of anxiety disorders
2. **PS8.2** Enumerate, elicit, describe, and document clinical features in patients with anxiety disorders
3. **PS8.3** Enumerate and describe the indications and interpret laboratory and other tests used in anxiety disorders
4. **PS8.4** Describe the treatment of anxiety disorders including behavioral and pharmacologic therapy
5. **PS8.5** Demonstrate family education in a patient with anxiety disorders in a simulated environment
6. **PS8.6** Enumerate and describe the pharmacologic basis and side effects of drugs used in anxiety disorders
7. **PS8.7** Enumerate the appropriate conditions for specialist referral in anxiety disorders

INTRODUCTION: THE FEAR RESPONSE

Fear is the normal neurophysiological reaction in response to any dangerous or threatening stimulus. The fear response is necessary **for harm avoidance** (such as avoiding predators) and the **survival of the species** (and not going the 'DODO' way). Fear is considered a **primary emotion** and is regulated by a small almond-shaped brain structure known as the **amygdala**. Amygdala is a **part of the limbic system** and is regarded as **'the fear center of the brain'**. It is the extensive connection of the amygdala with other brain structures which starts fear response and results in peculiar bodily changes in response to fearful stimuli (Fig. 9.1).

A dangerous stimulus is perceived **via special sense organs** and the information about the stimulus is sent to various **primary sensory cortices** (parietal, occipital, and temporal cortices) and thereafter to the **sensory association cortex** (situated at the confluence of these above cortices). After processing the information in the association cortex, a signal is sent to the **amygdala.** A signal is also sent to the hippocampus to activate any memory about the fear stimulus.

Amygdalar activation is necessary and sufficient to start a fear response. The activated amygdala now sends a signal to the **orbitofrontal cortex** where the subjective sensation of fear is perceived resulting in a feeling of dread (**cognitive appraisal of fear**). Signals from the amygdala are also sent to the **hypothalamus** (humoral control center) which mediates the **hormonal response** of fear (increased catecholamine and glucocorticoid levels). Amygdala-mediated activation of brainstem nuclei such as **locus coeruleus and parabrachial nuclei** results in **autonomic responses** of fear such as palpitation, perspiration, muscle tension, shakiness of hands, shortness of breath, etc. The person

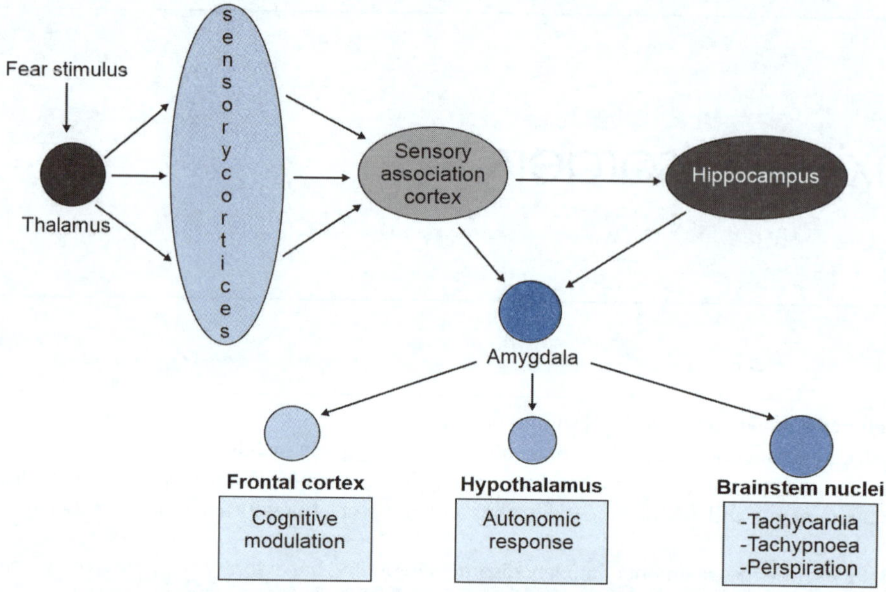

Fig. 9.1: Information flow in the fear circuit of the brain.

may face the danger and be ready to fight or may avoid the danger by fleeing from the situation which is famously known as the **'fight and flight response'**.

ANXIETY DISORDERS

Anxiety disorders are psychiatric conditions arising due to **abnormal activation of the fear circuit (abnormal fear response).** These conditions vary from one another in presentation depending upon the context in which the fear circuit has been activated.

Depending on the **clinical presentation** anxiety disorders can be categorized as:

1. **Generalized anxiety disorder**
2. **Panic disorder and**
3. **Phobic anxiety disorders**

Epidemiology

Anxiety disorders are one of the **most common psychiatric illnesses in the community** and studies have found that one in every four people is suffering from some type of anxiety disorder. Females are more prone to develop anxiety disorders than males and prevalence is higher among lower socioeconomic groups. The presence of any type of anxiety disorder significantly impairs the day-to-day functioning of an individual and hence needs to be diagnosed and treated effectively.

Etiology

1. **Psychodynamic theories** of anxiety disorders emphasize **unconscious conflict** as the basis of anxiety. Conflicts in the unconscious arise due to clashes between the **repressed desires and wishes** of the Id and the controlling effects of the Superego.
2. **Behavioral theorists** argue that anxiety is a **learned behavior** that is acquired with experience during childhood through the process of **conditioning. Punishment and**

criticism by parents and authority figures play an important role in the development of anxiety and neurosis in children. Similarly, children also learn these behaviors from anxious parents **via imitation.**

3. **Biological theories** emphasized abnormal neurotransmitter-mediated modulation of the fear circuit as the basis of the development of anxiety disorders. **Abnormal activation of the amygdala** lies at the cornerstone of the development of anxiety disorders and the pattern of amygdalar activation also determines the type of anxiety neurosis. This abnormal activation of the amygdala may be due to abnormal levels of modulating neurotransmitters such as **GABA, glutamate, serotonin, norepinephrine,** etc which stems from genetic risk factors and environmental effects.

GENERALIZED ANXIETY DISORDER (GAD)

GAD is a fairly common psychiatric illness with onset in late adolescence and early adulthood with a female predisposition. A case of GAD presents with the following symptoms

1. Apprehension
2. Excessive worry about future untoward events
3. Palpitation, tremors, shortness of breath, and excessive sweating
4. Increased muscle tension with an 'on-edge' feeling
5. Sleep disturbance, especially difficulty in falling asleep due to excessive worry
6. Poor coping with day-to-day stress and
7. Predominant irritable mood most of the time

For a diagnosis, these symptoms must be present for most of the day and almost every day **for a period of 6 months** and must cause significant impairment in day-to-day activities.

Neurobiology

The above-mentioned symptoms of GAD arise due to abnormal **low-level persistent activation of the fear circuit** without any fear-inducing stimulus. This abnormal activation might be due to neurotransmitter imbalance in the fear circuit such as decreased levels of serotonin, GABA, noradrenaline, etc. This low-level persistent activation of the fear circuit leads to excessive worry, apprehension, and other objective symptoms of GAD.

Complications

Long-standing GAD can lead to the following complications:

1. Secondary depression and suicidal tendency
2. Substance abuse such as abuse of alcohol to get rid of anxiety symptoms
3. Weight loss (long-standing GAD can lead to weight loss)
4. Panic attacks
5. Poor day-to-day functioning

Differential Diagnosis and Suggested Investigations

1. Hyperthyroidism is to be ruled out with routine thyroid profile tests in all cases of anxiety disorders.
2. Anaemia can mimic symptoms of GAD for which a complete blood count is often indicated.

3. For cardiac ailments, ECG should be performed in all cases of GAD.
4. For frequent hypoglycemia, testing for blood sugar levels is mandatory.

Treatment

The treatment approach involves **pharmacotherapy and psychotherapy**. Medications are the mainstay of treatment and SSRIs are the first line of drugs for GAD. Among all the SSRIs, evidence in favor of **paroxetine and escitalopram** is more robust as compared to sertraline and fluvoxamine. **Escitalopram** is preferred over paroxetine because of fewer sexual side effects and less incidence of discontinuation symptoms. However, it should be remembered that **SSRIs take 2–3 weeks** to exert their actions. This period can be managed by **coprescribing benzodiazepines** such as clonazepam and etizolam along with SSRIs for 2–3 weeks and then tapering down their doses and stopping the benzodiazepines. Unsatisfactory response to SSRIs invites adding other anxiolytics such as:

1. **Propranolol** effectively controls objective symptoms of GAD such as palpitation, tremor, perspiration, etc.
2. Low dose **quetiapine and**
3. **Pregabalin**

The psychotherapeutic approach includes behavioral therapy such as **breathing exercises, JPMR** (Jacobson Muscle Relaxation Technique**), meditation, and aerobic exercises**. Combining behavioral therapy with medications yields the best results.

PANIC DISORDER

A panic attack is characterized by **sudden onset extreme fearfulness** with a feeling of **impending doom or death** or going mad accompanied by palpitation, excessive sweating, and shakiness of hand and wobbly legs. The person generally runs away from the place where the attack has occurred (flight response). Many describe panic attacks as **having a heart attack**. Each attack is generally **preceded by a sensory aura** or a sense of discomfort starting from the legs or hands and the person can sense the impending attack.

Panic disorder is characterized by **two or more panic attacks** within a period of 1 month with the apprehension of having further attacks. Panic disorder is a psychiatric illness arising due to **sudden and excessive activation of the amygdala** and the fear circuit. It may be hypothesized as seizure activity arising within the amygdala leading to its sudden and excessive activation. Just like a seizure, every attack generally **lasts for 2–5 minutes**. In panic disorder, an attack can occur anywhere and anytime. The panic disorder must be differentiated from the following conditions presenting with similar symptoms

1. **Mitral valve prolapse** and echocardiography may be done to rule out this condition.
2. **Pheochromocytoma** is a tumor of the adrenal medulla which might present with features of an adrenergic burst. Ultrasonography of the abdomen is done to rule out the adrenal tumor in case of doubt.
3. **Hypoglycemic attacks and**
4. **Thyroid crisis,** thyroid function is done to rule out hyperthyroidism.

Treatment

Medications are the mainstay of treatment for panic disorder. SSRIs are the first-line medications with **paroxetine and escitalopram** preferred over other SSRIs. Short-acting benzodiazepines such as **etizolam and clonazepam** are prescribed as and when required basis which the patient can take on sensing an attack. Patients not responding to SSRIs can be put on a trial of SNRIs such as venlafaxine or desvenlafaxine. Poor response to these drugs invites add-on therapy with pregabalin or gabapentin. **Psychotherapy** for panic disorder includes **breathing exercises** and muscle relaxation techniques.

PHOBIC ANXIETY DISORDERS

A phobia is defined as an **excessive and irrational fear** of harmless objects or circumstances. These objects and circumstances are perceived as harmless by others and do not evoke any fear but induce extreme fearfulness and avoidance by the patients suffering from a phobia. When phobic stimuli are encountered, these patients feel extremely fearful with palpitation, tremor, excessive sweating, and shortness of breath which are typical of the fear response. The phobia can be **explained by classical conditioning** in which a harmless stimulus is conditioned with a harmful stimulus (generally in childhood) leading to the **activation of the fear circuit by this conditioned harmless stimulus** even in the absence of the naturally harmful stimulus (see chapter 2). However, the patient usually cannot remember the situation in which this conditioning has occurred.

Depending on the circumstances, **specific phobias** can be grouped into the following **four categories.**

1. **Animal types** such as fear of dogs (cynophobia), spiders (arachnophobia), and horses (equinophobia)
2. **Situational types** such as fear of closed spaces (claustrophobia), of heights (acrophobia), etc.
3. **Natural environmental types** such as fear of thunderstorms (astraphobia), fear of woods (dentophobia), etc.
4. **Blood and injury types** such as fear of blood (hemophobia) and of needles (trypanophobia).

Agoraphobia is a special type of phobic disorder in which the patient is afraid of any situation where **escape from or finding help is difficult** and presents as a fear of open places, crowded places, staying home alone, traveling alone, etc. The patient feels helpless in these situations and begins to panic. The patient may experience symptoms similar to panic attacks in such situations.

Another very common phobic disorder is **social phobia or social anxiety disorder** which is defined as a fear of social situations or public places where there is a **possibility of being scrutinized** by others. In such situations, the patient is constantly worried about **negative evaluations** by others or doing something which will cause embarrassment. Social phobia is highly disabling and patients suffering from this condition cannot express their talent at its full potential.

Treatment

Psychotherapy is the first line of management for specific phobias. Gradual and repetitive **exposure to phobic stimuli** with prior relaxation (with a breathing exercise or with benzodiazepines) leads to desensitization to these harmless stimuli and they will no longer evoke the fear response. This process is known as **systematic desensitization**. Another psychotherapy technique is **flooding** in which the patient is directly exposed to the phobic stimulus and forced to bear with the fear without avoidance which ultimately results in the resolution of symptoms and **deconditioning**. **CBT** is another psychotherapeutic technique used for phobic disorders, especially agoraphobia and social phobia.

Medications for phobic disorders are **SSRIs and SNRIs**. SSRIs such as paroxetine and escitalopram are first-line medications but usually take 2–3 weeks to exert their effects. This period can be covered with short course benzodiazepines such as clonazepam and etizolam.

Family Education in Cases of Anxiety Disorder

Psychoeducation about the nature of anxiety disorders is of utmost importance. Family members should understand that anxiety is an illness and the patient has no control over it. Furthermore, they are also taught about the need for treatment, good compliance, and the duration of treatment. Family members are also counseled regarding emotional and financial support to the patient.

Conditions for Referral to a Psychiatrist in Case of Anxiety Disorder

1. Cases not responding to initial treatment
2. The emergence of secondary depression with suicidal tendency
3. Complete impairment in socio-occupational activity due to anxiety disorder
4. Those requiring psychotherapy or counseling
5. The emergence of secondary substance abuse behavior

SUMMARY

1. Fear is the normal physiological reaction in response to any threatening stimulus and is mediated by the amygdala and its connections with other brain areas (the fear circuit). Amygdala is also known as the fear center of the brain.
2. Abnormal activation of fear circuits can lead to the occurrence of fear response without any relevant stimulus and presents as anxiety disorders. Presenting features depends upon the pattern of activation of the fear circuit.
3. Anxiety disorders are classified as generalized anxiety disorder, panic disorder, and phobic anxiety disorders. PTSD was earlier classified under anxiety disorders, however, has been grouped under stress-related disorders.
4. GAD presents with low-level anxiety symptoms such as apprehension, tremors, perspiration, sleep disturbances, etc with symptoms persisting throughout the day, almost every day for a period of 6 months. GAD is thought to be due to low-level persistent activation of the fear circuit.
5. Panic attacks present with sudden onset excessive fearfulness with a feeling of impending doom or death. Two or more panic attacks within a period of 1 month with the apprehension of having further attacks are features of panic disorder.
6. A phobia is defined as an excessive and irrational fear of harmless objects or situations. Specific phobias are of 4 types: animal type, situational type, natural environmental type, and blood-injury type. Social phobia and agoraphobia are special types of anxiety disorders associated with a host of similar situations.
7. Management of anxiety disorders is mainly behavioral. Relaxation therapy for GAD and panic disorder and systematic desensitization for phobic disorders are treatments of choice. Medications such as SSRIs, beta blockers, buspirone, etc. are reserved for cases not responding to behavioral therapy. Combining medications with behavioral therapy yields better results than individual treatment alone.

BIBLIOGRAPHY

1. Steimer T. The biology of fear- and anxiety-related behaviors. Dialogues in clinical neuroscience, 2002; 4(3):231–49.
2. Tyrer, Peter. Classification of Anxiety. The British journal of psychiatry: the journal of mental science. 1984;144:78–83. 10.1192/bjp.144.1.78.
3. Gale C, Davidson O. Generalised anxiety disorder. BMJ. 2007 Mar 17;334(7593):579–81.
4. Taylor CB. Panic disorder. BMJ. 2006 Apr 22;332(7547):951–5.
5. Eaton WW, Bienvenu OJ, Miloyan B. Specific phobias. The Lancet. Psychiatry, 2018;5(8):678–686.
6. Bandelow B, Michaelis S, Wedekind D. Treatment of anxiety disorders. Dialogues in clinical neuroscience, 2017;19(2):93–107.

Chapter 10

Obsessive–Compulsive Spectrum Disorders

INTRODUCTION

Many varied yet related disorders are grouped under the obsessive–compulsive spectrum disorders which share the core 'obsessive–compulsive' features. Apart from sharing obsessive–compulsive features, they are also similar in patient characteristics, course of the illness, underlying neurobiology, and response to treatment. Being a spectrum it has two ends: a compulsive end, and an impulsive end. At the compulsive end of the spectrum are disorders characterized by excessive sensitivity to life risk and subsequent harm avoidance behaviors and disorders included are OCD, body dysmorphic disorder, illness anxiety disorder, anorexia nervosa, etc. (Fig. 10.1). At the impulsive end of the spectrum are disorders characterized by poor impulse control with

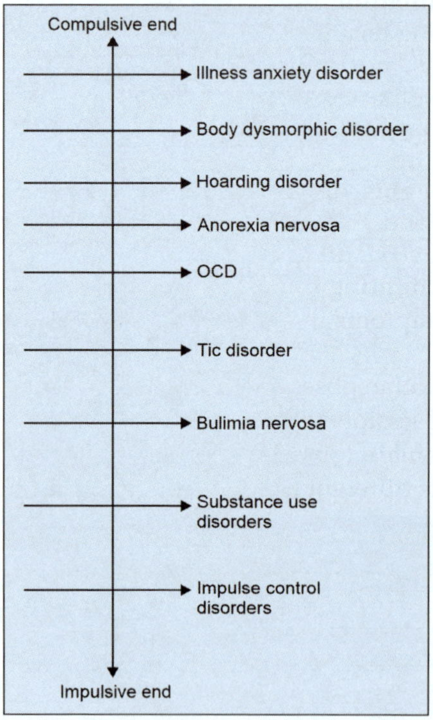

Fig. 10.1: Various disorders in the impulsive-compulsive spectrum.

risk-taking behaviors and include pathological gambling, trichotillomania, kleptomania, pyromania, sexual compulsion, binge eating disorder, etc. Here we will discuss some common disorders in OC spectrum disorders.

OBSESSIVE–COMPULSIVE DISORDER

OCD is a fairly common psychiatric illness **characterized by repetitive intrusive thoughts and compulsive acts**. It is a highly debilitating illness causing significant impairment in the socio-occupational well-being of the patient. Symptoms of OCD generally appear in late adolescents or early adulthood, are more common in females than males, and follow a **lifelong waxing and waning course (symptom severity goes up and down over a period of time)**.

Clinical Presentation

OCD is characterized by the presence of obsession and compulsion. Obsession is defined as **repetitive intrusive thoughts, impulses, or images** that come into the mind even if there is resistance to stop them causing significant distress. These thoughts are generally recognized by the patient as his thoughts and are not inserted by an outside agent. In OCD, the patient finds **these thoughts irrational, unwanted, and excessive** and tries to stop them but without any success. Obsessions are **ego-dystonic** means they are highly annoying and **cause subjective discomfort**. Common themes of obsessions in a case of OCD are (Table 10.1):

1. **Obsession of dirt**, thoughts coming into mind that hand or other body parts are still dirty even after repetitive washing.
2. **Obsession of contamination**, repetitive thoughts of getting infected with virus or bacteria after touching harmless household objects.
3. **Obsession of doubts**, not getting enough confidence of completion even after completing a task (like closing the door, turning the gas off).
4. **Obsessive sexual thoughts**, discomforting ideas of incest, or sexual thoughts involving religious figures.
5. **Obsessive violent thoughts**, discomforting ideas, images, or thoughts of harming a family member or a friend.
6. **Obsession with symmetry and orderliness.**
7. **Obsessive counting (counting footsteps, electric poles, etc.)**

All these obsessive symptoms in cases of OCD can be grouped into **four domains** as follows:

1. **Contamination domain** (an obsession with dirt and contamination)
2. **Symmetry domain** (obsession with symmetry, orderliness, and obsessive counting)
3. **Forbidden thought domain** (obsessive sexual or violent thoughts) and
4. **Hoarding domain** (it is different from the other three domains)

Table 10.1: Common obsessions and associated corresponding compulsions

Obsessions	*Compulsion*
Obsession of dirt	Repetitive cleaning rituals
Obsession of contamination	Hand washing, use of sanitizer
Obsession of doubt	Repetitive checking
Violent and sexual thoughts	Praying (mental compulsion)
Obsession with orderliness	Rearranging

Compulsions are **repetitive acts (physical or mental) performed by the patient to reduce the discomfort associated with obsessions**. A person with an obsession with dirt and contamination often washes his hands repeatedly and is involved in repetitive cleaning rituals, obsession with doubts leads to compulsive checking (repetitive checking of door padlock or gas bolt). To get rid of sexual or violent obsessive thoughts about religious figures, the person may repeatedly pray to god (**mental compulsion**). Compulsive acts reduce the discomfort temporarily but obsessive thoughts would come after some time and compulsive acts are **repeated again and again**. This vicious **cycle of obsession–discomfort–compulsion followed by obsession** is known as the **OC cycle**. The patient finds these obsessive thoughts and compulsive acts **illogical and excessive** but still will not be able to control them. These patients spend a good amount of time engaging in compulsive acts to get rid of their irrational obsessive thoughts and often get annoyed and irritated.

Apart from obsession and compulsion, patients of OCD often complain about anxiety which is inherent to OCD. However, the **anxiety in OCD is more like a subjective discomfort or distress** rather than like true anxiety as seen in other anxiety disorders. Many patients also suffer from somatic symptoms like tingling or burning sensation or pain symptoms. **Sleep disturbance** is frequently associated with OCD because of obsessive thoughts coming into the mind while the patient tries to sleep.

Few patients with OCD (mostly those with sexual or violent obsessive thoughts) often present with **psychotic features like ideas of persecution and ideas of reference**. These patients often have poor insight into their illnesses. Earlier a diagnostic entity known as **schizo-obsessive disorders** was assigned to this category of patients. Currently, it is recognized as a sub-type of OCD only.

Etiology

The exact cause of OCD is not known. The following theories try to explain the origin of obsessions and associated compulsions.

1. Psychodynamic Theory

As per **Freud's psychodynamic theory**, OCD is the result of **fixation in the later anal stage (anal masochistic stage)** of psychosexual development. Because of **harsh toilet training,** there might be fixation in this stage and the child develops the **defense mechanism of reaction formation and undoing** to deal with the strict toilet rules of toilet training imposed by parents. Under the reaction formation as a defense mechanism, the child **develops excessive cleanliness** in response to the dirt inside the body (holding stool in the anal masochistic stage).

2. Genetics

OCD is found to run in families. Family studies and twin studies have established the genetic basis of OCD with a **heritability of 45–65%.** Search for candidate studies has implicated various genes, the most prominent of which is the **serotonin reuptake transporter (SERT) gene**.

3. Social Learning Theory

As per behavioral theorists, compulsive behaviors are **learned from parents and significant others**. Maintenance of cleanliness and orderliness and strictly following rules and social norms are praised in certain cultures (especially in Asian cultures). The presence of obsessive and compulsive behavior in parents or significant others is learned by the patient during childhood.

4. PANDAS

Pediatric autoimmune neuropsychiatric disorders associated with **streptococcal infection (PANDAS)** often present with OC symptoms. Because of this association, an **autoimmune response to streptococcal infection** was implicated in the etiology of OCD. However, these symptoms are short-lived and subsequent researchers have denounced this hypothesis.

Neurobiology

The basic problem in patients of OCD is the patient's inability to inhibit an ongoing thought or action leading to repetitive obsessive thoughts and subsequent compulsive behaviors. A neural network known as the cortico-striato-thalamo-cortical (CSTC) loop is tasked with the modulation of an ongoing thought process and the consequent action. FMRI studies have revealed **hyperactivity** of structures forming the **CSTC loop** in cases of OCD (Fig. 10.2). Hyperactivation of the CSTC loop is thought to be due to **the** poor inhibitory action of OFC on the CSTC loop due to **decreased level of serotonin** neurotransmitter in the frontal cortex. This is the basis of treatment of cases of OCD with serotonergic drugs such as SSRIs and clomipramine. Recently, other neurotransmitters such as **glutamate** (increased glutamate activity in CSTC loop) and **dopamine (**dopamine hyperactivity**)** have also been implicated in some cases of OCD. This is the basis of augmentation of cases of OCD not responding to first-line drugs with **antipsychotics** drugs such as risperidone, haloperidol, or amisulpride or anti glutamatergic drugs such as **acetyl-cysteine** or **memantine** (**ketamine** is in experimental stage).

Comorbidity

OCD is frequently associated with other **OCD spectrum disorders** such as tic disorder and eating disorders. **Anxiety** is considered an inherent symptom of OCD and previously OCD was included in anxiety neurosis (as in ICD-10). However, neuropsychiatric studies have established OCD as a different entity resulting from an abnormality in the CSTC loop and no abnormalities in a fear circuit have been noted in OCD (in contrast to cases of anxiety disorders). Long-standing OCD can result in **secondary depression** because of the severe distress associated with it. Few cases of OCD often present with **psychotic symptoms** such as delusion of reference and persecutory ideas. Previously the term

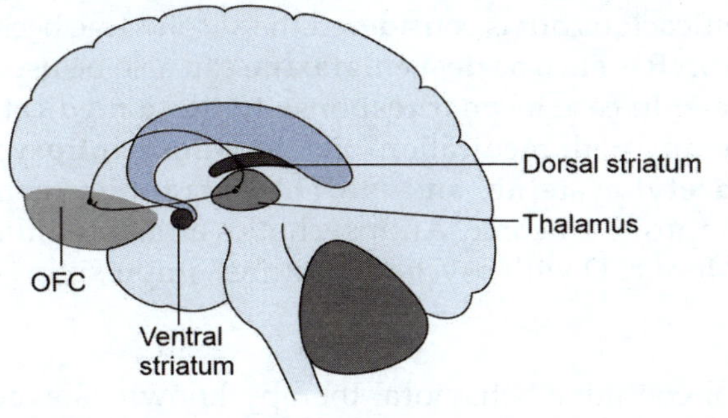

Fig. 10.2: CSTC loop involved in obsessive–compulsive disorder.

schizo-obsessive was used to denote these patients, but subsequently, this diagnostic entity was dropped both from ICD and DSM.

Course and Prognosis

OCD is a lifelong illness and follows a waxing-waning course over time which means symptoms may diminish for some time and then exacerbate for a few weeks or months and again come down but symptoms never resolve completely. Symptoms generally get aggravated during periods of psychological stress. With treatment, around 30% of cases improve significantly, 40% of cases improve moderately while the remaining 30% are resistant to standard treatment which is known as resistant cases of OCD. Long-standing OCD can lead to the following complications.

1. Secondary depression
2. Death by suicide
3. Excoriation of hands
4. Social isolation
5. Poor functioning in life

Diagnosis

Diagnosis of OCD is **mainly clinical**. As per ICD-10, the **presence of obsession and compulsion is sufficient** for the diagnosis of a case of OCD. As per DSM5, these symptoms must **cause significant distress or impairment in the social-occupational functioning** of the individual. However, new onset OCD symptoms in old age generally indicate an organic cause in which cases brain imaging studies are crucial to rule out organicity. DSM-5 also includes specifiers for the level of insight present in a case of OCD, e.g. OCD with good/fair insight or with poor/absent insight.

Treatment

Management of OCD is challenging, especially for patients with poor insight and with other comorbidities. Psychotherapeutic approaches such as **exposure and response prevention (ERP)** are first-line management approaches. However, combined treatment with medication and psychotherapy is most effective.

1. Pharmacotherapy

SSRIs are considered first-line medications for the treatment of OCD. Among all the SSRIs, **fluvoxamine and fluoxetine are the most efficacious** because of their strong serotonin reuptake-blocking activity. Among TCAs, **clomipramine** is approved for OCD and is quite efficacious but is considered the second line because of its unwanted side effects profile. **SNRIs such as desvenlafaxine** can also be used when the response to SSRI is inadequate. In case **of poor response to these medications, augmentation or replacement therapy** with medications like **low-dose antipsychotics (risperidone or amisulpride), acetyl-cysteine, and NMDA antagonist memantine**, usually in combination, can improve outcome. Antipsychotics and anti-glutaminergic drugs are specially indicated for OCD with psychotic features, impulsivity, and aggression.

2. Psychotherapy

A particular type of cognitive behavioral therapy known as **exposure and response prevention** is particularly designed for cases of OCDs and is highly effective. In ERP, the patient has been exposed to anxiety-provoking obsessive situations (like dirt) and advised to bear with it without yielding by engaging in compulsive activities (hand washing). With time, the discomfort due to obsession will increase to the maximum but if the patient remains adamant without yielding then the discomfort would gradually decrease and become bearable after a few sessions. The exposure to obsession-provoking stimuli should be gradual. **ERP is highly effective and when combined with pharmacotherapy yields the best results.**

EATING DISORDERS

Eating disorders are psychiatric illnesses **characterized by abnormal eating behaviors** associated with **disturbance in thought processes, perception of body image, and emotional regulation**. **Primary eating disorders** include **anorexia nervosa, bulimia nervosa,** and **binge eating disorder**. Other eating disorders such as **pica** (ingestion of non-food items) and **rumination disorders** are associated with an intellectual disability or other conditions and are considered different from primary eating disorders.

Currently, there is a paradigm shift in the classification of Eating disorders and these disorders are included in **obsessive–compulsive spectrum disorders**. Anorexia nervosa falls at the compulsive end of the spectrum as it is associated with an obsession with low body weight and thinning and harms avoidance behavior; binge eating disorder (impulsively eating a large amount of food) falls at the impulsive end of the spectrum while bulimia nervosa falls in between.

Etiology

The exact etiology of eating disorders is not known. The **biopsychosocial model** emphasizes **genetic risk,** abnormal **psychological development in childhood,** and **socio-cultural influences** as the factors contributing to the development of eating disorders.

There is a definite **genetic risk** for the development of eating disorders as evident from family studies and twin studies. Eating disorders run in families and first-degree relatives are at increased risk of developing eating disorders. In cases of identical twins, if one twin has the disorder then the risk in the other twin is more than 50%. Genome-wide association studies have identified single **nucleotide polymorphism** in genes encoding proteins involved in the **regulation of appetite** such as **ghrelin, orexin A and B, leptin, etc**.

Abnormal psychological development due to sexual or physical abuse or problematic parenting contributes to the development of eating disorders to a great extent. These factors impair the ability to regulate emotion which is one of the important aspects of eating disorders.

Societies and professions where weight loss and thinness are admired and encouraged are also risk factors for the development of eating disorders, especially anorexia nervosa. Cases of anorexia nervosa are quite common in professions such as **dancing, modeling, and athletics** which put a great emphasis on the maintenance of low body weight.

Anorexia Nervosa

Clinically it is the most important eating disorders. The term anorexia nervosa means **loss of petite which is of nervous origin**. The prevalence of anorexia nervosa is about 7–10 times more in girls than boys with onset in the late teenage period or early adulthood.

Cases of anorexia nervosa present with an obsession with thinness and maintenance of **extremely low body weight with extreme fear of gaining weight**. This is due to the patient's altered **perception of body image**. Even if they are extremely thin they perceive themselves as overweight with the need to further shed some weight. This altered perception of body image with fear of gaining weight is the core feature of anorexia nervosa.

Depending upon the eating behavior anorexia nervosa can be categorized into two types.

1. **The restricting type** is characterized by **restrictions on food and calorie intake**. These patients are very cautious regarding the amount of calorie intake and are obsessed with calorie counts. They eat very little even if they are hungry. They are obsessed with food and recipes and make elaborate food for others but they eat little. Some even play with food by arranging food items, cutting them into small pieces, and carrying eatables in their bags. When eating with others they often secretly discard food, others unknowing.
2. The other category is the **binge eating-purging type**. In this type, there is no restriction on food intake and in fact, they **impulsively eat a large amount of food in a binge pattern**. After these binge eating episodes, they feel fearful about gaining weight and feel guilty about their lack of control over their feeding. Subsequently, they indulge in **compensatory purging behavior** such as self-induced vomiting, taking a laxative or diuretics, and excessive water to purge out the food eaten. Some of them also indulge in **excessive physical exercise to lose weight**.

Apart from psychiatric symptoms such as altered body image perception, obsession with thinness, and fear of gaining weight, anorexia nervosa also presents with **medical problems** secondary to starvation and low-fat content in the body. Physical examination reveals extreme emaciation, lackluster skin, and body hair, soft silky lanugo hair all over the body, bradycardia, and hypothermia. They also complain about **amenorrhea** (secondary to low body weight), infertility, generalized weakness, muscle ache, etc. Purging type also presents with dental problems (enamel erosion due to gastric acid regurgitation), halitosis (bad breath), and symptoms of GERD.

Other psychiatric disorders may be present in patients with anorexia nervosa. **Depression** is often associated with AN. **Anxiety disorders**, personality disorders (**borderline or OC personality**), body dysmorphic disorder; **OCD,** etc. are other associated comorbidities. Suicidal risk and suicidal behavior must be assessed in all patients of anorexia nervosa.

Complications

Medical complications in cases of anorexia nervosa arise due to starvation and purging behavior. Many patients are anemic and **prolonged anemia can lead to heart failure**. Decreased bone mass density and **osteoporosis** may lead to frequent fractures of limb bones or the spine. Frequent self-induced purging can result in **hypokalemia** and irregular cardiac rhythm and death due to sudden cardiac arrest. Regurgitation of gastric acid can cause **esophagitis** and Mallory–Weiss tears. So, overall mortality in anorexia nervosa is high either due to medical complications or suicide.

Treatment

1. **Psychotherapy** has proven efficacy in restoring body weight and can normalize the altered body image and associated emotional disturbances. **Cognitive behavioral**

therapy is aimed at correcting altered body image perception and emotional dysregulation. Supportive psychotherapy with family involvement (**Maudsley family therapy**) can restore body weight in 70–90% of cases.

2. **Medications** can help improve emotional regulation. SSRIs such as **fluoxetine** are frequently prescribed and have shown moderate efficacy. Fluoxetine also improves depression, impulsivity, and anxiety. SSRIs combined with antipsychotics (olanzapine) yield better results. **Olanzapine** improves appetite, can potentially correct disturbed body image, and can improve other comorbid psychiatric illnesses. However, medications are a second-line management approach, and psychotherapy should be considered first. Combining psychotherapy with meditation gives the best result.

Bulimia Nervosa

Bulimia nervosa or simply bulimia is an eating disorder **characterized by binge eating episodes followed by compensatory behaviors to avoid weight gain**. However, **body weight in bulimia is more or less preserved** and body image disturbance is seldom present. Fear of gaining weight is also a core feature of bulimia nervosa and these patients indulge in purging behavior to avoid weight gain after a binge eating episode**. Binge eating means eating a large amount of food** until interrupted by someone else or their stomach starts hurting. Binge eating episodes in these patients are followed by guilt feeling and fear of gaining weight. This leads to **compensatory behavior** like self-induced vomiting and purging behavior to get rid of the eaten food in the body. Some patients abuse laxatives and diuretics as means of purging. Many do hard physical exercise to avoid weight gain. However, unlike anorexia nervosa, **obsession with thinness and maintenance of very low body weight is not present**; they just avoid gaining weight beyond normal.

Patients suffering from bulimia often have **problems regulating emotions**. Impulsivity and guilt feeling are frequently present. Many patients also suffer from ongoing **depression and anxiety disorders**. Personality problems, especially **borderline personality disorder** are seen in many cases as comorbid illnesses.

Complications in bulimia nervosa are mainly due to compensatory purging behavior. Self-induced vomiting can result in **dental erosion, chronic pharyngitis, esophagitis, and Mallory–Weiss tears**. Frequent vomiting and abuse of diuretics can result in electrolyte imbalances such as **hypokalemia.** Hard knuckles and fingers are often noticeable in these patients due to self-induced vomiting by inserting fingers into the mouth. Death can occur due to electrolyte imbalance, aspiration of gastric content, and cardiac complications due to hypokalemia.

Treatment involves **supportive psychotherapy** with family involvement (Maudsley family therapy) and medications. Medications such as **fluoxetine** can help improve impulsivity, depression, and anxiety symptoms. A combination of medications with psychotherapy yields better results.

Binge Eating Disorder

Binge eating disorder is the most common eating disorder **characterized by compulsive eating of large amounts of food** till one feels uncomfortably full (binge eating). After binge episodes, the person feels guilty about a **lack of control over their eating behavior**. However, they **do not indulge in compensatory behavior** like self-induced vomiting or purging as the fear of gaining weight is conspicuously absent. Persons suffering from binge eating disorder often eat in secrecy and feel embarrassed of their eating behavior and lack of control over it. These persons frequently gain a lot of weight due to a lack of compensatory behavior and feel ashamed about it.

Many patients when presenting themselves in clinics are visibly depressed. Along with **depression**, **impulsivity** in other areas such as compulsive buying and spending, frequent **explosive behavior**, and **self-harm behavior** are often present. **A borderline personality disorder** is another condition comorbidly associated with binge eating disorder. Many think of committing suicide and few do so.

Treatment involves cognitive behavioral therapy (**dialectical behavioral therapy**), family therapy, and medications. SSRIs such as **fluoxetine** help in improving impulsivity and depressed mood. Stimulants like methylphenidate can improve impulsivity and decrease appetite and promote weight loss. Similarly, the anticonvulsant **topiramate** is also useful as it stabilizes mood and impulsivity and it also decreases appetite and promotes weight loss.

Differentiating features of all three types of eating disorders discussed above are depicted in Table 10.2.

OTHER EATING DISORDERS

PICA

PICA is characterized by the **ingestion of non-food substances** such as mud, dirt, chalk, plastic beads, paper, etc. PICA is commonly seen in patients with **intellectual disabilities** but can also be seen in normal persons suffering from **iron deficiency anemia** or those with emotional dysregulation. Ingestion of nonfood substances can lead to many complications such as **intestinal obstruction** (due to ingestion of plastic beads), **worm infestation**, **chronic poisoning** (lead poisoning can be caused due to ingestion of flakes of lead paint), etc. Treatment is by correction of iron deficiency anemia and behavior therapy.

Rumination Disorder

It is characterized by the **regurgitation of gastric content** (semi-digested food) into the mouth followed by **chewing and reingestion**. It is seen exclusively in patients with intellectual disabilities.

Table 10.2: Difference between various eating disorders

Eating disorder	*Thought*	*Perception*	*Emotion*	*Behavior*	*Complications*
Anorexia nervosa	Obsession with thinness	Disturbed body image perception present	Fear of gaining weight	Food restriction or binge eating-purging behavior	Anaemia, osteoporosis, electrolyte imbalance, hypothermia
Bulimia nervosa	Nil	Seldom present	Fear of gaining weight	Binge eating and purging behavior	Electrolyte imbalance, dental erosion, oesophagitis
Binge eating disorder	Nil	Absent	Guilt feeling	Only binge eating, no purging	Weight gain, metabolic syndrome

Night Eating Syndrome

Night-eating syndrome is characterized by **daytime anorexia, evening hyperphagia, and insomnia**. These patients eat very less during the daytime but ingest a large amount of food after the evening meal. They frequently wake up at night and engage in eating food which happens mostly in REM sleep. Many of these patients suffer from depression, poor emotional regulation, and obesity. Treatment is with SSRIs such as **fluoxetine**, often combined with **topiramate** which suppresses appetite and promotes weight loss.

Tic Disorder

Tic is defined as a **sudden, brief, repetitive contraction of a group of muscles** that produces visible motor activities or vocalization. It presents with **sudden, brief, and involuntary motor movements or vocalization**. Even if these movements or vocalizations are involuntary, the patient **can control them for some time** but eventually, it fails and tics will come after some time. There is a **sense of urge and building-up of discomfort before the act**. This **discomfort is relieved after the act** (movement or vocalization) which is often short-lived and discomfort will build up once again after some time. Therefore, tics are repetitive (occur many times during daytime) and chronic in nature. The frequency of tics decreases when the person is relaxed or is engaged in other activities and disappears completely when the person goes to sleep. When the person is anxious, in distress, or under the scrutiny of others, Tics frequency increases drastically. The onset of the disease is mainly in childhood (5–7 years of age) and in many cases gradually subsides as the person reaches adulthood. Prevalence is more in boys than in girls.

Both motor and vocal tics are further divided into **simple or complex tics**. Simple tics involve less number of muscles or the production of simple sounds and serve no purpose. Examples of **simple motor tics** include eye blinking, head jerking, facial grimacing, etc. **Simple vocal tics** include throat clearing, groaning, screaming, etc. Complex tics on the other hand are more noticeable and apparently purposeful. **Complex motor tics** may present as frequent touching, jumping, waving of hands, etc. **Complex vocal tics** are rare albeit interesting. Few patients with complex vocal tics may repeat the words of others **(echolalia)** or their own words or sentences **(palilalia).** An extreme case is a **coprolalia** where the patient produces **obscene and abusive words or language** involuntarily.

Tourette syndrome is a rare type of tic disorder presenting with a complexity of motor tics and vocal tics. To diagnose a case of Tourette syndrome, **at least 4 motor tics and one vocal tic** must be present for a period of **1 year**. Motor tics might be changing in nature and might involve different muscle groups during the course of the illness.

Tic is a **neurodevelopmental disorder** arising from abnormal wiring of neural circuits during the developmental period and subsequent altered information processing. Abnormal information processing in the CSTC **loop (cortico-striato-thalamo-cortical loop)** is responsible for the development of tic disorder (as in the case of OCD). Basic abnormality lies in basal ganglia such as the **caudate nucleus and putamen**, which are a part of the striatum, as revealed by structural and functional imaging studies (voxel-based morphometry and fMRI). It is hypothesized that there are abnormal **focal dopaminergic discharges in the basal ganglia** which produce repetitive motor movements or vocalization, both of which are due to abnormal muscle contractions. This is the basis of targeting **dopamine activity** with dopamine receptor blockers (antipsychotics) as a treatment modality for tic disorder.

Treatment

Antipsychotics with strong dopamine-blocking activities (**haloperidol or risperidone**) are frequently prescribed as they are quite efficacious. However, these medications should be given in **low doses** which are sufficient enough to suppress the tics only as they are associated with side effects like weight gain and EPS. Apart from antipsychotics, **centrally acting alpha2 agonists (clonidine and guanfacine)** also have proven efficacy and are first-line drugs for tics with ADHD features.

A special type of psychotherapy known as **habit reversal technique (HRT),** similar to ERP in OCD, has been developed as a treatment for tic disorder. It involves engaging oneself in other activities to keep him distracted to suppress the urge for motor movement or vocalization. This leads to the building of the discomfort to a level maximum but with persistence, it gradually wanes down and the patient does not feel compelled anymore to carry out the movement. HRT is highly efficacious in controlling tics.

IMPULSE CONTROL DISORDERS

Introduction

Impulsivity is defined as performing an **action without any forethought** or making a decision without thinking about the consequences. According to Barratt, impulsivity has **three-dimensional aspects**: **motor dimension** (action without thinking), **cognitive dimension** (quick cognitive decision-making), and **non-planning factors**. Impulsivity is common during childhood and adolescent periods but control over impulsivity is gradually attained over time. Impulsivity is also an important feature of many psychiatric illnesses such as ADHD, conduct disorder, ASPD, and an eating disorder. However, impulse control disorders are a constellation of illnesses presenting primarily with failure to control impulsivity in different contexts which define these illnesses.

Neurobiology

The connection between the **anterior cingulate cortex (ACC)** and **ventral striatum** (in contrast to OCD where the dorsal striatum is involved) **forming the CSTC loop** is responsible for impulse control (Fig. 10.3). The **top-down inhibition** arising from ACC imparts the desired control over the impulsivity. **Poor top-down inhibition** due to cortical hypoactivity leads to poor cognitive control over impulsivity and poor forethought into the actions. This **poor top-down inhibition** is thought to be due to **decreased level of serotonin neurotransmitter**. Conversely, the CSTC loop can be activated by excessive activity of the ventral striatum which consists of nucleus accumbens and habenular nuclei (**bottom-up activation**) which can override normal top-down inhibition. This excessive bottom-up activation is thought to be due to **excessive glutaminergic or dopaminergic activity** in the ventral striatum.

Group of Disorders

These are a group of disorders that share similar clinical characteristics, neurobiology, and genetic predispositions. These disorders share the following **clinical features:**

1. **An urge or appetite** builds up before the action (**craving**)
2. **Lack of control** over acting on the impulsive urge (**action**)
3. **A feeling of satisfaction** or relaxation after acting on the impulse (**hedonic pleasure**)

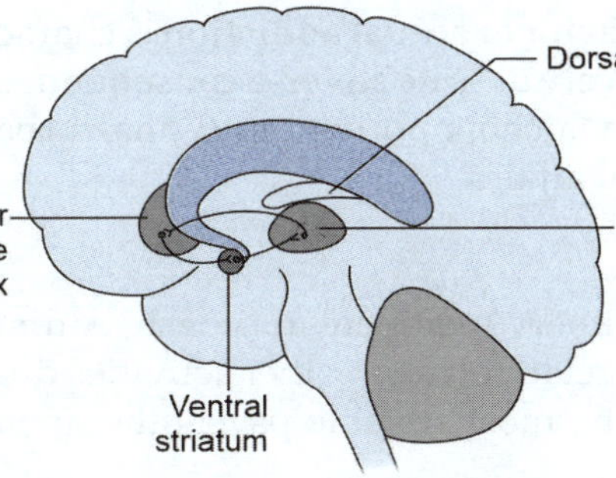

Fig. 10.3: CSTC loop involved in impulse control.

The disorders grouped under impulse control disorders are described in short as follows:

1. **Trichotillomania (TTM)** is characterized by **repetitive hair-pulling** from the scalp, eyebrows, or other hairy parts of the body causing noticeable hair loss. Because of this **noticeable hair loss** from the scalp or other parts, these patients feel embarrassed and avoid socialization which causes significant functional impairment. The vast majority of patients are female and many are suffering from low self-esteem or other psychiatric illnesses such as anxiety and OCD.
2. **Kleptomania,** which is mostly seen in females, is characterized by **compulsive stealing** of petty items not needed for personal use. These patients cannot resist the impulse to steal and get a sense of satisfaction or relaxation from stealing.
3. **Pyromania** is characterized by **recurrent indulgence in fire-setting behavior** which is deliberate and purposeful to gain satisfaction only. Pyromania is seen mostly in adolescent boys. This fire-setting behavior may lead to dangerous accidents.
4. **Compulsive buying or oniomania,** which is also seen predominantly in women, is characterized by **repetitive indulgence in compulsive buying** of less expensive items in an excess amount that one does not need or cannot afford. This behavior causes significant financial and interpersonal problems and other socio-occupational distress. The purchased items are seldom used and are generally returned to the store by family members.
5. **Intermittent explosive disorder (IED)** is characterized by the **sudden onset of out-of-context aggression on minor provocations**. This aggression is directed toward people or properties and causes significant distress in day-to-day activities. Aggressive episodes are short-lived and there is a feeling of guilt in the patient for lack of control over his action.
6. **Pathological gambling** is characterized by **compulsive indulgence in gambling behavior** despite the behavior causing significant financial, marital, or legal problems. The behavior generally appears in late adolescence and takes years to cause socio-occupational problems. Pathological gambling is considered a **behavior addiction** and is mostly seen in men.
7. **Pathological skin picking** is characterized by the **picking of skin from the face or other body parts** resulting in tissue damage and scarring. This condition is also seen predominantly in females and causes significant distress in day-to-day life. Many patients also have comorbid psychiatric illnesses such as mood disorder, borderline personality disorder, and substance abuse disorders.

8. **Compulsive sexual behavior or sexual addiction** is characterized by **engagement in sexual activities repetitively despite adverse consequences**. These behaviors include excessive indulgence in watching pornography, masturbation, going to prostitutes, or repetitive extramarital affairs.

Treatment

1. **Psychotherapy** is the primary treatment approach. **A distraction strategy** in which the patient is advised to get involved in other activities during impulse builds (**habit reversal technique**) is the most suitable psychotherapeutic approach for impulse control disorders.
2. No medication has been approved by the FDA for the treatment of impulse control disorder. **Fluoxetine** has some efficacy in controlling impulsivity and is indicated in many cases of ICDs. **Mood stabilizers** such as lithium and sodium valproate may be effective in intermittent explosive disorder. **Atypical antipsychotics** such as risperidone and amisulpride are used in TTM. **Opioid antagonist** naltrexone is specially indicated for pathological gambling

SUMMARY

1. The OC spectrum runs from the compulsive end to the impulsive end. OCD, hoarding disorder, body dysmorphic disorder, etc lie at the compulsive end, while impulse control disorders, binge eating disorder, etc lie at the impulsive end of the spectrum.
2. OCD is one of the commonest psychiatric illnesses presenting with obsessions and compulsions as clinical features. Obsessions are repetitive and intrusive thoughts, impulses, or images that come into the mind even if there is resistance to stop them and cause significant distress. Compulsions are physical or mental actions performed to alleviate the distress associated with obsessions.
3. The basic neurological abnormality in OCD is abnormal activation of the CSTC (cortico-striato-thalamo-cortical) circuit due to abnormally low levels of serotonin or increased levels of glutamate neurotransmitter.
4. OCD if left untreated can cause significant impairment in day to day functioning of the individual and can also lead to secondary depression and suicide.
5. Treatment of OCD can be done with pharmacotherapy and psychotherapy. SSRIs such as fluvoxamine and fluoxetine are the mainstays of treatment. Cases not responding to SSRIs can be prescribed clomipramine which is more efficacious although causes more side effects. The psychotherapy of choice for cases of OCD is exposure and response prevention or ERP.
6. Tic disorder, which is also included in the OC spectrum disorder presents with abnormal involuntary movements of a group of muscles leading to abnormal movement of vocalization. Consequently, tic can be motor tic or vocal tic. Tourette syndrome is a special type of tic disorder presenting with at least 4 motor tics and one vocal tic. Vocal tic in Tourette syndrome can present with coprolalia (involuntary utterance of obscene language).
7. Impulse control disorders present with repetitive indulges in certain activities despite known adverse consequences. Common ICDs include trichotillomania, pyromania, kleptomania, oniomania, sexual compulsion, etc.

BIBLIOGRAPHY

1. Allen A, King A, Hollander E. Obsessive-compulsive spectrum disorders. Dialogues in clinical neuroscience, 2003;5(3):259–71.
2. Brock H, Hany M. Obsessive-Compulsive Disorder. [Updated 2022 Feb 10]. In: StatPearls [Internet]. Treasure Island (FL): StatPearls Publishing; 2022 Jan.

3. Macmaster FP, Rosenberg DR. Glutamate and the Treatment of Obsessive-Compulsive Disorder. Psychopharm review: timely reports in psychopharmacology and device-based therapies, 2010;45(5):33–40.
4. Pittenger C, Kelmendi B, Bloch M, Krystal JH, Coric V. Clinical treatment of an obsessive-compulsive disorder. Psychiatry (Edgmont (Pa.: Township)), 2005.;2(11):34–43.
5. Allen A, King A, Hollander E. Obsessive-compulsive spectrum disorders. Dialogues in clinical neuroscience, 2003;5(3):259–71.
6. Morris J, Twaddle S. Anorexia nervosa. BMJ (Clinical research ed.), 2007. 334(7599), 894–8.
7. Jain A, Yilanli M. Bulimia Nervosa. [Updated 2022 Apr 30]. In: StatPearls [Internet]. Treasure Island (FL): StatPearls Publishing; 2022 Jan.
8. Iqbal A, Rehman A. Binge Eating Disorder. [Updated 2022 May 1]. In: StatPearls [Internet]. Treasure Island (FL): StatPearls Publishing; 2022 Jan.
9. Mittal SO. Tics and Tourette's syndrome. Drugs Context. 2020 Mar 30;9:2019-12–2.
10. Schreiber L, Odlaug BL, Grant JE. Impulse control disorders: an updated review of clinical characteristics and pharmacological management. Frontiers in Psychiatry, 2011;2:1.
11. Talha Tahir, Melanie Mitsui Wong, Muhammad Maaz, Roshan Naufal, Rabia Tahir, Yedishtra Naidoo, Pharmacotherapy of impulse control disorders: A systematic review, Volume 311, Psychiatry Research, 2022.

Chapter 11

Stress-related Disorders

Competency achievement: Students should be able to
1. **PS9.1** Enumerate and describe the magnitude and etiology of stress-related disorders
2. **PS9.2** Enumerate, elicit, describe, and document clinical features in patients with stress-related disorders
3. **PS9.3** Enumerate and describe the indications and interpret laboratory and other tests used in stress-related disorders
4. **PS9.4** Describe the treatment of stress-related disorders including behavioral and psychosocial therapy
5. **PS9.5** Demonstrate family education in a patient with stress-related disorders in a simulated environment
6. **PS9.6** Enumerate and describe the pharmacologic basis and side effects of drugs used in stress-related disorders
7. **PS9.7** Enumerate the appropriate conditions for specialist referral in stress-related disorders

INTRODUCTION

Stress is a well-known contributor to the development of psychiatric illnesses. However, not all individuals are equally prone to develop psychiatric illnesses when exposed to stress. This vulnerability to stress depends upon an individual's genetic makeup, coping skills, psychological development, and support system. The onset and amount of stress also determine the type of illness. In this chapter, we will discuss some common psychiatric illnesses that are precipitated by some overwhelming stress or any significant change in life. These stressful events are exceptionally severe and can cause distress in any individual when exposed to such stress, such as disaster, combat, rape, torture, etc. Illnesses grouped in this category are:
1. Acute stress reaction
2. Post-traumatic stress disorder
3. Adjustment disorder and
4. Prolonged or complicated grief

ACUTE STRESS REACTION

When an individual is exposed to any **sudden and significant stress**, he may develop an **illness** known as an acute stress reaction (ASR). Symptoms of ASR must appear within 3 days of exposure to the stressful event and must subside within a month. The type of stress preceding the development of ASR is significant enough to **threaten the survival of the person or threatens his integrity** such as:

1. **Threat to survival** (natural disaster, war, terrorist attacks, etc.)
2. **Threats to personal integrity** such as rape, torture, slavery, etc.
3. **Threat to loved ones** like death of close family members or friends, sudden onset major injury or illness, etc.

Clinical Presentation

After the exposure, the individual develops **a state of dissociation characterized by confusion, impaired response to external stimuli, numbness, and disorientation.** This initial state of **'daze'** is often followed by dissociative stupor or agitation, restlessness, or a fugue-like state. Symptoms of autonomic hyperactivity such as anxiety, perplexity, startling, and insomnia are often present. The onset of symptoms is rapid and follows the event almost immediately and resolves within hours to days (symptoms generally resolve within 3 days in most cases and must resolve within 1 month).

Complications

1. **PTSD**: Persons with acute stress disorder are at the **highest risk of developing PTSD** and treatment should be initiated as early as possible to prevent progression to PTSD.
2. **Suicidality**: Patients with ASR are at high risk of suicidality. It is mandatory to assess the risk of suicidal tendencies in all patients of ASR.
3. **Substance abuse**: Many patients after experiencing a traumatic event develop substance abuse behavior such as alcoholism and opioid abuse to get rid of negative emotions associated with the trauma.

Differential Diagnosis

A case of ASR should be differentiated from the following illnesses which also present with similar symptoms:

1. **In acute and transient psychotic disorder**, symptoms are less severe and reality testing is impaired in ATPD.
2. **Mild traumatic brain injury:** The patient may be confused with impairment in consciousness.
3. **Complex partial seizure**
4. Substance intoxications such as cannabis and LSD.

Suggested Investigations

1. Complete blood count with differential counts
2. Liver and renal function tests to rule out encephalopathy
3. CT or MRI scanning of the brain to rule out head injury
4. Urine drug analysis to rule out drug intoxication
5. EEG, when the complex partial seizure is suspected

Treatment

Treatment should be initiated at the earliest in cases of ASD to prevent progression to PTSD and to prevent the possible emergence of substance abuse behavior or suicide. **Psychotherapy is the treatment of choice for these patients**. Specific psychotherapeutic approaches in these patients are:

1. **Trauma-focused CBT** helps in mitigating negative emotions and attitudes associated with the traumatic event. This technique is effective in preventing the progression to PTSD.

2. **Desensitization** involves gradual exposure of the individual to trauma-related stimuli (both real and imaginary). This technique is based on the principles of fear extinction and is particularly effective in decreasing the severity of symptoms in patients with ASD.

The pharmacological approach has limited scope in the treatment of ASD. **SSRIs** such as paroxetine and fluoxetine are considered first-line medications with limited success. Benzodiazepines should be avoided as they can worsen symptoms. **Alpha1 antagonists** such as **prazosin** are specifically effective in mitigating anxiety, nightmares, and flashbacks and also in preventing the progression to PTSD.

POST-TRAUMATIC STRESS DISORDER

Post-traumatic stress disorder (PTSD) can follow any **highly stressful traumatic events** which threaten a **person's survival** such as motor vehicular accidents, war, natural disasters, etc, or his **integrity** such as rape, torture, long-standing abuse, etc. Persons at risk of developing PTSD are children, refugees, soldiers, and persons employed in disaster management task forces. The prevalence of PTSD is around 5–10% after exposure to acute trauma and women are more prone to develop PTSD than men.

PTSD was earlier included under anxiety disorder as it occurs due to the **formation of strong abnormal emotional memory** of these events **involving the amygdala** and fear circuit. Any clue which evokes memories of the event can activate a fear response leading to the characteristic symptoms of PTSD. However, PTSD occurs in response to some extremely stressful events and is hence included under stress-related illnesses in DSM5.

PTSD presents with a confluence of symptoms which can be grouped into the following headings:

1. **Re-experiencing the event** in the form of **nightmares or flashbacks**. Flashbacks are spontaneous dissociative episodes during which the patient re-experiences the traumatic event almost as vividly as the actual event. Flashbacks are also associated with feelings of depersonalization and derealisation.
2. **Hyper-arousal symptoms** are characterized by excessive vigilance, startling, palpitation, emotional numbness, and insomnia.
3. **Avoidance of any stimulus** that can evoke the memory of the event.

Complications

PTSD is associated with significant distress and if not treated can lead to following complications:

1. Suicide
2. Substance abuse behavior
3. Anxiety neuroses and
4. Depression

Prevention

PTSD can be prevented following any traumatic event with the help of **psychotherapy which teaches adaptive coping skills.** Medications such as **prazosin** given for a few days just after the event can also prevent the development of PTSD.

Treatment

Treatment of PTSD is challenging both for the treating psychiatrist and the patient. Psychotherapy involving **relaxation techniques and coping skills training** helps mitigate symptoms of PTSD. When medications are considered, SSRIs are considered as drugs of choice and quite efficacious in case of PTSD.

ADJUSTMENT DISORDER

Adjustment disorder presents with significant emotional and behavioral problems following some **important change in life causing significant emotional distress** and impairment in the socio-occupational well-being of the patient. **Any changes in the life of a person disrupting social relations due to death or separation or social integrity due to migration and refugee status can induce symptoms of adjustment disorder**. Adjustment disorder is a relatively new diagnostic entity that first appeared in DSM-III and was further elaborated in DSM-IV.

The condition presents with depressive symptoms often associated with anxiety, anger, frustration, etc. The person feels frustrated: neither being able to plan nor being able to linger in the current situation. Some patients also feel the urge to act violently and aggressively, although actual aggression is rare in adults. However, adolescents may develop antisocial behaviors such as stealing and aggressive and destructive behaviors.

For a diagnosis of adjustment disorder, these **symptoms must appear within 3 months** following a stressful change in life. These symptoms must cause significant distress and impairment in the socio-economic functioning of the individual. Generally, symptoms of adjustment disorder resolve within 6 months of the removal of the person from the stressful situation. However, in protracted cases, symptoms can last for more than 6 months.

Adjustment disorder significantly increases substance abuse behavior and about 60% of patients with adjustment problems indulge in some form of substance abuse behavior. Other psychiatric complications associated with adjustment disorder are secondary depression, anxiety disorders, and suicidal tendencies.

Treatment of adjustment disorder is mainly psychological. **Solution-focused therapy** is aimed at teaching the person how to effectively handle the current difficulties by developing positive coping skills. Other psychotherapeutic approaches helpful in adjustment disorder are **interpersonal psychotherapy**, **marital counseling**, **brief psychotherapy,** etc. Medications such as SSRIs, mirtazapine, and vortioxetine may help mitigate anxiety and depressive symptoms associated with adjustment disorder.

PROLONGED GRIEF

Grief is the normal emotional reaction following the death of a loved one and is evident by feelings of sadness, teary eyes, insomnia, and preoccupation with the memories of the person. Normal grief reaction has the following 5 stages:

1. Denial and isolation
2. Anger
3. Bargaining
4. Depression and
5. Acceptance

On the other hand, **mourning is the customary ritualistic activity** carried out by family members and friends following the death of a person. **Bereavement** is the combined aspects of grief and mourning.

Grief reaction is universal after the death of a loved one and symptoms generally resolve within weeks to months following the incidence. However, **sometimes grief reactions can persist beyond the normal period in which case it is known as prolonged grief or complicated grief.** It is considered a disorder when it significantly impairs day to day functioning of the individual. Risk factors for the development of prolonged grief are:

1. Sudden unnatural death
2. Vulnerable persons (women, children, dependent persons, etc)
3. Death of a person with strong emotional bonding (e.g. death of a spouse, death of a young child)

Clinical Presentation

Prolonged grief is characterized by persistent preoccupation with or persistent longing for the deceased. Along with this, the patient also presents with persistent sadness and guilt feeling, emotional numbness, a feeling of emptiness, etc. These symptoms must cause significant impairment in the socio-occupational functioning of the individual.

Treatment

Complicated grief is treated by a specific psychotherapeutic approach known as **complicated grief therapy** which promotes adjustment to the loss. Another therapy effective in complicated grief is CBT. Medications such as SSRIs and mirtazapine are also helpful in mitigating distress and depression associated with prolonged grief.

Conditions for Specialist Referral

1. Patients presenting with suicidal tendency
2. Cases not responding to initial treatment
3. Cases requiring psychotherapy or counseling
4. Cases of PTSD with secondary depression
5. Cases of prolonged grief with secondary depression or secondary substance abuse behavior.

SUMMARY

1. Stress is a well-known contributor to the development of many psychiatric illnesses, especially neurotic illnesses. Certain stressful events if significant enough in terms of impact or duration can lead to certain illnesses known as stress-related disorders which include acute stress reaction, PTSD, adjustment disorder, and prolonged grief.
2. Acute stress which threatens the survival of an individual or his loved one or threatens his integrity can lead to the development of acute stress reaction. It is characterized by dissociative symptoms, extreme anxiety, numbness, and a state of 'daze' or mental fogging. Acute stress reaction develops within 3 days of exposure to the stressful event and generally resolves by itself within a period of 1 month. However, in cases where coping skills are poor, it may progress to PTSD.
3. Post-traumatic stress disorder or PTSD is a long-lasting form of acute stress reaction. It is characterized by a triad of symptoms: Re-experiencing the event in the form of flashbacks or nightmares, avoidance of any stimuli that might rekindle the memory of the actual event, and hyper-arousal symptoms such as hyper-vigilance, startling, sleep disturbance, and numbness. PTSD is difficult to treat once symptoms start. CBT, exposure therapy, and supportive psychotherapy are treatments of choice for PTSD. Medications such as SSRIs may help in the treatment of depression secondary to PTSD.

4. Adjustment disorder presents with significant emotional and behavioral problems following some **important change in life causing significant distress** and impairment in the socio-occupational well-being of the patient.
5. Prolonged grief is characterized by persistent preoccupation with or persistent longing for the deceased after the death of a loved one. It is common after sudden unnatural demise, the death of a child, or the death of a person with special importance in life.

BIBLIOGRAPHY

1. Fanai M, Khan MAB. Acute Stress Disorder. [Updated 2022 Jul 12]. In: StatPearls [Internet]. Treasure Island (FL): Stat Pearls Publishing; 2022 Jan.
2. Meiser-Stedman R, McKinnon A, Dixon C, Boyle A, Smith P, Dalgleish T. Acute stress disorder and the transition to posttraumatic stress disorder in children and adolescents: Prevalence, course, prognosis, diagnostic suitability, and risk markers. Depress Anxiety. 2017 Apr; 34(4):348–55.
3. Mann SK, Marwaha R. Posttraumatic Stress Disorder. [Updated 2022 Feb 7]. In: StatPearls [Internet]. Treasure Island (FL): Stat Pearls Publishing; 2022 Jan.
4. O'Donnell ML, Agathos JA, Metcalf O, Gibson K, Lau W. Adjustment Disorder: Current Developments and Future Directions. Int J Environ Res Public Health. 2019 Jul 16;16(14):2537.
5. World Health Organization (WHO). The ICD-10 Classification of Mental and Behavioural Disorders. Genève, Switzerland: World Health Organization. 1993.
6. Szuhany KL, Malgaroli M, Miron CD, Simon NM. Prolonged Grief Disorder: Course, Diagnosis, Assessment, and Treatment. Focus (Am Psychiatr Publ). 2021 Jun;19(2):161–72.

Chapter 12

Somatoform Disorders

Competency achievement: Students should be able to

1. **PS10.1** Enumerate and describe the magnitude and etiology of somatoform, dissociative, and conversion disorders
2. **PS10.2** Enumerate, elicit, describe, and document clinical features in patients with somatoform, dissociative, and conversion disorders
3. **PS10.3** Enumerate and describe the indications and interpret laboratory and other tests used in somatoform, dissociative, and conversion disorders
4. **PS10.4** Describe the treatment of somatoform disorders including behavioral, psychosocial, and pharmacologic therapy
5. **PS10.5** Demonstrate family education in a patient with somatoform, dissociative, and conversion disorders in a simulated environment
6. **PS10.6** Enumerate and describe the pharmacologic basis and side effects of drugs used in somatoform, dissociative, and conversion disorders
7. **PS10.7** Enumerate the appropriate conditions for specialist referral in patients with somatoform dissociative and conversion disorders

DISSOCIATIVE AND CONVERSION DISORDERS

DISSOCIATIVE DISORDERS

Introduction

The conscious part of the mental psyche (also known as the **ego**) controls **self-identity, awareness** of self and surrounding, and **memory**. Consciousness acts as a glue to paste all our memories episodically to make a mental diary of our past life, which may be called a mental **autobiography**. Furthermore, memory, self-identity, and self-awareness are integrated by the conscious part of the ego and are under voluntary control. Any painful event or experience can trigger the separation of any of these conscious functions from the rest of the conscious apparatus and that function will be no more under our conscious control (Fig. 12.1). The process by which any of these functions get separated from the conscious apparatus is known as **dissociation**. Dissociation is nothing but a defense mechanism employed by the ego itself to get rid of excessive anxiety caused by a stressful event by using the libidinal energy associated with it to separate one of the conscious functions (memory, awareness of self/surrounding, and self-identity) from the conscious apparatus. This dissociation of a conscious function from the rest of the mental psyche helps mitigate the anxiety associated with the painful event.

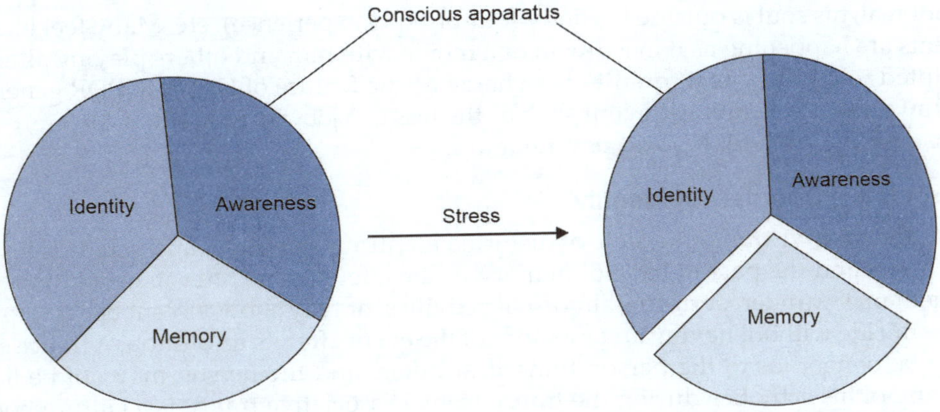

Fig. 12.1: Mechanism of dissociation (Representational).

Depending upon the conscious function that has been separated from the rest of the consciousness, dissociation can present with impairment of memory known as **dissociative amnesia, disturbance in self-identity** (dissociative identity disorders), and impaired awareness of self and the surrounding (**depersonalization/derealization disorder**).

Dissociative Amnesia

Dissociative amnesia or **psychological memory loss** is the most common of all dissociative disorders and presents with the inability to remember details surrounding a stressful event. Memory loss is extensive enough to be explained by normal day-to-day forgetfulness. Loss of memory is generally patchy and mostly related to some stressful event; however, sometimes can be extensive and the person cannot remember anything about the past (retrograde amnesia). Accordingly, dissociative amnesia can of the following 4 types:

1. **Localized amnesia** is when only the memory surrounding a stressful event is lost.
2. **Generalized amnesia** is when all the memories before the event are lost (analogous to retrograde amnesia).
3. **Systematic amnesia** is when memories pertaining to a person or an object or a situation are lost.
4. **Continuous amnesia** is when the patient cannot remember events following a stressful event (analogous to anterograde amnesia).

Dissociative fugue is a special type of dissociative amnesia in which the person wanders aimlessly ending up in a distant place, assumes a new identity, remains there for some days, and returns without having any memory of the event. It is generally seen in persons with ongoing financial, familial, or social stress. Basic self-care like eating, hygiene, and grooming are maintained during the stay.

Depersonalization and derealization

Depersonalization and derealization **(DPDR)** is a **complex dissociative phenomenon** involving awareness of self and the surrounding. Depersonalization means **detachment from self** and derealization means **detachment from the surrounding** environment. The patient presents with a feeling of unreality such as the world around them is unreal, he is not real; his soul is outside his body (out-of-body experience), etc. Many feel like the events are happening as if in a dream or a movie with him and others playing already-scripted roles. This **'as if' quality** is a characteristic feature of DPDR. DPDR generally **follows a severe traumatic event** such as the loss of a job, an accident or torture, or the consumption of **cannabis and psychedelics**.

Dissociative Disorders of Identity

1. **A dissociative trance** is a state of distorted identity, perception, and behavior lasting for hours and the person has no memory of the altered state after its resolution. The patient may wander, performs abnormal activities, or may show violent behavior such as homicide without having any memory of the event after its resolution. A trance state may be dangerous to the person himself or others and the person may not be liable for any of his activities during the trance state. Dissociative trance is a culture-bound syndrome and presents differently in different cultures (such as *amok* in Malaysia, ***latah*** in Indonesia and other Southeast Asian countries, ***pibloktoq*** among Eskimos, and ***ataque-de-nervios*** in Hispanic America). In the Indian subcontinent, it takes the shape of **possession syndrome**.
2. **Dissociative possession** presents with a sudden change in identity and the person assuming the identity of a **deity, a religious figure** (goddess *Kali* or *Durga*), or a spirit, showing behaviors about the assumed identity, talking in their tone and demanding to be worshipped and to be consoled with animal sacrifice. The episode is short-lived and the person reverts to his original identity after some time. It is considered a **culture-bound syndrome** and is predominantly found in societies with strong cultural and religious beliefs. The victims are generally females from low socioeconomic backgrounds and those undergoing chronic stress or identity crisis in society.
3. **Dissociative identity disorder (DID):** It is commonly known as **multiple personality disorder**. DID is one of the most interesting, albeit controversial, psychiatric conditions thanks to its frequent portrayal in movies and cinemas often in an overdramatic manner. It is a very rare psychiatric condition in which the person often has **two or more different personalities** each with a distinct memory, attitude, and behavior. Each of these personalities is unaware of the existence of the others. Personality swapping generally occurs when the person is exposed to extreme stress. Persons with DID frequently have had problematic childhood with a history of sexual or physical abuse. Extreme stress and anxiety at the time of exposure to these events lead to the splitting of the personal identity and ego into two or more distinct forms to cope with the stress.

CONVERSION DISORDERS OR FUNCTIONAL NEUROLOGICAL SYMPTOM DISORDERS

Introduction

Under dissociative disorder, we learned that **dissociation** involves the separation of **psychological functions** from the conscious apparatus. Similarly, there are few physical functions under our conscious control such as voluntary motor function and sensory functions. When one of these **physical functions** gets separated from the conscious apparatus following a stressful incident then the presentation mimics some serious neurological conditions such as paralysis, blindness, or seizure. It seems as if the **libidinal energy** associated with the stress is converted into symptoms of some neurological conditions, hence the term **conversion** is applied for these presentations. The underlying mechanism for both dissociation and conversion are the same and many authorities consider them as different presentations of the same illness. A case of conversion disorder may present as one of the following illnesses.

1. Psychogenic Loss of Motor Functions

In this category, the patient presents with a loss of control over voluntary motor movements. Complete or partial loss of limb movement (**paraplegia and paraparesis respectively**), and loss of movements of one side of the body (**hemiplegia)** are common. The presentation is in the form of a patient's idea of the disease and frequently it is found that a family member or close relative is suffering from a similar medical illness (from where they got the idea of the illness albeit unconsciously). Detailed neurological examination and necessary laboratory investigations are mandatory to rule out any possible organic cause for the illness.

Other presentations in this category are gait disturbance of psychogenic origin (***astasia abasia***), psychogenic tremor, and psychogenic loss of speech **(psychogenic aphasia)**.

2. Psychogenic Loss of Sensations

Psychogenic **blindness is** the most common presentation in this category. The patient complains of an inability to visually recognize objects shown to him and also cannot recognize his family members. Interestingly, the patient even cannot recognize his family members by their voices (the patient is psychologically blind!). However, the patient's day-to-day activities like finding the way to the bathroom, avoiding obstacles in the path, etc remain undisturbed. The person also shows little concern about the loss of vision or other sensations (***la belle indifference***). Few patients also present with **psychogenic anesthesia** (loss of bodily sensations). **Psychogenic deafness** (hearing loss) and **psychogenic anosmia** (loss of sense of smell) are rare presentations.

3. Psychogenic Seizure

Psychogenic seizure is also known by other names like **pseudoseizure or pseudo-convulsion**. It presents as episodes of the **apparent loss of consciousness** and abnormal movements of hands and legs which are confused with the presentation of a seizure episode. Each episode lasts for 5–10 minutes but sometimes can even last for hours. Pseudo-seizure is differentiated clinically from true seizures by probing for **stigmata of true seizure** like the presence of aura, tongue bite, injury due to fall, urinary or fecal incontinence, post episodic confusion, etc all of which are conspicuously absent in cases of pseudoseizure. In case of any confusion, EEG can help in differentiation.

4. Psychogenic Stupor

The patient presents with an **apparent loss of consciousness** with poor response to external stimuli. The patient often **resists the forceful opening of eyes** by the examiner. Supraorbital or sternal pain stimulus can awaken the patient from an apparent stupor. Vital examination findings like heart rate, blood pressure, and plantar reflexes are found to be normal. However, in all cases of suspected conversion stupors, possible medical conditions should be ruled out by careful examination, blood investigation, and brain imaging studies, if deemed necessary.

Table 12.1: Comparison between dissociative and conversion disorder		
Disorder	***Dissociative disorder***	***Conversion disorder***
Definition	Separation of a psychological function from the consciousness	Conversion of psychic anxiety into physical symptoms
Defense mechanism used	Dissociation	Conversion
Functions involved	Psychological functions such as memory, identity, and awareness	Physical functions such as motor function, sensory functions, etc.
La belle indifference	Present	Present
Antecedent stressor	Present	Present
Treatment	Psychoanalytic psychotherapy, family therapy (cutting down on secondary gain)	Psychoanalytic psychotherapy, family therapy (cutting down on secondary gain)

Diagnosis

Diagnosis is done clinically by ruling out any medical cause for the presentation. Medical investigations are indicated whenever there is any confusion.

La belle indifference is the lack of concern by the patient with dissociative and conversion disorders for her illness. Even if the presentation indicates a serious underlying medical illness, the patient shows little or no concern regarding his/her illness.

Dissociative and conversion disorders are induced by the ego unconsciously for primary or secondary gain in stressful situations (Table 12.1). **The primary gain** is the care the patient gets from family members and other caregivers by inducing a seemingly severe medical condition albeit unconsciously. **Secondary gain** is the exemption of the patient from duties, personal obligations, and responsibilities because of the illness. However, this occurs without any conscious effort on the part of the patient which differentiates it from factitious disorder and malingering. In **factitious disorder,** a physical or mental illness is consciously and deliberately induced for **primary gain** (to get care and attention) while in **malingering** an illness is deliberately feigned for **secondary gain** (to avoid trial or work).

Etiology

Stress is considered the primary factor provoking dissociation and conversion. The **Ego** uses the defense **mechanism of dissociation** or conversion to cope with severe anxiety or stress. Childhood history of sexual or physical abuse or ongoing familial or interpersonal conflicts is frequently found in these disorders.

Biology of Dissociation

(Ketamine is a general anesthetic agent also known as **dissociative anesthesia**. It can induce a state similar to **dissociative trance** with poor response to external stimuli, lack of sensation, and loss of the memory of the event. Ketamine is an **NMDA antagonist that acts** by inhibiting NMDA receptors in the GABAergic interneurons in the cerebral cortex leading to **excessive cortical activation** which induces a trance-like state.)

Studies have suggested that **excessive cortical activation** is the underlying mechanism for dissociation in dissociative disorders. As we know that the basic function of the cerebral cortex is to inhibit the subcortical structures, hence excessive cortical activation can lead to **loss of information sharing** between the cortex and subcortical structures like the thalamus. This loss of information exchange can result in a lack of perception of sensation, loss of voluntary motor functions, and memory formation presenting with symptoms of dissociative or conversion disorders.

Suggested Investigations

Dissociative and conversion disorders are diagnoses of exclusion and laboratory investigations and imaging studies are often indicated to rule out any organic cause. Suggested investigations vary from case to case and depend upon clinical presentation.

1. Complete blood count as a routine test
2. Serum electrolyte levels to rule out electrolyte imbalance in cases presenting with paralysis (hypokalemia often presents with recurrent paralysis)
3. EEG to differentiate true seizure from pseudoseizure
4. Imaging studies (MRI and CT scanning) in cases presenting with amnesia, paralysis, and sensory disturbances.

Treatment

Psychotherapy is the primary therapeutic approach for a case of dissociative and conversion disorders. **Psychoanalytic psychotherapy** aims at resolving unconscious conflict and alleviating anxiety. **Cognitive behavioral therapies** also focus on altering maladaptive thinking patterns in the case of dissociative and conversion disorders. **Family therapy** is directed at **cutting down the secondary gain** and regulation of **expressed emotion** which is responsible for the recurrence of dissociative episodes.

SOMATIC SYMPTOM DISORDER

Somatic symptom disorder presents with **bodily symptoms** (somatic symptoms) which cannot be explained by any general medical condition. These symptoms are associated with **excessive worry, anxiety, and/or preoccupation** and cause significant impairment in the socio-occupational functioning of the individual. In the current edition of DSM (DSM-5), somatoform disorder, pain disorders, somatization disorder, and undifferentiated somatoform disorders are included under the umbrella term **'somatic symptom disorder'**. DSM-5 also states that the person may or may not be having some underlying medical condition, but that cannot explain the symptoms themselves or the amount of suffering (due to the severity of symptoms or the preoccupation and worry) associated with it.

Clinical Presentation

Somatic symptom disorder presents with bodily symptoms which **suggest an underlying serious general medical condition**. These symptoms are always associated with **excessive worry, anxiety, or preoccupation**. However, the patient generally has none or even if they have any general medical condition, that cannot explain the severity of symptoms or the amount of worry or preoccupation associated with it.

Somatic symptoms are complained by these patients concerning the following systems.

1. **Pain symptoms** such as pain over multiple parts of the body, headache, low back pain, joint pains, etc.
2. **Neurological symptoms** such as tingling, numbness, paraesthesia, burning or hot sensations, etc.

3. **Gastrointestinal symptoms** such as poor appetite, the sensation of fullness of the stomach, frequent diarrhea or constipation, dyspepsia, etc.
4. **Sexual symptoms** like white discharge, burning micturition, pain during menstruation, etc. in females and erectile dysfunction, premature ejaculation, and decreased libido in males.

Onset is generally after the age of 30 years and females are more prone to develop somatic symptom disorder than males. It generally follows a stressful event; however, many patients generally deny having any stress. This condition is usually associated with other psychological symptoms like anxiety, depression, and sleep disturbance.

Etiology

The exact cause of somatic symptom disorder is not known. History of trauma during childhood such as abuse (sexual or physical), broken family, problematic parenting, or parental relationship put a person at the highest risk of developing somatic symptom disorder in the future. Histrionic and antisocial personality disorders are associated with increased risk of somatic symptom disorders. Family studies and twin studies have revealed genetic risk to some extent and heritability is 7–30 percent. Ongoing stress is by far the most important factor contributing to the development of this condition.

Pathophysiology

Patients with somatic symptom disorder generally have a **heightened perception of somatic sensa**tions. Heightened perception of somatic sensations may be due to **abnormal gating of sensory stimuli** in the sensory pathway. This might be due to decreased levels of monoamine neurotransmitters such as **serotonin and norepinephrine** or endogenous morphine (endorphin, enkephalin, and dynorphin). Decreased levels of noradrenaline are responsible for somatic symptoms while serotonin is responsible for worry and preoccupation associated with it. The role of endogenous morphine is poorly supported by studies.

Diagnosis

DSM-5 requires the presence of somatic symptoms associated with excessive worry, anxiety, or preoccupation for a **period of 6 months** or more for a diagnosis. These symptoms must cause significant impairment in the socio-occupational functioning of the individual. The patient may or may not have an underlying general medical condition, but that does not explain the severity of symptoms or the amount of worry and preoccupation associated with it. In DSM-5 earlier diagnoses such as somatization disorder, pain disorder, and undifferentiated somatoform disorder are merged under this condition.

Comorbidity

Depression is most commonly associated with somatic symptom disorder and many patients also complain of prominent **anxiety symptoms**. Other psychosomatic disorders like irritable bowel syndrome, fibromyalgia, and tension-type headache may be comorbidly associated with this condition.

Differential Diagnosis

The somatoform disorder must be differentiated from the following illnesses

1. Conversion and dissociative disorders
2. Fibromyalgia
3. Irritable bowel syndrome
4. Connective tissue disorders

Treatment

The management approach to somatic symptom disorder consists of psychotherapy, pharmacotherapy, or a combination of both. Pharmacotherapy combined with psychotherapy yields the best results as compared to individual treatment approaches.

1. Pharmacotherapy

Medications which increase serotonin and norepinephrine levels in the CNS are effective in somatic symptom disorder. **Tricyclic antidepressants** such as amitriptyline, nortriptyline, and dosulepin are first-line medications. However, these medications are associated with troublesome anticholinergic and antihistamine side effects. Newer drugs like **SNRIs** (venlafaxine, desvenlafaxine, and duloxetine) yield a good response with fewer side effects. Add-on therapy with pregabalin or memantine improves response to first-line medications and **pregabalin** also improves sleep and anxiety symptoms.

2. Psychotherapy

Psychodynamic psychotherapy aims at resolving subconscious conflicts and was employed in earlier days. However, in recent times **CBT** has replaced psychoanalytic psychotherapy as the standard psychotherapeutic approach. CBT aims at correcting the abnormal thoughts and perceptions associated with bodily sensations. The therapist helps the patient develop coping skills to cope with stress in day-to-day life and manage anxiety, worry, and preoccupations. CBT is highly effective in somatic symptom disorder, but it yields the best results when combined with medications.

Conditions for specialist referral in cases of dissociative, conversion, and somatic symptom disorders are as follows:

1. When there is doubt regarding the diagnosis of pseudoseizure and a true seizure cannot be ruled out.
2. A patient presenting with repeated episodes of dissociation or conversion.
3. Chronic cases of conversion disorders, especially those with motor symptoms such as paralysis and paraparesis.
4. Somatic symptom disorders with secondary depression.
5. Cases not responding to initial treatment.
6. Cases requiring psychotherapy and counseling.

SUMMARY

1. Some psychological functions such as memory, awareness of self and surroundings, and self-identify, and a few physical functions such as perception and voluntary motor activities are under the conscious control of the mind.
2. Dissociative disorders present with the separation of any of the conscious psychological functions from the rest of the consciousness. Consequently, the dissociative disorder presents with dissociative amnesia, depersonalization-derealisation disorder or DPDR, and dissociative disorders of identity.

3. Conversion disorders present with the conversion of anxiety associated with distress to some physical illness involving perception or motor activity. The presentation can vary from psychological blindness to psychological loss of motor functions leading to paralysis.
4. Psychogenic epilepsy and hyperventilation syndrome are complex conversion disorders presenting with a confluence of symptoms.
5. Both conversion and dissociation are defense mechanisms employed by the ego to deal with anxiety associated with some stressful life events. Both these disorders involve primary, secondary, and tertiary gains and are characterized by la belle indifference which means a lack of concern by the patient for his/her illness.
6. Both dissociative and conversion disorders are treated by psychotherapy such as psychoanalytic psychotherapy and CBT.
7. Somatic symptom disorder presents with widespread somatic symptoms including pain symptoms, gastrointestinal symptoms, and sexual and neurological symptoms.
8. Treatment of somatic symptom disorders involves both psychotherapy and pharmacotherapy. TCAs and SNRIs are frequently prescribed to deal with somatic symptoms.

BIBLIOGRAPHY

1. World Health Organization. The ICD-10 classification of mental and behavioral disorders: Clinical descriptions and diagnostic guidelines. Geneva: World Health Organization, 1992.
2. Gillig PM. Dissociative identity disorder: a controversial diagnosis. Psychiatry (Edgmont (Pa.: Township)), 2009;6(3):24–9.
3. Angelica Staniloiu, Hans J. Markowitsch. Dissociative Amnesia – A Challenge to Therapy. International Journal of Psychotherapy Practice and Research, 2018;1(2):34–47.
4. Sadock and Pedro Ruiz. Kaplan and amp; Sadock. Synopsis of Psychiatry: Behavioral Sciences/ clinical Psychiatry. Eleventh edition. Philadelphia: Wolters Kluwer, 2015.
5. Ali S, Jabeen S, Pate RJ, Shahid M, Chinala S, Nathani M, and amp; Shah R. Conversion Disorder-Mind versus Body: A Review. Innovations in clinical neuroscience, 2015;12(5-6):27–33.
6. Souza RS, Hooten WM. Somatic Syndrome Disorders. [Updated 2022 May 2]. In: StatPearls [Internet]. Treasure Island (FL): StatPearls Publishing; 2022 Jan.

Chapter 13

Personality Disorders

Competency achievement: Students should be able to
1. **PS2.4** Describe the principles of personality development and motivation
2. **PS11.1** Enumerate and describe the magnitude and etiology of personality disorders
3. **PS11.2** Enumerate, elicit, describe, and document clinical features in patients with personality disorders
4. **PS11.3** Enumerate and describe the indications and interpret laboratory and other tests used in personality disorders
5. **PS11.4** Describe the treatment of personality disorders including behavioral, psychosocial, and pharmacologic therapy
6. **PS11.5** Demonstrate family education in a patient with personality disorders in a simulated environment
7. **PS11.6** Enumerate and describe the pharmacologic basis and side effects of drugs used in the treatment of personality disorders
8. **PS11.7** Enumerate the appropriate conditions for specialist referral in cases of personality disorders

PRINCIPLES OF PERSONALITY DEVELOPMENT

INTRODUCTION

Personality is the enduring and pervasive **pattern of thinking, emotion, and behavior** a person shows while interacting with his surrounding. There are two important defining features associated with personality; the term **enduring** signifies a temporal component that refers to the fact that these thought, emotion, and behavioral patterns are long-lasting and present throughout life after their consolidation in the late teenage period. The other term is **pervasive** which indicates that these patterns are expressed in all contexts of life (social, occupational, and interpersonal context).

THEORIES OF PERSONALITY

Some theories of personality try to evaluate various aspects of personality and are known as **descriptive theories** while others try to explain the basis of their expression and are known as **explanatory theories** (Fig. 13.1). Descriptive personality theories such as **type and trait theories** solely emphasize the nature and characteristics of personality while explanatory theories such as **psychodynamic, behavioral and humanistic theories** try to explain why a person behaves in the way as defined by his personality.

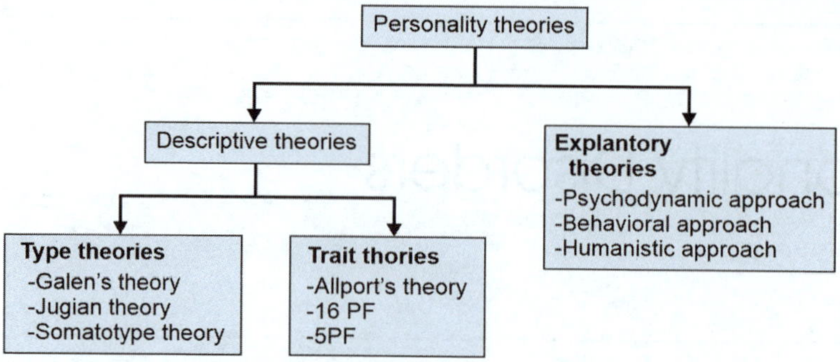

Fig. 13.1: Theories of personality

DESCRIPTIVE THEORIES OF PERSONALITY

TYPE THEORIES

Type theories try to **put individuals in various groups or categories** with each group or category defined by certain characteristic features. The type approach is the earliest in this field and dates back to the early Christian era. One of the major disadvantages of this type of approach is that it does not consider personality as unique by putting individuals into groups. Some of the famous type theories are mentioned below.

Galen's Type Theory

Galen, a Greek philosopher, tried to categorize individuals into **4 groups based on the 4 vital body fluids** known as humor**: blood, black bile, yellow bile, and phlegm**. He suggested that the thought, emotions, and behavior of an individual are determined by the relative amounts of this humor in the body and consequently determine the personality of the individual. He described 4 different personality types as follows:

1. **Sanguine or blood-like:** These individuals are warm, jovial, and optimistic. They are often considered the 'life of the party' by others.
2. **Melancholic:** These individuals are cold, sad, and pessimistic and yet are thoughtful and artistic. This group is diagonally opposite to the sanguine type.
3. **Phlegmatic:** They are flexible, relaxed, and easygoing. They are often considered likable and lovable individuals by others.
4. **Choleric:** These individuals are irritable, impulsive, egoistic, and determined. This type is opposite to the phlegmatic type.

This theory of humorism was debunked with the advent of the germ theory of diseases which suggests that human diseases are caused by microorganisms rather than some vital body fluid imbalance. Therefore, any role of vital body fluids or humor in determining human personality was questioned.

Sheldon's Somatotype Theory

In the early 1940s, Sheldon typified individuals based on the **characteristics of body features** into the following 4 types.

1. **The ectomorphs:** Bodies of these individuals are mostly derived from ectoderm. Hence, they are **skinny and lanky with big brains**. These individuals are intelligent and artistic but at the same time are anxious and prone to develop schizophrenia and neurotic illnesses.

2. **The mesomorphs:** These individuals are muscular with a **broad upper body structure** (muscles and bones are derived from mesoderm). These individuals are aggressive and competitive and tend to be impulsive and messy.
3. **The endomorphs:** They have a **pear-shaped body with central obesity** and short hands and legs. They have big stomachs and big hearts, hence are warm, relaxed, jovial, and loveable. These individuals are prone to develop mood disorders such as depression and BPAD.

Jungian Type Theory

Carl Gustav Jung was a colleague of Freud and worked with him in the initial part of his career. Jung first categorized individuals into **extroverts and introverts** based on how they energize themselves. Extroverts energize themselves by going out and mixing with people while introverts energize themselves by withdrawing and spending time alone. Later, he further categorized both extroverts and introverts based on how they gather information into **sensing and intuitive types**. Sensing individuals gather information from outside by using their senses (sense organs) while intuitive persons gather information by looking into their inner world and listening to their intuition. These types are further divided into **thinking and feeling types** depending upon how they make decisions: thinking individuals listen to their minds while feeling individuals listen to their hearts. Therefore, according to Jungian type theory, **a total of 8 personalities are possible**.

Later, **Katharine Cook Briggs and her daughter Isabel Brigg Myers** introduced another dichotomous function in the Jungian type based on how a person executes his functions: **judging or perceiving function.** Judging individuals are highly organized, plan ahead and stick to their plan throughout the course of action. On the other hand, perceiving individuals are more flexible and open to changes from time to time during the execution of their works. To conclude, by combining these 2 dichotomous functions with 8 Jungian types, it is possible to build **16 personality types** as indicated in the **Myers–Briggs type indicator** (a personality test based on this theory).

Personality Type A and Type B

This classification was proposed by two cardiologists **Friedman and Roseman** based on a person's ability to **handle stress** and his proneness to develop **cardiovascular conditions** such as hypertension and myocardial infarction.

1. Individuals with **type A personalities** are competitive, assertive, and dominant. They seem to be always in a hurry and are restless and often get irritated and have a difficult time relaxing. They are more prone to develop cardiovascular illnesses.
2. On the contrary, individuals with **type B personalities** are cool, calm, and easygoing. They are flexible and often get a sense of completion. They are less prone to develop cardiovascular illnesses.

TRAIT THEORIES

Trait theories emphasize **various aspects or facets of the personality of an individual** rather than grouping them into types. These facets or aspects of personality are **known as traits**. The trait approach is more scientific and practical than the group approach as it gives importance to the individuality and uniqueness of the personality of a person. Famous trait theories are mentioned below.

Allport's Trait Theory

Gordon Allport was the first to put forward a comprehensive trait theory in 1927. He collected all the words which describe the personality of a person and divided them into three important categories of traits.

1. **Cardinal traits** are those traits that describe a person wholly. Phrases such as ***'A Gandhian'*** or ***'Hitler-like'***, etc. describe the total aspects of the personality of an individual and are considered cardinal traits by Allport. Cardinal traits are rare and not seen in the majority of persons.
2. **Central traits** are traits that describe a major part of an individual's personality. Such traits as 'warm' or 'irritable' or 'helping', etc. describe the major aspect of a person's personality and are considered central traits by Allport.
3. **Secondary traits** describe discrete aspects of personality and different secondary traits are expressed while dealing with different situations. For example, someone's likes and dislikes about various food, clothing, etc. represent secondary traits. Secondary traits must be included to get a complete picture of a person's personality.

(One of the major disadvantages of Allport's trait theory is the exhaustive list of secondary traits. Some secondary traits are in fact different expressions of a single dimension. For example, secondary traits such as 'love to go out', 'like to talk', 'like to make friends', 'like to party', etc. are different expressions of a single personality dimension known as extraversion.)

Dimensional Approach

Raymond Cattel was the first to apply a statistical model known as **factor analysis**, to group various similar traits into a few broad dimensions and put forward the first-dimensional approach known as the **16 personality factor or 16PF**.

Later, **Paul Costa and Robert McCrae** further narrowed down the personality traits into **5 broad dimensions** and put forward their famous **5-factor personality model (5PF in short)**. Currently, 5PF is the most widely accepted and practical personality model, and its principles are widely used in the assessment of personality. Each dimension in the 5PF model is a spectrum that runs from the higher extreme to the lower extreme and a person can fall anywhere in between. These traits are **openness to experience, conscientiousness, extraversion, agreeableness, and neuroticism,** and are described below. 5PF is also known as the **OCEAN model** (taking initials of every dimension as shown in Fig. 13.2).

1. **Openness to experience** signifies how eager a person is in exploring new places and things. Those at the higher end are extremely curious and take interest in a wide variety of topics while those at the lower end are cautious and conventional.
2. **Conscientiousness** refers to the work ethic of a person. Those at the higher end in this dimension are highly organized and work hard while those at the bottom end are messy and impulsive.
3. **Extraversion** is the dimension that signifies a person's involvement with the external world. Those at the higher end are outgoing and highly social while those at the bottom end are withdrawn and homebound.
4. **Agreeableness** signifies a person's regard for the opinion of others. Those at the higher end are empathetic, considerate, and give importance to other people's opinions while those at the lower end are egoistic, and critical and give value to their opinions and needs only.

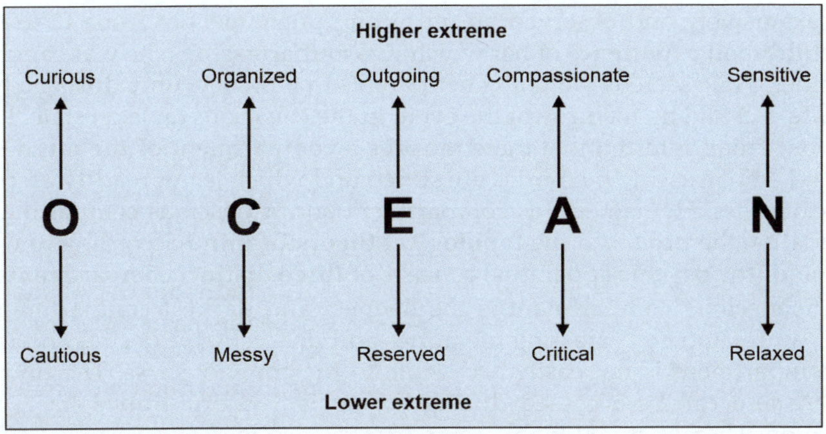

Fig. 13.2: Personality dimensions in 5PF (OCEAN) personality model. O: Openness to experience; C: Conscientiousness; E: Extraversion; A: Agreeableness; N: Neurotism

5. **Neuroticism** is the dimension that refers to the emotional regulation capability of an individual in a reverse pattern. Individuals at the higher end are highly emotional and sensitive and have poor emotional regulation, often getting irritable and depressed. Those at the lower end are calm and relaxed and do not easily get emotional at the time of distress.

EXPLANATORY THEORIES OF PERSONALITY

These theories are explanatory in nature. They delve into the developmental aspect and try to explain the basis of personality expression. Famous explanatory models are described below.

PSYCHODYNAMIC THEORY OF PERSONALITY

The psychodynamic theory of personality is based on **Freud's principles of psychoanalysis** which are described in detail in this topic.

What is Psychoanalysis?

Psychoanalysis is the brainchild of **Sigmund Freud**. He developed this method as a modality of treatment for neurotic disorders such as hysterical neurosis. Psychoanalysis is based on such theoretical foundations as the **structure of the mind** (conscious, subconscious, and unconscious), **ego psychology** (id, ego, and superego), **object relations theory**, **free association,** and **hypnosis**. Although these concepts are interesting, they are still difficult to understand.

Life of Sigmund Freud

Freud was born in **Moravia, Freiburg, a small** town in the former **Austrian Empire** (now in the **Czech Republic**) in 1856 in a Jewish family. He was trained as **a neurologist** and used to practice in **Vienna** but after the Nazi takeover of Austria, he fled to the UK and died in 1939 in exile. While still in **Vienna** his mentor **Josef Breuer** assigned him an interesting case famously known as **'the case of Anna O'**.

'Anna O' is the pseudonym given by Breuer to his patient named **Bertha Pappenheim**. She was suffering from **hysteria** as the disease was called in those days. Freud studied the case extensively and observed an intriguing phenomenon: Anna O used to tell about a **childhood experience** of her which was **embarrassing** (she was caught by her elder brother while secretly watching her parents in intimacy) only during a **hypnotic trance state,** but had no memory of the event in the conscious (awake) state. From this observation, Freud inferred that there must be a **compartment of the mind** in which painful and embarrassing memories are stored and which is **not readily accessible** to the consciousness. He named this compartment an unconscious **compartment**. With this foundation, he proposed the **topological theory of mind** according to which the human mind (the psychic apparatus) consists of **three distinct compartments**.

1. **The unconscious compartment** is the **deepest and darkest compartment** which stores painful and embarrassing memories and unacceptable desires and impulses. This compartment is not easily accessible to the consciousness. The unconscious compartment can be accessed during hypnosis, hysteric trance state, and free association. Themes stored in this compartment also **feed our dreams**.
2. The **preconscious compartment** is the compartment lying in between the unconscious and conscious compartment. In this compartment are stored such memories which are not readily accessible but **can be retrieved by giving subtle clues,** e.g. we might not always be aware of the fact that Columbus discovered America but if a question is presented then this information is readily retrieved.
3. The **conscious compartment** is part of the mental psyche which makes us aware of the **ongoing events** occurring at present. It is also part of the mental psyche which controls all our **conscious functions** such as perception, motor activities, and self-identity.

According to Freud, these psychic compartments are tightly separated from one another without any information easily jumping from one compartment to another. This poses a fundamental problem as during the actual occurrence of the event the memory is in the conscious compartment and subsequently pushed to the unconscious compartment if it is painful and embarrassing, and subsequently stored there. Therefore, there must be **a dynamic force or process of mind** which has access to all these three compartments and actively shifts painful memories from the conscious to the unconscious compartment. Freud named this dynamic process as Ego. To resolve the origin and characteristics of the Ego, Freud came up with an ingenious theory, famously known as the **structural theory of mind**.

Structural Theory of Mind

To resolve the above-mentioned conflict, Freud introduced the concept of **the id, ego, and superego** which are components of the structural theory of mind. He proposed that it is the ego that is involved in shifting the memories of painful experiences from the conscious compartment to the unconscious compartment. Now the question is from where ego comes? Freud argued that ego comes from the id, the mental apparatus present at the time of birth. The components of the structural theory of mind are as follows (Fig. 13.3).

1. Id

When a child is born, the mental psyche (mind) is full of unconscious **basic drives** such as hunger, thirst, and aggression. The energy associated with these basic drives is known as libido. This part of the mental psyche which is full of basic drives (libido) and

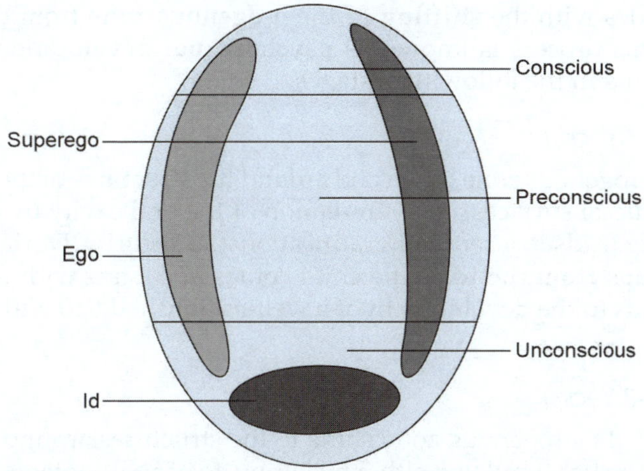

Fig. 13.3: Dynamic and static components of the psychic apparatus.

completely buried in the unconscious compartment is **known as the id**. The demands of the Id need to be fulfilled immediately; hence, it is said to function on the **pleasure principle**. When its demands are not fulfilled immediately, it expresses its displeasure in the form of aggression (crying).

2. Ego

When the Id comes in **contact with reality** as the child grows and is exposed to the environment, a part of the id comes to realize that not all its demands can be fulfilled immediately. Gradually, with this awareness, a part of the Id starts working on reality principles. This part of the id which starts **working on the reality principle** comes to be known as ego. The ego is spread across the conscious, preconscious, and unconscious compartments of the mental psyche. The primary function of the ego is to **delay or deny the demands of the id** in response to external opportunities. All the conscious functions such as **perception, motor activities, memory, and self-identity** are under the conscious control of the ego. The ego also **handles anxiety** arising from painful experiences and unacceptable desires by employing defense mechanisms known as ego defenses.

3. Superego

Superego is that part of the mental psyche which **deals with morality**. As the child gradually comes in contact with **significant others** (parents, teachers, and elders) a part of the mental psyche starts imbibing moral values and norms and comes to be known as the superego. Morality is gradually imbibed into the superego via introjections of qualities of the significant others.

Ego ideal is a special part of the superego which deals with **positive aspects of morality** such as 'it is good to help the poor', 'respect elders', etc. Superego always comes in conflict with the demands of the id and tries to suppress them, but ego comes to its rescue and strikes a balance between the demands of the id and denial of the superego.

Psychosexual Stages of Development

Development of the ego from the id and subsequent development of the superego occur in a stage-wise manner as the child grows. This stage-wise **development of psychic**

apparatus coincides with the **shifting of the erogenous zone** from one body part to another, hence this process is known as **psychosexual development**. Psychosexual development occurs in the following 5 stages:

1. Oral Stage (0–1 Years)

In this stage, the erogenous zone lies in and around the structures of the **oral cavity** such as lips, tongue, buccal surfaces, etc. Stimulation of the oral cavity by certain activities like **breastfeeding** leads to a sense of gratification and security. During this stage, **ego gradually develops from the id** as the child comes in contact with reality. Adequate breastfeeding leads to the development of a well-established ego with a good sense of security.

2. Anal Stage (1–3 Years)

In the anal phase, the erogenous zone shifts to the structures around **the anal cavity**. These structures can be stimulated either by letting go of anal contents or holding them back for a prolonged period which dilates the anal cavity. Accordingly anal stage can be divided into two substages: the **anal sadistic phase** and the **anal masochistic phase**.

The anal **sadistic phase** is the first substage in which sexual gratification is obtained by **repeatedly passing stool**. This action is considered **sadistic behavior** of the child toward the mother. In this stage, the **ego fully develops** and takes its final shape. Stress and conflict in this phase can lead to poor development of ego resulting in the development of **externalizing behaviors** such as irritable mood, temper tantrums, aggression, etc.

The anal masochistic phase follows the anal sadistic phase and in this phase sexual gratification is obtained by holding a stool for a prolonged period and this stage **coincides with toilet training**. In this phase, the child develops a sense of control over his actions for the first time in his life. **Superego starts developing** in this phase by internalizing of characteristics of significant others such as parents, teachers, and elders in the family.

3. Phallic Stage (3–6 Years)

In this stage, the erogenous zone shifts to the **underdeveloped genital organs** (penis in boys and clitoris in girls) also **known as the phallus**. Some important events in this phase occur, the most significant of which is the **development of attraction** by the child toward the parent of the opposite sex known as the **oedipus complex** in the case of boys (and the **electra complex** in the case of girls).

The boy child develops sexual attraction toward the mother but feels a sense of competition from the father. As the father is more powerful and masculine, the boy becomes apprehensive that he might castrate him; this is known as **castration anxiety**. Castration anxiety is resolved by **internalizing** the characters of the father by the child which may make him acceptable to his mother. This internalization of characteristics of the fathers leads to the **development of a mature superego**. A similar phenomenon also happens in the case of a girl child and is known as **'penis envy'**.

4. Latent Stage (6 Years to the Onset of Puberty)

This stage is not associated with any erogenous zones**. No significant psychological developmental** milestone occurs in this stage hence the name latent stage.

Table 13.1: Psychosexual stages of development					
Stages	***Timing***	***Erogenous zone***	***Major events***	***Dev. of psychic apparatus***	***Defense mechanism***
Oral	0–1 years	Oral cavity	Breastfeeding	Ego starts developing	Psychotic defenses
Anal	1–3 years	Anal cavity	Toilet training	• Ego matures • Superego starts developing	Immature defenses
Phallic	3–6 years	Underdeveloped sexual organs	Oedipus complex	Superego matures	Neurotic defenses
Latent	6 years to puberty	None	None	---	None
Genital	After puberty	Mature sexual organs	Attraction toward the opposite sex	---	Mature defenses

5. Genital Stage (after Puberty)

After puberty the erogenous zone of the body shifts to the **fully developed sex organs**. This phase is associated with the development of **sexual attraction toward a person of the opposite sex.** As the child reaches this stage, both ego and superego are fully developed with imbibitions of rational and logical **thinking** (Table 13.1).

Concept of Fixation

When a child is **exposed to any significant stressful event** during psychosexual development, **fixation may occur** in the stage in which the stress has occurred. Fixation does not mean that psychosexual development will not proceed further. The development will normally proceed through all the stages, but whenever the person is exposed to any stress in adulthood he will behave as if he is still stuck in the fixated stage. Fixation also means that the child will employ the **defense mechanisms specific to the fixated stage** to deal with day-to-day activities. Fixation also **determines the specific personality traits** the child will develop in the future. These aspects have been described elaborately under ego defenses and personality.

Ego Defenses

Ego defenses are mechanisms **employed by the ego to deal with stress in life**. Stressful experiences in life lead to the formation of painful memories which create severe anxiety if we remain aware of them. It is the function of the ego to push these painful memories to the unconscious compartment and make them stored there forever. However, these memories always attempt to intrude into the conscious compartment by breaching the barrier. To prevent the intrusion of these painful memories and unacceptable impulses into the consciousness, Ego employs a certain defense mechanism. **Repression is the primary defense mechanism** employed during childhood for this purpose. However, in adulthood, if the person is further exposed to a similar stressful event then repression fails to withhold these memories back in the unconscious making them prone to intrude into the conscious compartment which can cause anxiety and distress. In this situation, Ego employs **secondary defense mechanisms** to send these memories back into the unconscious and keep them imprisoned in it. Secondary defense mechanisms are of various types and what type of defense will be used by the Ego depends upon the **stage of fixation**.

Classification of Defense Mechanisms

George Eman Vaillant categorized ego defense mechanisms into the following 4 groups (Fig. 13.4):

1. Psychotic Defenses

When these defense mechanisms are used the person shows **psychotic behaviors such as delusions and hallucinations**. These defenses are associated with the oral stage of psychosexual development and include:

a. **Denial** is characterized by the complete denial of the facts to get rid of the anxiety associated with them.
b. **Distortion is** characterized by distorting reality for personal soothing.
c. **Projection** involves projecting the thoughts and images associated with a stressful experience into the outer world to reduce the anxiety associated with it.

2. Immature Defenses

When these defense mechanisms are used the person **behaves like an immature individual.** These are associated with the anal sadistic stage of psychosexual development and include:

a. **Acting out** involves the sudden expression of emotion via explosive behaviors without giving any forethought to it.
b. **Blocking** means complete avoidance of any contact with a stressful event or experience.
c. **In passive-aggressive behavior**, aggression is expressed in the form of disobedience, obstruction and procrastination.
d. **Splitting** means all or none attitude, the individual considers others as all good or all bad. Seen in persons with borderline personality disorder.

3. Neurotic Defenses

The use of these defenses can lead to the **development of neurotic illnesses** such as conversion disorder, somatoform disorders, OCD, etc. These are associated with anal masochistic phage and phallic phage and include

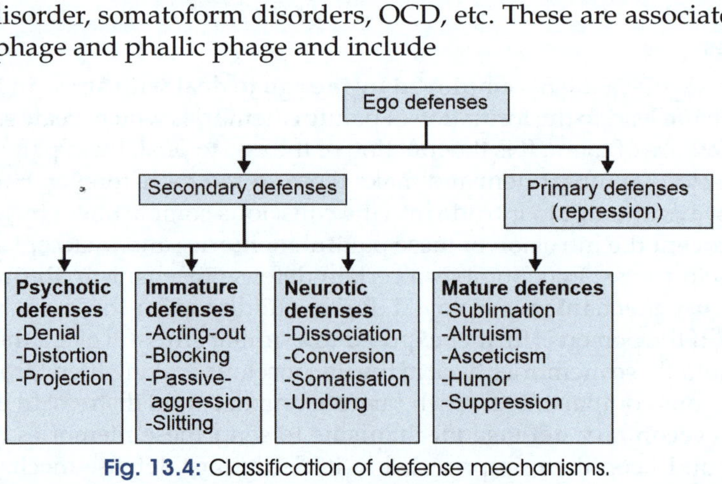

Fig. 13.4: Classification of defense mechanisms.

a. **Dissociation** involves the separation of a conscious function such as memory, identity, self-awareness, etc. from the rest of the consciousness.
b. **Conversion** means a transformation of libidinal energy associated with stress into symptoms of seemingly serious medical illnesses.
c. **Somatization** involves the conversion of libidinal energy into somatic symptoms such as pain, tingling, burning sensation, etc.
d. **Reaction formation** is the development of behaviors that are opposite of the true self. It is seen in obsessive-compulsive personality disorder.
e. **Undoing** involves engaging in behaviors that lessen the distress associated with an experience. It is also in OCD.

4. Mature Defenses

When a person reaches the genital phase of psychosexual stages of development **without any fixation, he** can employ mature defense mechanisms to deal with anxiety in day-to-day situations. The behaviors arising from employing mature defenses are socially acceptable and sometimes revered in society and make a person a **mature human being**. These include

a. **In sublimation**, libidinal energy is invested in personal achievement and the development of some artistic qualities.
b. **Asceticism** involves the renunciation of material pleasure and the pursuit of spiritualism.
c. **Altruism is when** the libidinal energy associated with some painful experience is invested for the betterment of mankind.
d. **Humor** involves dealing with anxiety-provoking situations in sarcastic and humorous ways.
e. **Anticipation** means expecting some undesirable consequences in the future and being prepared for them.
f. **Suppression** is the **only conscious ego defense mechanism** and involves conscious suppression of memories of some painful experiences.

Ego Defense Mechanism and Personality

Personality is defined as the pattern of thinking and behavior a person shows while interacting with the environment. Every person has a unique distinctive personality which depends upon the pattern of defense mechanisms used by the person to deal with the environment and which defense mechanisms the person uses depending upon the stage in which the fixation has occurred. In most cases, fixation does not occur and psychosexual development is complete in which case the person can use all the defense mechanisms in his repertoire. Individuals who have completed all the stages of psychosexual development without fixation usually show flexible behavior with a mature personality profile. Excessive use of defense mechanisms about any single stage (such as psychotic, immature, or neurotic defenses) leads to the development of personality disorders.

BEHAVIORAL THEORY

Behavioral theorists such as **BF Skinner** reject the psychodynamic principles of unconscious forces, psychosexual stages, and fixation, citing that these principles are entirely subjective in nature and cannot be verified experimentally. Rather, they proposed that behaviors that define personality are learned through experiences. This behavior learning can happen via **classical conditioning, operant conditioning, or via social learning**. Behaviorism also rejects any role of cognition (thought process) and emotion in shaping the personality of an individual. Behavioral theories are explained in detail in **Chapter 2**.

HUMANISTIC APPROACH

The humanistic approach was developed in the 1940s by **Abraham Maslow and Carl Roger**. They rejected the application of findings from animal experiments on humans. According to humanists, humans are unique in their ability to think and consciously perceive the world.

According to Maslow's hierarchy of needs (refer to Chapter 2), after meeting all the basic needs, an individual strives for the highest need known as self-actualization. He argued that each human is born good and aspires to reach his full potential known as 'self-actualization '. While striving to achieve these needs we behave in a certain way that defines our personality.

Carl Roger argued that each individual has an ideal image of himself known as the **'ideal self'**. However, our true self may or may not match this 'ideal self'. When the true self is congruent with the ideal self then the individual displays a mature well adjusted personality. It is the incongruence between the true self and the ideal self that can lead to personality disturbances.

PERSONALITY ASSESSMENT METHODS

Personality assessment methods employ certain standardized tests which are based on various theories of personality to assess the personality of an individual. Out of a multitude of personality assessment tools, **projective tests** which are based on Freudian psychoanalytic theory, and **personality inventories** based on trait theories are the most widely used.

Commonly Used Personality Tests

A. **Projective tests** (these are based on the Freudian psychodynamic principles)
   1. Rorschach inkblot test
   2. Thematic apperception test or TAT
   3. Sentence completion test

B. **Personality inventories** (these are based on the trait theories)
   1. Minnesota multiphasic personality inventories of MMPI
   2. 16 PF questionnaire
   3. Neopersonality inventory based on the 5PF model

Rorschach Inkblot Test

The Rorschach inkblot test, developed by Swiss psychiatrist **Hermann Rorschach** in the year 1921, is the most widely used personality assessment tool and is based on Freudian principles of unconscious wishes and drives. It employs ambiguous stimuli to delve into the unconscious forces that define the true personality of an individual.

The Rorschach test consists of 10 cards, each printed with **bilaterally symmetrical inkblots** which serve as **ambiguous stimuli**. Out of the 10 cards, 5 are monochromatic (gray scale), two are gray and red in color while the remaining 3 are multicolored

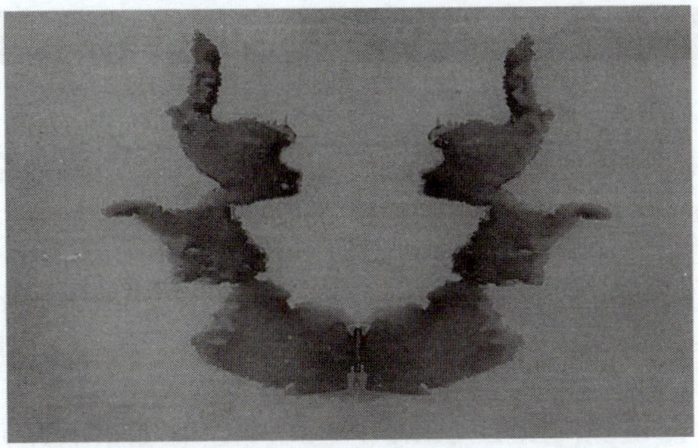

Fig. 13.5: A monochromatic Rorschach card.

(Fig. 13.5). These cards are presented to the examinee one by one and he is asked certain specific questions such as what he sees in the picture, why he thinks so, etc. Assessment is done by employing **Exner's comprehensive scoring system**, which takes into account various responses such as matching with popular responses, movement responses, color responses, and whole responses.

Thematic Apperception Test or TAT

TAT as a projective test was developed by **Murray and Morgan** in 1930 and is also based on Freudian principles of unconscious motives and drives. It employs cards printed with real-life scenarios which are **highly loaded with emotions** (Fig. 13.6). Each card is presented to the examinee and is asked to tell a story as vividly as possible which must have the following components: what led to the current situation (**the background**)? What is going on in the scene (**the body**)? What the characters are thinking and feeling (the test taker generally gives special importance to a single character known as **the hero**)? And what is going to happen next (**the outcome**)? Evaluation is done by analyzing these responses of the individual.

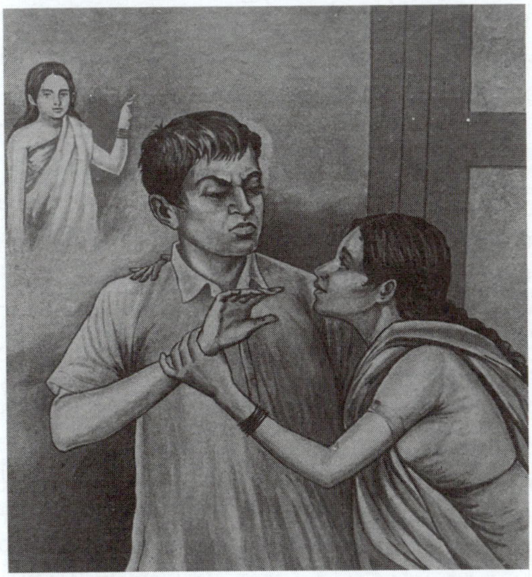

Fig. 13.6: A TAT card modified by Dr Uma Choudhury to suit Indian cultural contexts.

PERSONALITY DISORDERS

INTRODUCTION

Personality disorders are **maladaptive patterns of thinking and behavior** (maladaptive personality) that create problems in social, occupational, and interpersonal settings. However, the person lacks insight into the maladaptive pattern of his behavior and considers them as normal, and does not seek medical treatment. These behavioral and thinking patterns are also **ego-syntonic** which means that the person doesn't feel distressed regarding his behavioral and thought patterns.

Personality disorders are quite common in society and when psychiatric patients are taken into account, about 50–60% of them have underlying personality disorders which make them the most common psychiatric disorder in the clinical setting. The onset is generally in the late teens or early adulthood and remains throughout life, although generally becomes less severe after 40 years of age. Borderline personality disorder is the most important personality disorder from a clinical perspective.

ETIOLOGY

The exact etiology of personality disorders is not known. As per the psychoanalytic theory, personality disturbance stems from **fixation during psychosexual development**. Fixation at different stages manifests as separate disorders; dependent, obsessive-compulsive, and histrionic personality disorders are consequences of fixation at oral, anal, and phallic stages, respectively.

Exposure to sexual or physical abuse is another contributing factor in the development of personality disorder.

Genetic contribution toward the development of personality disorder is quite high, specifically in schizotypal, borderline personality disorder (BPD), and antisocial personality disorder. Search for candidate genes has implicated genes involved in the regulation of serotonin (5-HT), dopamine (DA), and noradrenaline (NA) neurotransmitter systems. Cultural factors also contribute to the development of personality disorders as evidenced by the different prevalences of personality disorders in different cultures.

CLASSIFICATION

The system of classification of personality disorders mentioned in ICD-10 and DSM-5 is widely used by clinicians. Although both these classification systems share most of the basic features, still there are some differences (e.g. schizotypal is grouped as a personality disorder in DSM-5 while in ICD-10 it is grouped as a category of schizophrenic illnesses). The classification system mentioned in **DSM-5**, which has categorized them into three different clusters is more comprehensive and is covered in this chapter

1. **Cluster A** is also known as a **'odd and aloof' personality disorder**. It includes paranoid, schizoid, and schizotypal personality disorders
2. **Cluster B** or **erratic, immature, or unstable personality disorders** which include histrionic, borderline, narcissistic, and antisocial personality disorders
3. **Cluster C** includes **anxious and fearful personality disorders**. Obsessive–compulsive, anxious-avoidant, and dependent personality disorders are included in this category.

CLINICAL PRESENTATION

Cluster-A Personality Disorders

These patients use psychotic defense mechanisms such as **denial, distortion, and projection** to deal with their environment. Excessive use of psychotic defenses makes them behave like psychotic persons.

1. Paranoid Personality Disorder

Pervasive and persistent **suspiciousness** with general **distrust** is the core features of paranoid personality disorder. These patients always look serious with poor emotional expression, do not trust anyone, and suspect everyone of malevolent intentions. Because of their **suspicious nature,** they frequently quarrel with others (hence known as **querulant personality**) and bear grudges against others for a long time.

2. Schizoid Personality Disorder

These individuals often remain **aloof and indifferent** with poor social interaction. They generally like their own company and do not try to establish social or personal relationships and show general aversions toward life goals. They are frequently seen sitting idly in a corner of the house with restricted facial expressions. Persons suffering from this personality disorder, although are socially inhibited, can contribute some creative and genius ideas to the society.

3. Schizotypal Personality Disorder

It is characterized by odd and **eccentric behaviors and thinking patterns**. They wear fancy clothes and tell odd and eccentric stories full of pseudophilosophical ideas. Their thinking pattern is considered illogical or implausible (**magical thinking**) for example one may claim that he can read others' minds. Even if they try to establish social and personal contacts they are generally avoided by others because of their eccentric behavior.

Cluster B Personality Disorders

Persons suffering from cluster B personality disorders use **immature defense mechanisms** such as projective identification, splitting, passive-aggressive behavior, acting out, etc. Because of this, these patients often show erratic and unpredictable behavior considered by others as immature.

1. Borderline Personality Disorder or Emotionally Unstable Personality Disorder

The main theme of this personality disorder is **the instability of emotion and interpersonal relations, impulsivity, and frequent mood swings**. Predominant presenting symptoms are mood swings, impulsivity, fear of abandonment, and self-harm behaviors. These patients suffer from a chronic inner feeling of emptiness and there is the persistent fear of real or imaginary abandonment by loved ones. There is persistent doubt about own identity, body image, and sexual orientation. These persons frequently show **self-harm behaviors** (wrist slitting, ingesting small amounts of less harmful poisons, etc) and **all/non-attitude toward others (splitting)**. In stressful situations, they might develop frank psychotic episodes or depression with active suicidal tendencies.

2. Histrionic Personality Disorder

The primary theme is being the **center of attraction** in every situation. To gain attention these patients often show **overly dramatic behavior**, wear revealing dresses, and display seductive body language. They have poor self-esteem and are highly suggestive. Their **facial expression is shallow** lacking emotional depth. These patients also frequently experience mood swings and emotional outbursts.

3. Narcissistic Personality Disorder

'Self-love' is the core feature of this personality disorder. These people love themselves so much that all their actions are meant for their **gain** only. They consider themselves superior and are in constant need of admiration. These people are preoccupied with power, success, and beauty. They appear overly charming and friendly at first interaction and often **manipulate people** for their selfish gain. They **show little empathy** toward the emotional needs of others and there is a lack of remorse for their actions.

4. Antisocial Personality Disorder

Breaking the laws and rules of society and general disregard for the rights of others is the core feature of this personality disorder. Risk-taking activities such as rash driving, gang activities, and gambling are common in ASPD. They often indulge in **criminal activities** (stealing, drug abuse, trafficking, rape, murder, etc) with multiple criminal charges against them. There is a **tendency to blame others** for their disruptive behavior and destructive actions. They also show little or **no empathy** for others and there is a **lack of remorse** or guilt feeling for their antisocial behaviors.

Cluster C Personality Disorders

Various ego defenses utilized by persons with cluster C personality disorders are somatization, reaction formation, isolation, etc.

1. Obsessive–Compulsive Personality Disorder

The persons with these personality disorders are obsessed with **cleanliness, orderliness, rules, regulations, and morality**. They are rigid and inflexible which causes significant interpersonal problems in the life of the individual. However, these behaviors **are ego-syntonic** which means these are not bothersome to the person himself but they are quite annoying for the family members and close relatives. Patients with OCPD often get irritated by other people when they interfere with their obsessive behavior. As in other personality disorders, insight into their problematic behavior is absent and they do not consider their obsessive behavior as unusual and uncalled for.

2. Anxious Avoidant Personality Disorder

Persons suffering from this personality disorder **get nervous easily in risky situations** and often avoid such situations. These persons are overly sensitive to negative evaluations by others. They generally spend most of their time in a home environment where they feel secure and avoid going out. In severe cases the person may become completely homebound avoiding going out, traveling alone, riding motorcycles, going to social situations, etc. These traits make the person's life confined and unproductive.

3. Dependent Personality Disorder

Persons with this personality disorder have low self-esteem and are dependent on family members and close relatives in taking all their life decisions. They seek help while making any kind of life decision like while taking admission to college, choosing an academic or job career, opening a bank account, etc.

Complications

The presence of personality disorders makes a person vulnerable to other major psychiatric illnesses. Schizotypal personality is considered a harbinger of **schizophrenia** and other psychotic disorders. Persons with cluster B personalities are particularly prone to develop **substance abuse disorders, depression, micropsychotic episodes, and mood disorders**. Similarly, persons with cluster C personality disorders frequently develop **somatoform disorders, anxiety disorders, and depression**. **Suicidal risk** is also significantly high in patients with personality disorders, especially in cluster B personalities.

Suggested Investigations in a Case of Personality Disorder

1. Complete blood count as a routine test
2. Thyroid function test in cases of borderline and anxious-avoidant personality disorders
3. EEG to rule out seizure disorder as long-standing seizure disorder can present with problematic personality traits
4. Brain imaging studies to rule out organic causes of personality dysfunction
5. Liver and kidney function tests before treatment with mood stabilizers

Treatment of Personality Disorder

Psychotherapy is the primary treatment approach for personality disorders. CBT or cognitive behavior therapy is the treatment of choice for personality disorders. A modified version of CBT known as Dialectical behavior therapy or DBT is specially designed for borderline personality disorder. Other psychotherapy approaches in this regard are Mentalization-based therapy (MBT) and Transference-focused psychotherapy (TFP).

These psychotherapy techniques teach the patient how to cope with stress and how to regulate emotions. There is substantial evidence in support of psychotherapy in improving mood swings, emotional regulation, self-harm behavior, and impulsive behaviors in patients with BPD.

Family Education

Family members are also educated regarding the nature of illness and the need for treatment. They should understand that the patient has a psychiatric illness and that her behaviors are not deliberate. They are also trained on how to handle mood swings, self-harm behaviors, and other impulsive behavior. Finally, they should be supportive of the patient in seeking and continuing psychiatric care.

Medications are secondary to psychotherapy and are indicated only for the treatment of comorbid conditions. Medications like **mood stabilizers, SSRIs, and antipsychotics** are prescribed for corresponding comorbid conditions. Fluoxetine improves depressive symptoms, mood swings, impulsivity, and self-harm behavior. Psychotic episodes are treated with low-dose second-generation antipsychotics such as olanzapine and risperidone.

Conditions for Referral to a Psychiatric Specialist

A patient with a personality disorder can be referred to a psychiatrist in the following situations:

1. Patients presenting with frequent self-harm behavior
2. Frequent episodes of aggression toward people or property
3. Those requiring psychotherapy
4. Patients presenting with frequent psychotic episodes
5. The emergence of secondary substance abuse behavior

SUMMARY

1. Personality is defined as the unique pattern of thinking, emotion, and behavior shown by a person while interacting with the environment.
2. Descriptive theories such as type and trait theories try to describe various aspects of personality while explanatory theories (e.g. psychodynamic, behavioral, and humanistic approaches) try to explain the development of personality.
3. Psychoanalysis is the technique of theoretical analysis of the mind and application of knowledge in the treatment of psychiatric illnesses. Sigmund Freud developed all the basic theoretical aspects of psychoanalysis such as structural and topological theories of mind, psychosexual stages of development, the concept of fixation, and defense mechanism. He also developed therapeutic aspects of psychoanalysis such as free association, catharsis, transference and countertransference, and techniques of conflict resolution.
4. Personality disorders are maladaptive patterns of thought, emotion, and behaviors that cause significant socio-occupational and interpersonal well-being of an individual.
5. DSM5 classifies personality disorders into 3 clusters: cluster A, cluster B, and cluster C. Cluster A include psychotic personality disorders such as paranoid, schizoid, and schizotypal personality disorders. Cluster B includes erratic personality disorders such as histrionic, borderline, antisocial, and narcissistic personality disorders. Cluster C includes neurotic personality disorders such as anxious-avoidant, dependent, and obsessive–compulsive personality disorders.
6. Treatment of personality disorder is mainly psychological such as CBT or a version of CBT known as DBT specifically designed for BPD. Medications are only used to treat comorbid psychiatric illnesses such as depression and psychosis.

BIBLIOGRAPHY

1. McLeod SA. Theories of personality. Simply Psychology, 2017.
2. Lim A. The big five personality traits. Simply Psychology. 2020, June 15.
3. McLeod SA. What are the most interesting ideas of Sigmund Freud? Simply Psychology, 2018, April 05.
4. George E. Vaillant. Ego Mechanisms of Defense and Personality Psychopathology. Journal of Abnormal Psychology, 1994. Vol. 103, No. 1.44–50.
5. Fariba KA, Gupta V, Kass E. Personality Disorder. [Updated 2022 Apr 21]. In: StatPearls [Internet]. Treasure Island (FL): StatPearls Publishing; 2022 Jan.
6. American Psychiatric Association. Diagnostic and statistical manual of mental disorders, 2013. (5th ed.)
7. Chapman J, Jamil RT, Fleisher C. Borderline Personality Disorder. [Updated 2022 May 2]. In: StatPearls [Internet]. Treasure Island (FL): StatPearls Publishing; 2022 Jan.

Chapter 14

Psychosomatic Disorders

Competency achievement: Students should be able to
1. **PS12.1** Enumerate and describe the magnitude and etiology of psychosomatic disorders
2. **PS12.2** Enumerate, elicit, describe, and document clinical features in patients with psychosomatic disorders
3. **PS12.3** Enumerate and describe the indications and interpret laboratory and other tests of psychosomatic disorders
4. **PS12.4** Describe the treatment of psychosomatic disorders including behavioral, psychosocial, and pharmacologic therapy
5. **PS12.5** Demonstrate family education in a patient with psychosomatic disorders in a simulated environment
6. **PS12.6** Enumerate and describe the pharmacologic basis and side effects of drugs used in psychosomatic disorders
7. **PS12.7** Enumerate the appropriate conditions for specialist referral in psychosomatic disorders

INTRODUCTION

The term psychosomatic has been derived from two words, **psyche (mind) and soma (body)**. Psychosomatic illnesses are illnesses presenting with **bodily (somatic symptoms)** suggestive of an underlying medical illness; however, **no pathology** is found which can explain these symptoms. Earlier, it was thought that mind and body are separate entities and do not affect each other (mind-body dichotomy). Gradually, it was realized that mind and body are complementary to each other and abnormality in one can affect the other. Psychosomatic illnesses are also known as **functional illnesses** as there is **no organic pathology** found to explain the symptoms. Following are some important examples of psychosomatic disorders described in this topic.

1. Irritable bowel syndrome
2. Fibromyalgia
3. Primary headache disorders and
4. Psychocutaneous disorders such as excoriation disorder, trichotillomania, psychogenic pruritus, etc.

Other common psychosomatic illnesses such as **stomach ulcers, asthma, hypertension, heart diseases, eczema, and psoriasis** are not covered here as they fall under the purview of other branches of medicine.

IRRITABLE BOWEL SYNDROME

Irritable bowel syndrome is a common **functional gastrointestinal disorder** presenting intermittent abdominal pain and change in bowel habits. Being a Psychosomatics disorder, the symptom severity in IBS is substantially affected by stress and other psychiatric conditions such as anxiety, depression, somatization, and mood disorders. With onset at different age groups, IBS is 2–3 times more common in females than males and follows a waxing and waning course over time.

Clinical Presentation

Intermittent non-localized abdominal pain is the characteristic feature of IBS. Along with pain, the patient may complain of **vague abdominal discomfort, bloating sensation, abdominal distension, indigestion,** etc. Pain generally gets relieved with the passage of stool. The second most important feature of IBS is the recent onset **change in frequency or form of stool**. Many patients with IBD also complain of psychiatric symptoms such as **anxiety, low mood,** and **somatic symptoms.**

Depending upon the predominant bowel habit IBS can be classified into:

1. IBS-C (constipation)
2. IBS-D (diarrhea)
3. IBS-M (mixed)
4. IBS-U (unspecified)

Diagnosis

Rome's IV criteria for IBS require the following symptoms to be present for at least 3 days a month for a period of at least 3 months

1. **Abdominal pain** which improves after defecation
2. Pain is accompanied by a **change in the form or frequency of stool**.

Etiology

The exact etiology of IBS is not known. **Genetic risk, altered food habits, viral infection,** etc are implicated. **Immune activation** in a genetically predisposed individual by a bout of viral infection is the most correlated event that leads to the onset of symptoms in most cases of IBS.

Pathophysiology

Various pathophysiological disturbances seen in IBS are **impaired bowel motility, increased visceral sensitivity, disturbed gut-brain axis,** etc. It is believed that these disturbances are initiated by an episode of viral infection or psychosocial stress in a genetically predisposed individual. An episode of viral infection can lead to abnormal **immune activation** and subsequent disturbances in gut motility and sensitivity. Stress also leads to abnormal activation of the HPA axis and subsequent immune dysregulation.

Differential Diagnosis

The presence of low-grade fever, unexplained weight loss, anemia, or the presence of blood in the stool should cast some doubts on the diagnosis of IBS. In the presence of any of the above symptoms, investigational work-ups are necessary to differentiate it from **inflammatory bowel disease** and **colon carcinoma**. Other differential diagnoses are **somatic symptom disorders** and **fibromyalgia**.

Suggested investigations

1. Complete blood count with differential counts
2. Serum C-reactive protein (CRP) level
3. Ultrasonography of abdomen
4. Upper GI endoscopy or colonoscopy

Treatment

The most important aspect of treatments is the patient's understanding of the disease and its association with stress and anxiety. A good doctor–patient relationship is of utmost importance in the long-term management of IBS. Both pharmacological and nonpharmacological approaches are tried depending on the predominant symptoms and their severity.

1. Nonpharmacological Treatment

Regular exercise, relaxation therapy, and balancing food habits can help resolve symptoms in mild to moderate cases. Stress reduction with aerobic exercise and mindfulness meditation can help restore the disturbed gut-brain axis. In IBS-D cases consuming food containing less **FODMAP** (fermentable oligosaccharides, disaccharides, monosaccharides, and polyols) is advised to decrease the frequency of diarrhea. Foods high on FODMAP are fermented in the colon, absorbing water and causing bloating and diarrhea. In IBS-C cases, **a high-fiber diet** and consuming **adequate fluid** can mitigate mild to moderate constipation.

2. Pharmacological

Pharmacological agents are employed to manage predominant symptoms on a case-to-case basis. Pain in IBS is managed with **antispasmodic agents** like clidinium bromide and dicyclomine, constipation with mild laxatives (lactose), and diarrhea with loperamide and probiotics. Apart from symptomatic management with these drugs, low-dose TCAs (amitriptyline and dosulepin) or SSRIs help manage stress, anxiety depression, and somatic symptoms in all cases of IBS.

FIBROMYALGIA

Fibromyalgia is a **disease of CNS** presenting with widespread **musculoskeletal pain**. Pain is often accompanied by fatigue, sleep disturbance, and cognitive impairment such as forgetfulness and impaired judgment and reasoning. Other psychiatric illnesses such as anxiety and depression are often seen comorbidly with this condition. Fibromyalgia is considered to be due to **abnormal pain processing** in the CNS. A clear understanding of its clinical presentation and pathophysiology is required for proper diagnosis and treatment.

Epidemiology

The prevalence of fibromyalgia is found to be around 5–6% in the general population. Females are overwhelmingly more prone to develop fibromyalgia than males. The usual age of onset in females is between 30 and 50 years of age. However, this condition can also be seen in children and men.

Clinical Presentation

Patients with fibromyalgia complain of **pain all over the body**. They suffer from constant dull aching pain over multiple parts of the body. Pain is accompanied by **generalized weakness, easy fatigability,** and **sleep disturbance**. Many patients complain of frequent headaches, chronic low back pain, irritable bowel, and sensitivity to cold and loud noises. Symptoms of **anxiety** and **depression** are common in patients with fibromyalgia. When examined, these patients are visibly depressed and a good clinician can infer their suffering by reading their facial expressions. **Cognitive impairment** in the form of impairment in attention concentration, memory, judgment-reasoning, and the mental clouding is common. This cognitive impairment in patients of fibromyalgia is known as '**fibro-fog**'.

Diagnosis

The pain must be widespread and debilitating and should be present for a period of at least 6 months for a diagnosis of fibromyalgia. The American Rheumatological Association has prescribed the presence of tenderness over at **least 11 out of 18 tender points** over the body and both sides of the body must be involved for a diagnosis of fibromyalgia. Along with pain, sleep disturbance, fatigue, and cognitive impairment may be present and these symptoms must cause impairment in the socio-occupational functioning of the patient.

Etiology

The exact cause of fibromyalgia is not known. Both **genetic predispositions and psychological factors** play significant roles. Many patients develop the disease after a **psychological or physical trauma** or following an episode of viral infection. The clustering of cases in families and first-degree relatives signifies a **strong genetic influence**. Polymorphism in genes regulating the monoamine **system** (serotonin, noradrenaline, and dopamine) is implicated in many studies. The presence of **single nucleotide polymorphism** in the gene encoding the **5HT2A receptor** increases the risk of developing fibromyalgia by many folds. The inheritance pattern is thought to be **polygenic.**

The onset of the disease after a viral infection gave rise to the **autoimmune hypothesis**. Production of these immunoglobulins is triggered by the infection and these immunoglobulins act on the CNS leading to monoamine imbalance and symptoms of fibromyalgia.

Psychological factors also play a significant role in the development of the condition. Childhood history of **abuse, neglect, and trouble parenting** poses a significant risk. The disease often follows a significantly stressful event, which can be psychological or physical.

Pathophysiology

Patients with fibromyalgia have a hyperactive cerebral cortex and **abnormal processing of pain** by the CNS.

Hyperactivity is seen in principal pain-processing areas of the brain, especially the insular **cortex**. This is thought to be due to **increased glutamate activity** in these areas and other parts of the brain. Cortical hyperactivity leads to **a decreased threshold for pain** and other sensations. Long-standing glutamate-induced neuronal hyperactivity can lead to atrophy of the cortex leading to impairment in cognitive functions. Drugs that antagonize this hyperactivity such as pregabalin and memantine can improve pain symptoms and cognitive symptoms in fibromyalgia.

Central processing of pain involves endogenous opioids and amine neurotransmitters, especially serotonin and norepinephrine. There is poor evidence in favor of opioid system dysregulation in fibromyalgia. Many studies have implicated **serotonin and norepinephrine depletion** in fibromyalgia leading to failure of gating of pain sensation. Decreased levels of these amines also lead to sleep disturbance, fatigue, depression, and anxiety seen in these patients. This is also the basis of the effectiveness of SSRIs, SNRIs, and TCAs as treatment of fibromyalgia.

Differential Diagnosis

Fibromyalgia must be differentiated from other connective tissue disorders such as **rheumatoid arthritis, SLE, Sjogren's syndrome, myopathies,** etc. for proper management.

One of the most challenging differential diagnoses is **chronic fatigue syndrome**. Chronic fatigue syndrome also presents with widespread pain, chronic fatigability, sleep disturbance, anxiety, and depression. However, patients with chronic fatigue syndrome are more concerned with weakness and fatigue than bodily pain symptoms.

Suggested Investigations

1. Complete blood count with differential count
2. Serum CRP level
3. Other specific studies to rule out connective tissue diseases such as CCP (cyclic citrullinated peptide) level to rule out rheumatoid arthritis, anti-DNA antibodies in suspected cases of SLE, etc.

Treatment

Early diagnosis and treatment are imperative for a good response to treatment and to prevent the development of complications like depression and anxiety disorders. Medications such as **TCAs, SSRIs, and SNRIs** are the first choice in this regard. Among TCAs, **amitriptyline and dosulepin (doxepin)** have good efficacy; however, are poorly tolerated due to anticholinergic and antihistamine side effects. Newer agents such as **duloxetine and venlafaxine (SNRIs)** have good side effects profiles and efficacy similar to TCAs. These medications improve pain symptoms, fatigue, sleep, and anxiety depression; however, have little impact on cognitive impairment. **Adjunctive treatment with pregabalin or memantine** can improve the response to first-line medications and also improve cognitive deficits.

Behavioral therapy such as regular aerobic exercise, remaining active during the daytime, and maintaining sleep hygiene can improve response to medications. Cognitive behavioral therapy also improves both somatic and cognitive symptoms in these patients.

PRIMARY HEADACHE DISORDERS

Headache can be due to some brain pathology (infection, injury, toxicity, or space-occupying lesions) in which case it is known as a **secondary headache**. Certain disorders present with headache as the most prominent symptom (along with other associated symptoms) and no obvious brain pathology can be found in these disorders. These disorders are known as **primary headache disorders** and include

1. Migraine headache
2. Tension-type headache (TTH) and
3. Cluster headache

MIGRAINE HEADACHE

Migraine is a CNS disorder presenting as episodes of **headache** with other **associated symptoms.** Headache in migraine can be **unilateral** (in about 70% of cases) or **bilateral** and is **pulsatile** in nature. Headache can be moderate to severe in degree and can last for 4–72 hours. The headache increases with activity and subsides on falling asleep. Along with headache, migraine also presents with other associated symptoms such as

a. **Aura (**abnormal visual or other sensory perceptions). Migraine associated with aura is known as **classical migraine**
b. **Photophobia**
c. **Phonophobia**
d. **Nausea or vomiting** with headache subsiding after vomiting.
e. Gastric discomfort
f. Cognitive impairment

Onset is generally in late adolescence or early adulthood. Incidence is similar in both males and females. Migraine is the most common primary headache disorder in the clinical setting while TTH is the most common in the community. Migraine episodes can be triggered by stress, sleep deprivation, dehydration, alcohol intake, etc.

Neurobiology of Migraine: Cortical Spreading Depression

Migraine is a disorder of the brain occurring due to **abnormal activation** of the cortical tissue. This abnormal activation of the cortex in migraine is known as **cortical spreading depression or CSD** (activation is followed by inhibition hence the name depression). The underlying mechanisms of origin of CSD are not known but are thought to be due to a **channelopathy** or some abnormally irritable cortical tissue known as focus.

The activation starts at the focus and gradually spreads throughout the cerebral hemisphere. When it involves only one hemisphere, the pain will be unilateral and when both hemispheres are involved then the pain will be bilateral. Pain starts only when the activation reaches a pain-sensitive structure in the brain (especially a blood vessel). During the spread of CSD from the focus of a nearby blood vessel, it only activates the neural tissue which presents as an aura. When CSD reaches the blood vessel it activates the **pain-sensitive C fibers** wrapped around it, causing dull aching pain. The contraction of outer longitudinal muscles dilates the blood vessel and further irritates these C fibers and when the heart pumps, further dilatation increases the pain, which explains the pulsatile nature of the headache.

As the activation reaches the base of the brain it irritates the 5th cranial nerve and the trigeminal ganglion leading to the decreased thresholds of the 5th nerves which cause photophobia. Similarly, irritation of the 8th cranial nerve causes phonophobia, and irritation of the vagus nerve arising from the brainstem causes gastric discomfort with subsequent nausea or vomiting.

Treatment of Migraine

Acute episodes of migraine are treated **with NSAIDs** such as ibuprofen, paracetamol, or naproxen. Non-responsive cases can be controlled with **NSAIDs** combined with **caffeine or ergotamine** (vasoconstrictors). Severe episodes of migraine headache only respond to **5HT2a/2d agonists** such as **sumatriptan and rizatriptan**.

Prophylactic Treatment

Prophylactic treatment is needed when migraine episodes are too frequent or too severe, causing impairment in the socio-occupational functioning of the individual. Five first-line medications used for prophylactic treatment of migraine are:

1. **Propranolol,** a beta blocker also has nerve cell stabilization property
2. **Sodium valproate,** a broad spectrum antiepileptic
3. **Topiramate,** a sodium channel blocker
4. **Flunarizine,** a calcium channel blocker
5. **Amitriptyline** acts by modulating pain pathway in the CNS on long-term therapy

Similar to epilepsy, prophylactic therapy should be continued for a period of 2–3 years and if further migraine episodes occur on completion of 3 years of prophylactic management treatment is for life.

TENSION-TYPE HEADACHE

Tension-type headache (TTH) is a primary headache disorder presenting with bilateral **mild-to-moderate headaches** with a characteristic **tension band-like sensation**. It is the most common type of headache in the community with a female predisposition. Headache episodes are seldom associated with photophobia or phonophobia but never both and nausea or vomiting is conspicuously absent. Acute episodes are treated with NSAIDs and **amitriptyline** is used for prophylactic therapy.

CLUSTER HEADACHE

It is a primary headache disorder presenting with episodes of unilateral **very severe headache** of gunshot quality around the orbit associated with features of **sympathetic hyperactivities** such as ipsilateral lacrimation, congestion, nasal stuffiness, facial flushing, and drooping of the eyelid. Episodes of headache occur frequently for a period of a few months spanned by event-free periods of a few years. Because of this **clustering of headache episodes,** it is named as such.

Treatment of acute episodes involves **inhalation of hyperbaric oxygen (100% oxygen)** which is the only effective treatment for acute episodes. Prophylactic treatment is done with **sodium valproate or verapamil** (a calcium channel blocker) but efficacy is somewhat moderate.

PSYCHOCUTANEOUS DISORDERS

Excoriation disorder or pathological skin picking presents with self-inflicted skin lesions. Body parts most commonly involved are the extensor surfaces of the limbs, vulvar and perianal regions. On examination, lesions over these areas can be found at various stages: the weeping stage, crusting stage, and scarring stage. Excoriation disorder is classified as impulse control disorder in DSM.

Psychogenic pruritus or functional pruritus is an itching condition triggered and maintained by psychological factors. No primary skin lesion is found associated with this condition. The itching gets aggravated during stress and is generally more evident when the patient is at rest. Psychogenic pruritus is rarely diagnosed in psychiatry clinics as most patients visit the dermatology clinic. Treatment includes psychotropic medications such as amitriptyline or SSRIs and psychotherapy such as cognitive behavioral therapy

Trichotillomania (TTM) is characterized by **repetitive hair-pulling** from the scalp, eyebrows, or other hairy parts of the body causing noticeable hair loss. Because of this **noticeable hair loss** from the scalp or other parts, these patients feel embarrassed and avoid socialization which causes significant functional impairment. The vast majority of patients are female and many are suffering from low self-esteem or other psychiatric illnesses such as anxiety or OCD.

Conditions for Specialist Referral

1. Doubtful cases requiring further evaluation
2. Cases not responding to initial treatment
3. Cases requiring psychotherapy and counseling
4. Patients who have developed secondary depression
5. Patients with suicidal tendencies

SUMMARY

1. Psychosomatic illnesses present with somatic symptoms which suggest some underlying pathology, however, no organic pathology is found which can explain these symptoms. It includes irritable bowel syndrome (IBS), fibromyalgia, primary headache disorders, and psychocutaneous disorders.
2. Irritable bowel syndrome or IBS presents with intermittent vague abdominal pain and discomfort, bloating sensation, and change in frequency or form of stool. IBS is also associated with other psychiatric illnesses such as depression, anxiety, mood swings, etc.
3. The pathophysiological disturbances seen in IBS are impaired bowel motility, increased visceral sensitivity, disturbed gut-brain axis, etc. in most of these cases an episode of viral infection leads to abnormal immune activation and subsequent changes in gut motility and sensitivity.
4. Treatment involves both pharmacotherapy and psychotherapy. Regular exercise, relaxation therapy, and balancing food habits (consuming food containing less FODMAP) may be effective in sine cases. Cases not responding to behavioral modification are treated with antispasmodic agents, probiotics, and TCAs.
5. Fibromyalgia is a disease of the CNS presenting with widespread musculoskeletal pain associated with fatigue, low mood, sleep disorders, and cognitive impairment which is thought to be due to abnormal pain processing in the CNS.
6. The pharmacological treatment of fibromyalgia involves the use of serotonergic and adrenergic medications such as TCAs and SNRIs. Behavioral therapy such as physical exercise and maintenance of sleep hygiene and CBT helps in improving response to drug treatment.
7. Migraine headaches, tension-type headaches (TTH), and cluster headaches are known as primary headache disorders as no CNS pathology is found which can explain headaches in these disorders. Migraine headache which is the most common primary headache disorder in the clinical setting presents with unilateral (or bilateral), mild-moderate pulsatile headache lasting for 4-72 hours associated with photophobia, phonophobia, and nausea and vomiting.
8. TTH is the most common type of primary headache disorder in the community setting and presents with mild-moderate bilateral headache with a pressure band-like sensation. Cluster headache on the other hand is a rare type of severe headache that occurs in a cluster over some time.
9. Psychocutaneous disorders include skin-picking disorder (pathological excoriation), psychogenic pruritus, and trichotillomania.

BIBLIOGRAPHY

1. Saha L. Irritable bowel syndrome: pathogenesis, diagnosis, treatment, and evidence-based medicine. World J Gastroenterol. 2014 Jun 14;20(22):6759–73.
2. Jahan F, Nanji K, Qidwai W, Qasim R. Fibromyalgia syndrome: an overview of pathophysiology, diagnosis, and management. Oman medical journal, 2012;27(3):192–5.
3. Bhargava J, Hurley JA. Fibromyalgia. [Updated 2022 May 1]. In: StatPearls [Internet]. Treasure Island (FL): StatPearls Publishing; 2022 Jan.
4. Bahra A. Primary Headache Disorders: Focus on Migraine. Rev Pain. 2011 Dec;5(4):2–11. doi 10.1177/204946371100500402. PMID: 26525886; PMCID.
5. Misery L, Dutray S, Chastaing M, Schollhammer M, Consoli SG, Consoli SM. Psychogenic itch. Transl Psychiatry. 2018 Mar 1;8(1):52.

Chapter 15

Psychosexual and Gender Identity Disorders

Competency achievement: Students should be able to
1. **PS13.1** Enumerate and describe the magnitude and etiology of psychosexual and gender identity disorders
2. **PS13.2** Enumerate, elicit, describe, and document clinical features in patients with psychosexual and gender identity disorders
3. **PS13.3** Enumerate and describe the indications and interpret laboratory and other tests used in psychosexual and gender identity disorders
4. **PS13.4** Describe the treatment of psychosexual and gender identity disorders including behavioral, psychosocial, and pharmacologic therapy
5. **PS13.5** Demonstrate family education in a patient with psychosexual and gender identity disorders in a simulated environment
6. **PS13.6** Enumerate and describe the pharmacologic basis and side effects of drugs used in psychosexual and gender identity disorders
7. **PS13.7** Enumerate the appropriate conditions for specialist referral in psychosexual and gender identity disorders

NORMAL SEXUAL RESPONSE

The human sexual response cycle as proposed by **William H Masters and Virginia E Johnson** involves the following 4 phases.

1. **The desire phase** involves the initiation of sexual desire and is initiated by physical stimulation such as kissing, foreplay, or via sexual fantasies and viewing exciting images or videos.
2. **The arousal phase** involves further excitement and an increase in heart rate, heavy breathing, and increased blood pressure. There is a change in skin color, increased tension in certain muscles, and increased blood flow to sexual organs.
3. **The orgasm phase** is characterized by the rhythmic contraction of pelvic muscles and the feeling of intense pleasure. In males, it ends with the discharge of semen, and in women with the contraction of vaginal muscles.
4. **The resolution phase** follows the phase of orgasm. The excitement gradually cools down and heart rate, respiration, and blood pressure gradually return to normal and the body relaxes.

Hormonal Control of Sexual Behavior

Sex hormones such as **estrogen and testosterone** have pivotal roles in sexual behaviors (desire and arousal) both in males and females. More importantly, it is the **ratio of**

estrogen and testosterone (high E and low T or low E and high T) that leads to sexual excitement, arousal, and erection. Sexual desire and arousal are mediated by **sympathetic activity in the brain** while an erectile response is mediated via **parasympathetic activity in the spinal cord**. **Dehydroepiandrosterone (DHEA)** is more potent in initiating sexual response while testosterone is responsible for the sustainment of sexual response.

Neurochemical Control of the Sexual Response Cycle

Monoamine neurotransmitters especially **noradrenaline and dopamine** have special roles in the initiation and maintenance of sexual response. Dopamine is responsible for the initiation of sexual desire and the reward and pleasure associated with sexual activities. Noradrenaline-mediated sympathetic activity has a primary role in arousal phage. Similarly, acetylcholine-mediated parasympathetic action leads to increased blood flow into the sexual organs resulting in erection and lubrication. In contrast, **serotonin has inhibitory effects** on sexual response and decreases libido, inhibits erectile response, and delays ejaculation.

SEXUAL DYSFUNCTIONS

The problem of sexual dysfunction in the community is quite high with a prevalence of about 40% in women and 31% in men. In men, the most common sexual dysfunction is premature ejaculation and in women, it is hypoactive sexual desire disorder. Depending upon the onset, duration, and cause, sexual dysfunctions are categorized as:

1. lifelong or acquired
2. Generalized or situational
3. Due to psychological factors or due to combined factors.

As per DSM5, for a diagnosis of sexual dysfunction disorder, a psychophysiological factor must exist, it must cause marked distress or interpersonal difficulty, and the problem is not due to another psychiatric illness.

Etiology

The causes of sexual dysfunction generally vary from person to person and are grouped as psychogenic factors and organic factors and more often a complex interplay between these two. Psychogenic factors are vast and can be:

1. **Individual factors** include depression, anxiety, frustration, guilt, etc.
2. **Interpersonal and relationship factors** such as relationship conflict, diminished trust, fear of intimacy, family system conflict, etc.
3. **Psychosexual factors** such as negative attitudes, performance anxiety, prior sexual trauma, restrictive religiosity, etc.

Organic factors include chronic illnesses (COPD, heart disease, etc), side effects of medications, endocrine factors such as hypothyroidism, and other medical and surgical illnesses.

CLINICAL PRESENTATION

Sexual Desire, Interest, and Arousal Disorders

1. **Hypoactive sexual desire disorder** is characterized by persistently or recurrently deficient (or absent) sexual fantasies and desire for sexual activity.

2. **Sexual aversion disorder** is defined as "persistent or recurrent extreme aversion to, and avoidance of, all (or almost all) genital sexual contact with a sexual partner."
3. **Male erectile dysfunction** is characterized by an inability to achieve a sufficient erection to engage in penetrative intercourse. Erectile dysfunction is historically defined by the term impotence but is seldom used in the medical realm because of the derogatory tone associated with it. It accounts for almost 50% of all cases of male sexual dysfunctions presented to the clinic. Erectile dysfunction can be psychological, organic, or combined. History of spontaneous erections, morning intumescences, complete erection during masturbation, or achieving erection with a different partner usually rules out organic causes.

Orgasm Disorder

1. **Female orgasmic disorder or anorgasmia** is characterized by an inability to achieve orgasm by masturbation or coitus after a normal sexual excitement phage. Orgasm can be achieved in females by both clitoris and vaginal stimulation.
2. **Delayed ejaculation** is characterized by achieving ejaculation during coitus with great difficulty, if at all. The incidence and prevalence of delayed ejaculation in men are much less than that of premature ejaculation and erectile dysfunction.
3. **Premature ejaculation** in men is characterized by achieving ejaculation before they wish to. PME is complained by about 30–40% of men attending a clinic for sexual dysfunction and is more common in educated men than uneducated ones. Premature ejaculation can be due to two factors.
   - Physiologic factor due to **short nerve latency time**
   - Psychogenic factors in which it is behaviorally conditioned

DSM-5 defines premature ejaculation as achieving ejaculation within 1 minute of penetration. It further categorized the problem into mild (ejaculation between 30 seconds and 1 minute of penetration), moderate (within 15–30 seconds), and severe (within 15 seconds of penetration).

Sexual Pain Disorder

1. **Dyspareunia** is defined by pain occurring before, during, or after sexual intercourse making intercourse unpleasant and unbearable. Dyspareunia is explained by the psychodynamic model according to which women exposed to sexual abuse or rape during childhood develop excessive anxiety about intercourse. Due to this tension and anxiety, they experience involuntary contraction of pelvic floor muscles causing pain during intercourse. Dyspareunia is also common in post-menopausal women due to vaginal dryness and in the postpartum period in which case it is temporary.
2. **Vaginismus** is characterized by contraction of the outer third of the vagina during sexual intercourse making penile insertion difficult or impossible.

Laboratory Investigations

Recommended laboratory tests for men and women presenting with sexual problems include:

1. Blood sugar level to rule out diabetes mellitus
2. Lipid profile
3. Hormonal profiles (e.g. thyroid function test, androgen level in males, estrogen level in females)

4. X-ray spine to rule out spina bifida.
5. Vaginal and vulval discharge microscopy and cultures.

Treatment of Sexual Dysfunctions

1. **Dual sex therapy** was developed by **Masters and Johnson** by taking into account both partners as a unit or dyad. The basic concept is that both partners in a marital relationship must be treated even if one partner is dysfunctional. Therapy involves round table sessions involving male and female therapists who discuss and clarify the problems to the couple and try to improve communication between the couple. They explain the physiological and psychological aspects of sexuality, teach specific sexual practices to be followed by the couple, and also teach specific exercises to improve sexual activity. The importance of foreplay, giving and receiving bodily pleasure by touch, sight, smell, etc, and giving sexual pleasure by manual and oral means are explained. Genital stimulation is eventually added and they are encouraged to try various positions without any pressure of orgasm. Gradually the couple gains confidence and learns to make the sexual act more pleasurable and excitable removing any psychological dysfunction.
2. **Specific techniques and exercises** are mostly prescribed for premature ejaculation and vaginismus.
   a. **The squeeze technique** is highly efficacious **in cases of PME,** in which the female partner is taught to squeeze the glans at the height of ejaculatory sensation which leads to decreased excitation and delaying of ejaculation. The squeeze technique is repeatedly employed for an adequate time to be effective. Another similar technique is the **stop–start technique** in which all stimulation of the penis is stopped at the height of ejaculatory pressure and stimulation is restarted after some time when the excitation is lowered. Both these exercises are highly efficacious in cases of PME.
   b. **Vaginal dilatation** using a finger or a dilator is prescribed **for vaginismus and dyspareunia.**
   c. **Self-stimulation methods** such as masturbation, especially using a vibrator are indicated for the **female orgasmic disorder**.
3. **Pharmacotherapy**
   a. **Phosphodiesterase inhibitors like sildenafil and tadalafil** are used to treat erectile dysfunction. These drugs increase the level of nitric oxide which in turn improves blood flow into the penile muscle tissue. Side effects are headache, flushing, and postural hypotension. These drugs do not cause erection in the absence of sexual stimulation.
   b. **Serotonergic drugs** such as SSRIs (fluoxetine and paroxetine) and TCAs are used to treat **premature ejaculation**.
   c. **Dopaminergic agents** such as L-DOPA, bromocriptine, and bupropion are indicated for improving libido and sexual performance.
   d. A **combination of estrogen and progesterone** is used in postmenopausal syndrome to increase libido and improve vaginal lubrication in females. Estrogen creams can also be applied locally to improve vaginal lubrication in these patients.

GENDER ASSIGNMENT, GENDER IDENTITY, AND SEXUAL ORIENTATION

Gender assignment is the process of **assigning a gender to a child at the time of birth** as male or female by inspecting the anatomy of external genitalia. As the child grows, he/she gradually perceives himself/herself as either male or female. This **perceived gender** by a person as either male or female irrespective of the gender assigned at birth is known as **gender identity.** Gender identity is generally **established by 3 years of age** and is difficult to change thereafter. Gender identity may or may not be congruent with one's assigned gender. This **incongruity** between assigned gender and perceived gender may result in **gender dysphoria also known as gender identity disorder**. **Transgender** and **gender queers** are individuals whose perceived gender is different from that of one assigned at birth.

Sexual orientation is determined by the nature of romantic attraction a person develops toward other persons. **Heterosexuality** is the romantic attraction of a person toward persons of the **opposite sex** (male–female attraction and *vice versa*) while **homosexuality** is the romantic attraction of a person toward persons of the **same sex** (male–male and female–female attractions). In this section, we will discuss **gender dysphoria** (also known as gender identity disorder) and **homosexuality**.

GENDER DYSPHORIA OR GENDER IDENTITY DISORDER

Gender dysphoria as per DSM-5 is defined as a "marked incongruence between their experienced or expressed gender and one they were assigned at birth". These individuals are known as **transgender or genderqueer** in society. The presence of gender dysphoria causes marked subjective discomfort and is also highly stigmatized in society. The prevalence of gender dysphoria is found to be between 0.5–1.3% in the community in various studies. The presence of gender dysphoria increases the risk of depression, suicidality, and substance abuse in these individuals.

Etiology

The exact etiology of gender dysphoria is not known. However, some important biological and environmental risk factors are discussed below.

1. Individuals with **adrenal hyperplasia or androgen insensitivity syndrome** are assigned a female gender at birth based on the appearance of external genitalia. However, as the child grows the person develops a sense of incongruence and belongingness to the opposite sex. This incongruence becomes well evident when puberty is reached.
2. There are studies that have linked **in-utero exposure to phthalates** (present in plastics and polychlorinated biphenyls) which increase the risk of development of gender dysphoria. Phthalates increase the level of fetal testosterone which may lead to masculinization of the brain.
3. Individuals with other **psychiatric illnesses**, especially schizophrenia and autism spectrum disorders are also at higher risk of developing gender dysphoria.
4. Studies have also found a link between **childhood abuse** (especially sexual abuse) and maltreatment and the development of gender dysphoria in adults.

Diagnosis

DSM-5 has laid down the following criteria for a diagnosis of gender dysphoria in adults-

A. A marked incongruence between one's experienced/expressed gender and assigned gender, of at least 6 months duration, as manifested by at least two of the following:
   1. A marked incongruence between one's experienced/expressed gender and primary and/or secondary sex characteristics.

2. A strong desire to be rid of one's primary and/or secondary sex characteristics because of a marked incongruence with one's experienced/expressed gender.
3. A strong desire for the primary and/or secondary sex characteristics of the other gender.
4. A strong desire to be of the other gender.
5. A strong desire to be treated as the other gender.
6. A strong conviction that one has the typical feelings and reactions of the other gender.

B. The condition is associated with clinically significant distress or impairment in social, occupational, or other important areas of functioning.

Treatment

Treatment of gender dysphoria should be initiated by an adequately trained team consisting of a mental health professional, an endocrinologist, and an experienced surgeon in this field. Treatment guidelines laid down by **The World Association of Transgender Health (WPATH)** should be followed in these cases. The treatment modality of gender dysphoria consists of counseling, hormonal therapy, and surgical therapy.

1. Psychological Counseling

Before starting hormonal or surgical therapy, proper counseling of the patient is necessary regarding individual expectations, risks, and benefits of therapy and fertility preservation. The expectations should be realistic and patients should be made aware that treatment will make the external appearance in congruence with their perceived gender and these changes are non-reversible. Another important aspect is the risks associated with hormonal therapy, as they may cause complications such as venous thromboembolism, decrease bone mineral density, and pubertal suppression. Furthermore, the individual may lose the ability to reproduce further.

2. Hormonal Therapy

The aim is to suppress internally produced hormones and to administer hormones externally to bring out the expected changes in external appearance. Hormonal therapy depends upon whether the perceived gender is female or male. In the case of transgender females, it is aimed at removing facial hair, developing breasts, and a female body contour. It is achieved with externally administered anti-androgens, progestins, and estrogens. In transgender males, the aim is to increase muscle mass, cessation of menses, deepening of the voice, and enlargement of the clitoris. This is achieved with testosterone injectables given at weekly intervals.

3. Surgical Therapy

Surgical therapy is categorized as 'top surgery' and 'bottom surgery'. In transgender females, top surgery includes breast augmentation surgery and bottom surgery includes gonadectomy and vaginoplasty. Similarly, in the case of transgender males top surgery includes the removal of breast mass and bottom surgery includes scrotoplasty (testicular implant), phalloplasty (penile implant), and metoidioplasty (clitoris is released from the attached ligament).

4. Family Education

Family members are counseled regarding the nature of the condition and the need for treatment. They are also counseled regarding the importance of emotional, social, and financial support to the individual. Furthermore, they are trained on how to cope with the stress and stigma associated with the condition.

HOMOSEXUALITY

Homosexuality means **same-sex attraction**. It refers to the erotic attraction of a person toward persons of the same sex and is realized either in fantasy, in sexual behavior, or in sexual contact with persons of the same sex. Men with a homosexual orientation toward other men are known as **'gays'** while their female counterparts are known as **'lesbians'**. Earlier, homosexuality was considered a disorder; however, subsequent scientific studies have established homosexuality as **a variant of normal sexual behavior** rather than a deviation from normal sexuality.

The sexual orientation of a person is determined by **neurohumoral factors** such as sexually differentiated hypothalamus and relative levels of the hormone **androgen.** All human beings by default are destined to develop as females. It is the presence of the **'y chromosome'** that leads to the secretion of high levels of **androgen** from the adrenal cortex during the early stage of development. This androgen **acts on the developing brain** leading to structural changes in certain brain areas such as the **hypothalamus and frontal cortex** which is known as **masculinization of the brain**. A masculinized male brain makes the person attracted to females and a lack of masculinization makes the person attracted to males. Abnormal masculinization in females and lack of masculinization in males due to defective neurohumoral control results in homosexuality. This process is genetically determined and has nothing to do with the will of the person.

Concept of Coming out

Homosexuals are often perceived differently in many societies and are **highly stigmatized**. Because of fear of **social alienation,** many homosexuals hesitate to express their sexual behavior. The term **'Coming out'** means liberally expressing one's sexuality without fearing social alienation and backlash. In many cultures and societies, homosexuality is still perceived as a taboo and many religious texts prescribe the death penalty for homosexual behavior. However, with modernization, especially in the west, homosexuals are increasingly being assimilated into mainstream society.

Psychiatric nosology has also evolved significantly concerning homosexuality. In 1973, homosexuality was removed from DSM (diagnostic and statistical manual) as a psychiatric illness. Similarly, it was also deleted as a diagnostic entity in ICD-10 published in 1992.

Conditions for Referral to a Psychiatrist

A case of psychosexual or gender identity disorder should be referred to a psychiatrist in the following cases:

1. Patients showing poor response to initial treatment
2. Cases requiring behavioral interventions
3. Patients with secondary depression due to psychosexual or gender identity problems
4. Patients with suicidal tendencies
5. Patients who have developed substance abuse behavior due to psychosexual or gender identity problems

SUMMARY

1. Human normal sexual response involves the desire phase, arousal phase, orgasm phase, and resolution phase. Each of these phases is mediated and modulated by hormones such as estrogen and testosterone, sympathetic and parasympathetic reflexes, and neurotransmitters such as dopamine and noradrenaline.
2. A case of sexual dysfunction can involve any of the above-mentioned phases and presents as hypoactive sexual desire disorder, sexual aversion disorder, erectile dysfunction, orgasm disorder, premature or delayed ejaculation, and sexual pain disorder.
3. Dual sex therapy developed by Masters and Johnson is the treatment of choice for many of these sexual disorders. Pharmacological agents such as sildenafil, serotonergic drugs, dopaminergic agents, and a combination of estrogen and progesterone are also indicated as specific therapy.
4. Gender assignment is the process of assigning a gender to a newborn by visualizing its external genitalia. Gender identity is the gender perceived by the individual himself as male or female. Incongruence between assigned gender and perceived gender can lead to gender dysphoria as seen in transgender and gender queers.
5. Homosexuality, which is considered a normal variation of sexuality, is the erotic attraction of a person toward individuals of the same sex. Homosexual men are known as gays and women are known as lesbians.

BIBLIOGRAPHY

1. Masters WH, Johnson VE. Reproductive Biology Research Foundation (U.S.). (1966). Human sexual response. Boston: Little, Brown.
2. Halvorsen JG, Metz ME. Sexual dysfunction, Part I: Classification, etiology, and pathogenesis. J Am Board Fam Pract. 1992 Jan-Feb;5(1):51–61.
3. Sadock BJ, Sadock VA, Ruiz P. Kaplan & Sadock's synopsis of psychiatry: Behavioral sciences/ clinical psychiatry, 2015. (Eleventh edition.). Philadelphia: Wolters Kluwer.
4. Avasthi A, Grover S, Sathyanarayana Rao TS. Clinical Practice Guidelines for Management of Sexual Dysfunction. Indian journal of psychiatry, 2017. 59 (Suppl 1), S91–S115.
5. Garg G, Elshimy G, Marwaha R. Gender Dysphoria. [Updated 2022 Jul 18]. In: StatPearls [Internet]. Treasure Island (FL): StatPearls Publishing; 2022 Jan.
6. American Psychiatric Association. (2013). Diagnostic and statistical manual of mental disorders (5th ed.).

Chapter 16

Psychiatric Disorders in Childhood and Adolescence

Competency achievement: Students should be able to

1. **PS14.1** Enumerate and describe the magnitude and etiology of psychiatric disorders occurring in childhood and adolescence
2. **PS14.2** Enumerate, elicit, describe, and document clinical features in patients with psychiatric disorders occurring in childhood and adolescence
3. **PS14.3** Describe the treatment of psychiatric disorders occurring in childhood and adolescence including behavioral, psychosocial, and pharmacologic therapy
4. **PS14.4** Demonstrate family education in a patient with psychiatric disorders occurring in childhood and adolescence in a simulated environment
5. **PS14.5** Enumerate and describe the pharmacologic basis and side effects of drugs used in psychiatric disorders occurring in childhood and adolescence
6. **PS14.6** Enumerate the appropriate conditions for specialist referral in children and adolescents with psychiatric disorders

INTRODUCTION

Child Development

Child development is the natural process of biological development and the **acquisition of social and adaptive skills** after birth. Biological development involves the acquisition of developmental milestone which is genetically hardwired it the child's genetic blueprints. This involves natural biological processes such as **myelination of nerves, synaptic pruning, and synaptic plasticity and is known as maturation**. Various environmental factors such as nutrition, infection, and injury, patenting quality, etc. have a remendous impact on this process of development.

Developmental milestones are grouped into the following headings.

1. **Gross motor milestones**
2. **Fine motor milestones**
3. **Language milestones and**
4. **Social milestones**

Gross motor milestones include neck holding, sitting, crawling, standing, walking, etc. Fine motor milestones include bidextrous grasp, pincer grasp, scribbling, writing, etc. Acquisition of these motor milestones is necessary for the m**aintenance of posture, basic survival, and self-care**. Delayed development of these milestones is an early **sign of intellectual disability.**

Language milestones include babbling, the production of monosyllabic sounds, ability to speak words and sentences. **Social milestones** include eye contact, social smile, stranger's anxiety, imaginative play, sharing of interest with peers, etc. Timely acquisition of these milestones is necessary for the **development of social and adaptive skills**. Delayed development of language and social milestones (with normal motor milestones) is an **early sign of autism**.

Attachment and Bonding

Attachment is the emotional connection the child develops toward the mother (or other caregivers) while **bonding** is the love and affection developed by the mother toward the child. Development of attachment starts at the time of birth with skin-to-skin contact. This process of development of an emotional connection between mother and child within a **critical period** just after birth is known as **imprinting**. Attachment grows stronger with eye-to-eye contact, breastfeeding, and caressing.

Piaget's Theory of Cognitive Development

Jean Piaget was a Swiss biologist who extensively studied **the development of intelligence (cognitive abilities)** in children. He worked at the University of Vienna and also at the Binet Institute of Psychology and formulated a comprehensive theory of cognitive development in children. He observed that children think differently from adults and gradually acquired cognitive skills in a **stage-wise manner**.

According to Piaget, children acquire the ability to understand the world and acquire intelligence in the following **4 stages:**

1. **Sensorimotor stage**
2. **Stage of preoperational thinking**
3. **Stage of concrete operations and**
4. **Stage of formal operations**

1. Sensorimotor Stage (0–2 Years)

A human baby is **born with some basic skills** such as motor skills, and observational skills through senses and reflexes. With basic observational skills, the child gradually acquires knowledge about the immediate environment and also explores it via basic motor skills such as grasping, mouthing, movement tracking, etc. With this, the child gradually **becomes aware of his own body** and the environment and can understand the separation between the two. One of the important cognitive skills acquired in this stage is **object permanence**: the knowledge that objects continue to exist even after they are removed from the child's environment. Separation and stranger anxiety appear only after the development of object permanence and also the child starts taking interest in peek-a-boo games. Gradually at the end of 2nd year of age, the child develops a **mental image of objects** and can imagine them just by hearing their name, a process known as **symbolization**.

2. Stage of Preoperational Thinking (2–7 Years)

In this stage, the child extensively **uses language and symbols** and develops **basic intuitive thinking**. However, the thought process of the child **lacks logic and reasoning**. One of the important aspects of this stage is known as **animistic thinking**; natural objects are thought of as living beings (on visiting the sea beach, the child may imagine that the sea is a monster who is howling and screaming). Only after acquiring these skills, the child develops a fear of the **Bogie man** and gets interested in stories involving fantasy. In this stage, the thought pattern of the child is **egocentric** which means he thinks of himself as the center of the universe and everything happening in the outside world must be related to him in some way. However, the child cannot understand the moral dilemma, i.e. what is good and what is bad.

3. Stage of Concrete Operations (7–11 Years)

In this stage, egocentric thoughts are replaced with **operational thoughts,** e.g. the child can view the world from another's perspective. He can now use limited logic and reasoning and can order and classify objects based on similarities and differences **(syllogistic thinking)**. The child develops the **idea of quantity** and understands the **concepts of conservation** (the quantity does not change even if the shape is changed) and **reversibility** (things can go from one state to another and come back again, e.g. ice and water).

4. Stage of Formal Operations (11 Years–Adolescence)

In this stage, the thought process of the child is **highly logical and systematic**. Now he can understand concepts and **develop abstract abilities**. With the ability to understand abstract concepts, he develops an interest in science, philosophy, religion, social justice, etc. The highest form of formal operation is known as **hypotheticodeductive thinking** by which a person can make the observation, draw inference and can formulate hypotheses, and can test it against reality. Not all persons can achieve this level of cognitive abilities.

AUTISM SPECTRUM DISORDERS

Autism spectrum disorders are characterized by impairment in social communication, reciprocal interaction, restricted interests, and repetitive behaviors. They are considered as neurodevelopmental disorders and are thought to be caused by genetic and environmental factors affecting brain development. The spectrum concept was first introduced in DSM5 and all previous **pervasive developmental disorders (PDDs)** such as autistic disorder or autism, Asperger's syndrome, childhood disintegrative disorder, and pervasive developmental disorder not otherwise specified (PDD–NOS) are included in this spectrum. Rett syndrome is considered a separate condition and not included in ASD.

ASD occurs across all racial, ethnic, and socioeconomic subgroups with an estimated prevalence of about 0.5–1.5% among children. ASD is more common in boys than in girls with a prevalence ratio of 4:1. This condition is also much milder in girls than in boys hence frequently missed and left untreated.

Clinical Presentation of Autism

Autism or autistic disorder is the commonest of all the disorders included in autism spectrum disorders. Recent retrospective studies have revealed that autistic features can be recognized by parents as early as 12–18 months of age in babies. However, diagnosis is usually delayed and made at 3–4 years of age in most cases. Lack of social smiles and poor eye contact are the earliest signs that generate concerns among parents. As the child grows other features of autism become apparent. Lack of **social interaction**, verbal and nonverbal **communication**, **restricted interests,** and **repetitive behavior** are core features of autism that become apparent by 3–4 years of age.

1. Social Impairment

Autistic children find it **difficult in approaching peers** to make friends and hence, **prefer loneliness**. They seem to be in their little world. There is an absence of sharing of interests and toys with other children, taking part in imaginative play and social games. There is difficulty in recognizing the facial expressions and emotions (happiness, fear, or disgust) of other children. Many are also rejected by their peers because of inappropriate and odd approaches and interests.

2. Communication Deficit

Communication difficulty is due to **poor language comprehension** and difficulty in the proper use of language. They show poor response when called by their name**, and use** stereotyped, repetitive, and idiosyncratic language due to problems in the use of excessive and pragmatic language. Apart from having verbal communication difficulty, there is also **difficulty in nonverbal communication**. There is a lack of pointing and looking toward a pointed object (instead they look at the pointing hand), an absence of sharing of interest with others, and responding to others' facial expressions appropriately.

3. Stereotyped Interests and Activities

These children show an interest only in specific limited types of toys, arrange them one after another in a line, watch only a few television shows, and turn them off and on even if requested not to do so. They are **preoccupied with sameness** (same menu and recipe, same style of arrangement of furniture in the home, etc) and often get upset when their environment is changed. This is due to **poor cognitive flexibility** and **poor adaptive skills**. Many children with autism show excessive sensitivity to sounds and touch. Few show stereotyped self-harm behaviors like head banging, nail-biting, and aggression toward peers.

Diagnosis Criteria for Autism as per DSM5

For a diagnosis of autism following diagnostic criteria should be met in a child.

1. **Impairment in social interaction and communication** involving the following three domains
   - Social and emotional reciprocal interaction
   - Nonverbal communication
   - Starting and maintaining social relationship
2. **Abnormal and repetitive behavior, interests, and activities** involving the following four domains (2 are required for diagnosis)
   - Stereotype speech and behavior
   - Resistance to change
   - Fixed interest and activities
   - Hypersensitivity to sensory inputs
3. Symptoms must start during the period of **childhood development**
4. Symptoms must cause **impairment in day-to-day activities.**

Etiology

Genetic and environmental risk factors that affect brain development can contribute to the development of ASD. A complex interplay between both genetic risks and environmental factors leads to abnormal brain development (abnormal cerebral architecture and neural connections). However, the exact etiology is not known.

1. Genetic Factors

Family studies, twin studies, and adoption studies have revealed significant genetic risks for the development of ASD. The **heritability** is found to be as high as **70%**. However, no single gene has been identified to be solely responsible, instead, **multiple genes** are implicated which contribute a small risk toward the development of the condition. Search for candidate genes has identified genes that are **involved in brain development,** neurotransmitter functions, and neural excitability. Many of these genes encode proteins that regulate neuronal migration during brain development, activity-dependent synaptic plasticity (synaptic pruning), and neurotransmitter functions. Abnormal expression of these genes may be due to transcriptional or splicing dysregulation or alteration in epigenetic mechanisms such as DNA methylation and histone acetylation.

2. Environmental Factors

Environmental factors include prenatal, perinatal, and postnatal factors that modulate genetic risk and contribute to the development of ASD. **Advanced maternal or paternal age** is considered a significant risk factor for ASD. Maternal infections such as **TORCH infections** or immune activation during pregnancy, pregnancy-induced diabetes mellitus, preterm delivery, low birth weight, and birth hypoxia all contribute to the development of ASD. All these factors negatively impact brain development in-utero or in the early childhood period. A much-hyped myth that vaccines or vaccine components (thiomersal) lead to the development of ASD has been disproven.

Neurobiology

Neuropathological studies have revealed **abnormal neural architecture** in the frontal or temporal cortex, abnormality in cerebellar architecture and connection, and abnormal connection in the limbic system. One of the most important pathological findings revealed in many studies is focal abnormalities in the laminar architecture of the cortical neurons in the frontal and temporal cortex. This might be due to an **abnormality in neural differentiation and neural migration** during the period of neural development (see Chapter 22). Another important neuropathological finding is excessive neuronal growth due to **a lack of pruning** (deletion of neurons and neural connection during brain development that occurs in every person in childhood) or an increase in extra-axial fluid in neural tissue. All these abnormalities hamper prudent information processing in the cerebral cortex and other areas of the brain which present difficulty in communication and social interaction.

Autism and Theory of Mind

Theory of mind is the ability of a person to **infer the intentions of others**. It is a necessary **cognitive function** that helps a person to understand other people's emotions and show empathy toward them. Theory of mind is a cortical function controlled by a network of neurons known as **mirror neurons,** in the frontoparietal lobes. An underdeveloped theory of mind has been demonstrated by various tests (Sally and Anne test) in children with autism. This makes the child deprived of the ability to understand other people's emotions and shows empathy toward them, making socialization and communication difficult for them.

Comorbidity

Intellectual disability is most commonly associated comorbidity in children with ASD. Around 60–70% of children with autism fall within the subnormal intelligence category. Features of **ADHD** especially hyperactivity and impulsivity are found in many children with ASD. Many children with ASD also develop symptoms of childhood depression. **Self-harm behaviors** such as head banging, nail-biting and irritability, temper tantrums, and aggression toward others are common in these children. **Sleep disturbance** (frequent awakening from sleep at night) is also common with autism.

Suggested Investigations

1. Complete blood count with differential count as a routine test
2. Thyroid function test to rule out hypothyroidism
3. Electroencephalogram (EEG) in cases where epilepsy is suspected
4. Brain imaging studies to rule out tuberous sclerosis in suspected cases
5. Chromosomal analysis in cases with comorbid intellectual disability.

Treatment

1. **Psychosocial and family therapy** is the mainstay of treatment for the core symptoms of ASD. The patient-centered approach is aimed at teaching social and communication skills. Social skill interventions such as peer-related mediation, social narratives, and video modeling are effective in patients with moderate to good cognitive skills. A treatment approach called **applied behavior analysis (ABA)** based on principles of operant conditioning is effective in controlling problematic behaviors. The basic principle is giving positive reinforcement (verbal praise, tokens, eatables, etc.) for good and productive behaviors. Psychosocial intervention is effective in improving social/communication skills especially when administered early.
2. **Pharmacotherapy:** Medications are only indicated **for associated symptoms** of ASD. Antipsychotics such as **risperidone, aripiprazole, and haloperidol** are effective in controlling irritability, temper tantrums, and self-harm behaviors. Antipsychotics are started at a low dose (risperidone 0.5 mg twice daily or haloperidol 0.25 mg twice daily) and the dose is increased gradually over some time. Medications are used only after 5 years of age to avoid undesirable side effects. **SSRIs such as fluoxetine** are prescribed to control stereotyped and repetitive behaviors. Many children with symptoms of ADHD need **stimulant medications** to control their hyperactivity and impulsivity. **Melatonin** is safe and effective in improving sleep in autism.

ATTENTION DEFICIT HYPERACTIVITY DISORDER

Introduction

Attention deficit hyperactivity disorder or ADHD is a **neurodevelopmental disorder** characterized by **hyperactivity, impulsivity, and inattention**. Onset is in childhood but the symptoms can persist into adulthood and in recent times adult-onset ADHD is increasingly being reported. ADHD symptoms can be disabling and can impact the child's social well-being and scholastic performance. A thorough understanding of ADHD symptomatology, etiology, and neurobiology is imperative for the proper diagnosis and treatment of the condition.

Clinical Presentation

ADHD presents with features of hyperactivity, impulsivity, and inattention. Features of **hyperactivity** include fidgetiness, not being able to sit still, running here and there as if driven by a motor, jumping and climbing, etc. Children with ADHD cannot sit silently in the classroom, frequently disturb others (pull others' hair, snatch their pens, etc), and may get involved in petty fighting. Similarly, features of **impulsivity** can present with interfering with others during conversation, frequently interrupting others, answering before the question is finished, not being able to wait for his/her turn, etc. These features of hyperactivity and impulsivity are quite noticeable and apparent and parents generally complain about these symptoms. On the other hand features of inattention are less apparent but more disabling and have a greater impact on academic functioning. ADHD child with **inattention** frequently misses a detail, does not listen when spoken to directly, forgets pen, pencil, and other personal belongings in the classroom, cannot carry out an activity requiring sustained attention (e.g. studying, writing, watching TV) for an adequate time and appears inattentive and daydreaming most of the time.

Hyperactive-impulsive features cause more behavioral problems while inattention leads to poor academic performance. Features of hyperactivity and impulsivity gradually subside as the child reaches adulthood but features of inattention persist. Therefore, adult patients with ADHD complain of poor attention span, lack of interest in tedious activities, and a feeling of inner restlessness.

Depending on the predominant symptoms, ADHD can be categorized into:

1. **Hyperactive–impulsive type**
2. **Inattention type** and
3. **Combined type**

Hyperactive–impulsive type presents with symptoms related to hyperactivity and impulsivity with less impairment in sustained attention. These children have more behavioral and social problems but academic performance is more or less preserved. On the other hand, the inattention type of ADHD has more impairment in sustained attention leading to poor academic performance. Inattention type also frequently goes unnoticed leading to delay in treatment or no treatment at all. The combined type presents with a mixture of symptoms of hyperactivity-impulsivity and inattention.

Diagnosis

Diagnosis of ADHD is mainly clinical and laboratory tests are seldom indicated. Diagnostic guidelines such as ICD-10 and DSM-5 require the **presence** of hyperactivity-impulsivity and inattention symptoms for a period of **at least 6 months.** These symptoms must be present in **more than one setting** (at home, in school, in the workplace, or social setting). Symptoms of ADHD must **appear before 7 years of age** in the case of children and before 17 years of age in adults for a diagnosis. These symptoms must cause significant **impairment in the socio-academic performance** of the child.

Etiology

The exact etiology of ADHD is not known. **Genetic factors** contribute to the maximum developmental risk; however, the exact mechanism remains a mystery. Family studies, twin studies, and adoption studies have revealed a **heritability of 60–90%.** Search for candidate genes has revealed the involvement of genes responsible for the regulation of neurotransmission functions such as **DRD4, DRD5, SNAP 25,** etc. Genome-wide association studies have implicated several loci on various chromosomes but no single locus is solely responsible for the development of the condition signifying a polygenic pattern of inheritance with each susceptible gene contributing a small risk toward the development of the condition. Chromosomal abnormalities such as deletion and duplications known as **copy number variants (CNV)** are frequently identified in these loci.

Apart from genetic factors, certain **developmental factors** (both physical and psychological) also contribute to neurodevelopment illnesses. Physical factors include **pregnancy complications** (maternal malnutrition, eclampsia or preeclampsia, maternal diabetes mellitus, etc) and **birth injuries**. Many studies have revealed a firm association between maternal **alcohol intake in pregnancy** and the development of ADHD. Psychological factors such as childhood abuse and troubled family environments also contribute to a good extent.

Neurobiology

ADHD is a neurodevelopmental disorder presenting with hyperactivity–impulsivity and inattention. Neurological abnormalities lie in the circuits controlling these activities. **Orbito-frontal cortex** which lies at the base of the frontal lobe is involved in **controlling impulsivity** and regulation of emotion. The abnormal connection of **OFC with the striatum (caudate nucleus)** is implicated in ADHD. Weakness of **top-down inhibition** (from OFC to striatum) leads to impulsivity and hyperactivity. Similarly, the anterior **cingulate cortex** is responsible for the regulation of attention and concentration. The abnormal connection of ACC with the ventral striatum is implicated in inattention in ADHD.

The **neurotransmitters dopamine and norepinephrine** act in a balanced way in the frontal cortex and help sustain focus on the ongoing activity. Dopamine helps in canceling out unwanted stimuli (noise) and nor-epinephrine helps in amplifying the signal in focus. An imbalance in these two neurotransmitters can lead to either excessive noise resulting in easy distraction or impaired amplification of the task on focus resulting in a lack of sustained attention.

Comorbidity

ADHD is frequently associated with other neurodevelopmental disorders. Children with **autism** frequently show symptoms of ADHD. Many cases of children with **intellectual disabilities** show symptoms of ADHD. Conversely, many children with ADHD show impaired performance in many cognitive functions and fall within a mild level of intellectual disabilities. Poor social skills and reciprocal interaction are also seen in children with ADHD. **Tic disorder**, another neurodevelopmental disorder, is also commonly associated with ADHD.

Complications

The presence of ADHD in childhood is the harbinger of other disruptive behavior disorders like **oppositional defiant disorder** and **conduct disorder**. When the child reaches adulthood he may indulge in **substance abuse** behavior or may show **antisocial behaviors.** Many adults with antisocial personality disorder have ADHD in childhood. Other psychiatric illnesses such as anxiety disorders or depression can appear secondarily in patients having ADHD in childhood.

Suggested Investigations

1. Complete blood count with differential count
2. Liver and renal function tests before starting medications
3. EEG when epilepsy is suspected
4. Chromosomal analysis in cases with co-morbid intellectual disability.

Treatment

Treatment of ADHD is imperative to improve socio-academic performance and prevent complications. Behavioral therapy is the primary mode of management and medications are indicated only when the symptoms are more impairing or behavioral therapy yields unsatisfactory results.

1. **Behavioral and family therapy** involves parental training to control impulsivity-hyperactivity and temper tantrums. Principles of operant conditioning are applied to control the behavior of children and make them more productive. **Patient-oriented psychotherapy** helps in improving coping skills and attention in studies and other activities. **Behavioral therapy** yields very good results in ADHD cases with mild to moderate symptoms.
2. **Pharmacotherapy: Medications** are indicated when the symptoms are severe or behavioral therapy fails to yield satisfactory results. Medications for ADHD are grouped into **stimulants and nonstimulant medications**. **Stimulant medications** such as **amphetamine and methylphenidate** are dopamine reuptake inhibitors that act by increasing dopamine levels in the frontal cortex. Increased dopamine level in the frontal cortex (OFC and ACC) helps in strengthening inhibitory signals to the striatum and thereby decrease hyperactivity-impulsivity and inattention. There is strong evidence for stimulants in improving social and academic performances. However, treatment with stimulants can lead to side effects such as stomach pain, poor appetite, and growth retardation. Stimulants are contraindicated in children with epilepsy and ADHD with comorbid tic disorder in which cases non-stimulant medications are preferred.

Nonstimulant medications include **atomoxetine, bupropion, clonidine, and guanfacine**. Atomoxetine, a NET (noradrenaline transporter) inhibitor, increases dopamine and nor-epinephrine levels in the frontal cortex. The action of atomoxetine in **improving attention** is more robust than its action on hyperactivity-impulsivity.

The antidepressant **Bupropion** is also effective in controlling symptoms of ADHD by its DAT (dopamine transporter) blocking activity and is the **drug of choice for adult ADHD** patients. The centrally acting **alpha-2 agonists**, clonidine, and guanfacine are also commonly prescribed in ADHD as second-line medications. Clonidine is non-specific but more efficacious while guanfacine is more specific for CNS but somewhat less efficacious than clonidine. These drugs are specially indicated in ADHD with comorbid tic disorder where stimulant therapy can worsen tic symptoms.

DISRUPTIVE BEHAVIOR DISORDERS

Disruptive behavior includes negative, disobedient, defiant, destructive, and rule-breaking behaviors. **Oppositional defiant disorder (ODD) and conduct disorder (CD)** are two important disorders in children and adolescents presenting with **disruptive symptoms.** Disruptive behaviors in children can have a significant impact on their social and familial well-being and academic performance. Many children with disruptive behavior disorders progress to develop **antisocial personality disorder (ASPD)** and indulge in **substance abuse and criminal activities**, becoming a burden for society and their families. ODD, CD, and ASPD are considered as presentations of a **spectrum of the same psychiatric illness** with ODD at the milder extreme and ASPD falling at the severest extreme.

CLINICAL PRESENTATION

Oppositional Defiant Disorder

The oppositional defiant disorder (ODD) presents with irritability, frequent temper tantrums, defiant and argumentative behavior, and vindictiveness. These children are always touchy and irritable and throw temper tantrums on minor provocations. The most important aspect of ODD is defiant and argumentative behaviors which are mostly directed toward authority figures such as parents and teachers. Children with ODD show a negative attitude and often defy or deny requests from parents and teachers. They frequently argue with parents and teachers on minor occasions and become resentful. There is a tendency to annoy others and make them upset. These children also blame others for their own mistakes and unruly behaviors. Such children bear grudges against others and become vindictive.

What makes ODD different from conduct disorder is an **absence of aggressive, destructive, and deceitful behavior.** Even if they are irritable and touchy they don't show aggression toward others or cruelty to animals. They don't get involved in the destruction of others' property or deceitful activities such as lying and stealing.

Conduct Disorder

Conduct disorder (CD) in children presents with more severe disruptive behavior than ODD. It falls at the far end of the disruptive behavior disorders spectrum, just below antisocial personality disorder. Conduct disorder is similar in presentation to ASPD but the major difference is, it is a problem of childhood and adolescent period and ASPD cannot be diagnosed in persons below 18 years old. Symptoms of CD can be categorized into 4 domains as follows:

1. **Aggressive behaviors** present with aggression toward other children in the form of bullying, initiating a fight for minor reasons, using weapons such as knives to inflict injuries, etc. They also show cruelty toward animals and beat and injure them for no reason.
2. **Destructive behaviors** are deliberate and wilful. These children often involve in deliberate fire-setting behavior to destroy others' property. Some also get involved in vandalism.
3. **Deceitful behaviors** such as lying to parents and others, stealing, breaking into others' houses, and shoplifting are also common.
4. **Rule-breaking behaviors p**resent with disregard for age-appropriate social norms and rules and regulations. They frequently run away from home, stay outside the home even at night, skip school (truancy), indulge in sexual activity at a young age, etc.

Children with conduct disorder are emotionally cold, lack remorse and don't feel guilty about their disruptive behavior. They frequently throw temper tantrums and easily get irritated and have low self-esteem. Many find it difficult to make friends because of peer rejection.

These children do not show interest in academic activities because of impaired cognitive functions (memory, learning, attention, concentration, etc). This may lead to **poor academic and professional achievements.**

Etiology

The exact cause of disruptive behavior disorders is not known. Psychological factors such as troubled childhood are the single most important risk factor.

1. Psychological Risk

Children with a history of sexual or physical abuse or torture are at the highest risk of developing disruptive behavior disorders. **Broken families, parental neglect, and troubled parental relationships** (divorce e, separation, etc) carry substantial risk.

2. Social Factors

Children from poor socio-economic backgrounds, disruptive neighborhoods, living in refugee camps, etc are also at risk of developing disruptive behavior disorders.

3. Genetic Risk

The presence of other externalizing disorders like ADHD, ODD, CD, ASD and substance abuse in first-degree relatives indicates a strong genetic predisposition. Twin studies have revealed the **genetic risk can be as high as 50%.** Search for candidate genes has identified the COMT **gene (catechol-o-methyl-transferase gene)** that is involved in monoamine regulation and is implicated in many cases. However, the inheritance pattern seems to be **polygenic in nature** rather than following a Mendelian pattern.

Neurobiology of Disruptive Behavior Disorders

The neurobiological abnormality of conduct disorder and ODD involves three interrelated domains: **punishment processing, reward processing, and cognitive control**. These patients have low punishment sensitivity due to **amygdalar hypoactivity** in response to negative stimuli. Amygdala hypoactivity might be due to **abnormal levels of serotonin** and **noradrenaline** in fear-processing neural circuitry. Because of low punishment sensitivity, these patients cannot anticipate the possible negative outcomes of their disruptive and rule-breaking behaviors.

These patients also have **low reward sensitivity** in response to incentives and sensational stimuli. This might be **due to low dopamine levels** and consequent **orbitofrontal cortex hypoactivity** and failure of sympathetic activity in response to rewarding stimuli. Poor reward processing makes these patients indulge in risky behavior like rash driving, gambling, drug abuse, and inappropriate sexual behavior to get the required sensation. **Poor cognitive abilities** also make these patients **low in empathy** and reciprocal emotion and consequent lack of remorse for their erratic and dangerous behavior.

Complications

Disruptive behavior in children and adolescents is considered the harbinger of **antisocial personality disorder in adulthood**. More than 50% of patients with conduct disorder develop ASPD when they reach adulthood. Many develop substance abuse disorder and other **behavioral addictions (like gambling)** later in life. Episodes of depression with self-harm behaviors and suicidal attempts are also common in patients with disruptive behavioral disorders. Disruptive disorder in children also leads to poor academic and personal achievement. These risks are far greater in patients with CD than with ODD.

Differential diagnosis

Conduct disorder and ODD may be confused with disorders presenting with erratic behavior in childhood like disruptive mood dysregulation disorder, intermittent explosive disorder, and manic episodes in childhood.

Treatment

Treatment of disruptive behavior disorders involves psychosocial interventions, medications, or a combination of both.

1. *Psychotherapy* is a first-line management approach in these disorders and involves patient-oriented therapy like CBT, **family-oriented therapies** such as positive parenting programs, or multidimensional approaches such as multisystemic therapy.
2. *Pharmacotherapy:* Medications are considered when psychosocial interventions yield unsatisfactory results. Medications frequently used and have supportive evidence in their favor are atypical antipsychotics (**risperidone**), mood stabilizers like lithium, antiepileptics (**sodium valproate**, carbamazepine, and oxcarbazepine), and stimulants (**methylphenidate**). Evidence is good in favor of atypical antipsychotics and stimulants either as monotherapy or combination therapy. Medications when combined with psychosocial interventions yield the best results.

ELIMINATION DISORDERS

ENURESIS

Enuresis is defined as the failure to achieve urinary continence past 5 years of age. It is a fairly common condition in children and carries significant psychological morbidly. The presence of this condition in a child is troublesome both for the child himself and his parents and caregivers. Boys are overwhelmingly prone to this condition as compared to girls.

Clinical Presentation

Enuresis presents with frequent bedwetting and/or wetting of clothes either voluntarily or involuntarily. In some cases, the only complaint is bed wetting, some present only with the voluntary or involuntary passage of urine in undergarments while rest of the cases present with both. Many patients with enuresis also complain of constipation or lower intelligence than their peers.

According to achievements of continence, enuresis is classified into the following two types

1. Primary enuresis-where urinary continence is never achieved
2. Secondary enuresis is where urinary continence is achieved at some point in time but is subsequently lost.

Diagnostic Criteria

For a confirmed diagnosis of enuresis, the child must be of more than 5 years of age. Incontinence (either bed wetting or wetting of clothes or both) must occur at least

2 times a week for a period of at least 3 months. DSM5 adds the following specifiers with the core diagnosis of enuresis.

- Diurnal only
- Nocturnal only
- Both diurnal and nocturnal

Etiology

In most cases, the exact cause of enuresis is not known. In known cases, the cause is either chronic constipation or delay of development milestones. In chronic constipation, the impacted stool causes dilatation of the rectum which presses on the bladder causing frequent incontinence.

However, in the majority of cases, the exact cause is not known. In these cases, poor arousal during sleep, delayed bladder maturation, decreased bladder capacity, and inadequate secretion of antidiuretic hormone (ADH) is implicated.

Assessment

Complete history and clinical examination with necessary laboratory investigations is needed in a case of enuresis. History of achievement of development milestones, toilet training, constipation, and sleep pattern (arousal from sleep) is taken to find any known cause.

Medical history such as any signs or symptoms of UTI, seizure, diabetes, etc. is assessed. Urinalysis to rule out UTI, EEG in suspected cases of seizure disorder, and blood investigation to rule out diabetes is mandatory.

From a surgical point of view USG of the bladder, uroflowmetry, postvoiding residual urine, etc is an important investigation to find any causative factors in cases of enuresis.

Complications

Enuresis is associated with significant medical and psychological morbidity. Repetitive wetting may lead to fungal infection and itching, UTI, and excoriation.

Psychological complications of enuresis include poor self-esteem due to frequent wetting of clothes, social embarrassment, being bullied by peers, etc. These factors lead to poor socio-academic performance.

Treatment

Treatment of enuresis includes both nonpharmacological and pharmacological approaches. Nonpharmacological approaches are considered as first choice and medications are added later in cases of poor response to behavioral therapy.

Nonpharmacological approach includes:

1. Reassurance to parents that most children achieve continence with the advancement of age.
2. Bell and pad method is the treatment of choice for enuresis. It involves putting an electronic device on the bed which is activated by bedwetting and arouses the child.
3. In cases of poor arousal from sleep, parents are asked to frequently arouse the child from sleep and make it void. Restriction of water intake before going to bed also helps in cases of poor arousal and decreased bladder capacity
4. The parents are asked to make the child hold urine from time to time which helps in cases where poor bladder maturity is suspected

Pharmacological Approach

Medications are considered a second-line treatment approach in cases of enuresis and are indicated only when behavioral therapy fails or yields an unsatisfactory response. Desmopressin and imipramine are approved by the FDA for this condition.

1. **Desmopressin** is a synthetic ADH analog and acts by decreasing urine output. It is usually given at night which decreases urine output at night and the subsequent need for evacuation. Desmopressin is the first choice in enuresis when medication is needed because of its higher efficacy and safety profile. About 60–70% of cases of children with enuresis respond to this drug.
2. **Imipramine** is the first drug approved for this condition. It is supposed to act by causing relaxation of bladder muscles and thereby causing increased bladder capacity and decreased need for voiding. Imipramine is less effective than desmopressin and can cause troublesome side effects such as sedation and lethargy. Many children also revert to their enuretic behavior once the drug is stopped.

ENCOPRESIS

Encopresis is defined as the failure to achieve fecal continence past the age of toilet training. The condition is not diagnosed before the age of 4 years as the age for achieving bowel continence varies from child to child. Encopresis is a rare but troublesome condition and carries high social stigma and psychological consequences. An empathetic approach toward the condition with detailed evaluation and assessment is needed for proper management of the condition.

The prevalence of encopresis is around 1% in children less than 10 years of age. It is overwhelmingly more common in boys than girls (around 80% of cases are boys). The condition gradually improves by itself with the advancement of age.

Clinical Presentation

A case of encopresis presents with frequent soiling of undergarments with stool passed involuntarily. Fecal soiling occurs mostly during daytime and nighttime incontinence is quite rare. Many children with encopresis also complain of chronic constipation. The stool passed is foul smelling with black tarry in consistency.

Apart from these symptoms, children with encopresis complain of poor self-esteem, depressive symptoms, and social anxiety. This is because of the social stigma associated with this condition. Many children refuse to go to school or social gatherings for fear of embarrassment which impairs their socio-academic activities.

Depending upon the achievement of fecal continence, cases of encopresis can be divided into:

1. Primary encopresis where continence is not achieved at all
2. Secondary encopresis where continence is achieved at some point in time and then is lost subsequently

Diagnosis

For diagnosis, the child must be more than 4 years of age and fecal incontinence must be present for a period of 3 months or more. Fecal incontinence presents with the passage of stool at inappropriate places either voluntarily or involuntarily. The condition must cause significant impairment in the socioacademic performance of the child.

Etiology

Encopresis may be secondary to chronic constipation (retentive encopresis)or may be due to some other causes (nonretentive encopresis). Chronic constipation is implicated in the vast majority of cases. In the rest of the cases Hirsprung disease, myopathies involving external anal sphincter or pelvic floor muscles, spinal cord pathology, and cerebral palsy are implicated.

Pathophysiology

Constipation is present in the vast majority of cases of encopresis (around 80% of cases). These children have had an episode of constipation at the time of toilet training with subsequent painful bowel movements. Such conditions may arise in children because of a less fibrous diet or poor water intake which makes the stool hard and compact causing bowel movement difficult and painful. After such an experience, the child becomes fearful of bowel movement and generally suppresses the urge to pass stool by forcibly contracting the gluteal muscle. This causes chronic constipation with impaction of stool in the sigmoid colon. Fecal impaction and subsequent dilatation of the colon leads to a lack of urge to pass the bowel. As the impacted stool piles up, soft semi-formed stool starts leaking out through the gap between the impacted stool and the bowel wall causing frequent soiling, and at some point in time, the entire bowel content is expelled out involuntarily.

Complication

Encopresis has many medical and psychological complications. Frequent soiling of undergarments may cause itching leading to excoriation and skin infection or UTI. Psychological complications include low self-esteem, being bullied by peers, social anxiety, and depression. Many children suffering from encopresis who present to the clinic are visibly disturbed and depressed.

Treatment

Treatment of retentive encopresis involves two stages: Fecal dis-impaction followed by maintenance therapy. Fecal dis-impaction can be done by oral root or anal root. Oral root for disimpaction involves the use of laxatives such as lactose or Dulcolax while anal disimpaction involves the use of an enema. Some cases may require manual disimpaction. After fecal disimpaction, the child is put immediately under maintenance therapy.

Maintenance therapy involves dietary modification, behavior modification, and the use of laxatives. The child is put on a balanced diet with high fiber content with plenty of water intake to prevent constipation. Behavior therapy involves pelvic floor exercises to gain control over the sphincter muscles and reassurance and positive feedback from parents and caregivers. The use of laxatives should be considered in all cases to prevent constipation. Osmotic laxatives such as lactulose or magnesium hydroxide or polyethylene glycol are preferred.

There is no consensus on the treatment of non-retentive encopresis as a cause that can vary from patient to patient. These cases are carefully evaluated and treated on a case-to-case basis.

Conditions for Referral to a Psychiatrist

1. Uncontrolled behavioral problems like aggression and violence.
2. Patients requiring further evaluation, e.g. in suspected cases of epilepsy or intellectual disability.
3. Poor response to initial treatment.
4. Patients requiring behavioral interventions and family therapy.
5. Parents wanting a second opinion by a psychiatrist.

SUMMARY

1. Autism spectrum disorders, of which autism is the most common, are neurodevelopmental disorders characterized by impairment in social communication, reciprocal interaction, restricted interests, and repetitive behaviors.
2. The complex interplay between both genetic risks (genes involved in brain development, neurotransmitter function, and neural excitability) and environmental factors (Advanced maternal or paternal age, maternal infection such as TORCH infections, low birth weight, and birth hypoxia) leads to abnormal neural development giving rise to autism.
3. Treatment includes psychosocial intervention (teaching social and communication skills via peer-related mediation, social narratives, video modeling, applied behavior analysis for problematic behaviors, etc) and Pharmacotherapy (risperidone, aripiprazole, and haloperidol to control irritability, temper tantrums, and self-harm behaviors and SSRIs such as fluoxetine to control stereotyped and repetitive behavior).
4. Attention deficit hyperactivity disorder or ADHD is a neurodevelopmental disorder characterized by hyperactivity, impulsivity, and inattention which can impair the social and academic well-being of a child.
5. Genetic factors (genes responsible for the regulation of neurotransmission such as DRD4, DRD5, SNAP 25, chromosomal abnormalities such as deletion and duplications known as copy number variants) and developmental factors (both physical and psychological) also contribute to neurodevelopment illnesses.
6. Treatment of ADHD involves behavioral modification (parental training to control impulsivity-hyperactivity and temper tantrums, patient-oriented psychotherapy helps in improving coping skills and attention in studies and other activities) and pharmacotherapy (stimulant medications such as amphetamine and methylphenidate and nonstimulant medications including atomoxetine, bupropion, clonidine, and guanfacine).
7. Untreated cases can lead to the development of ODD, conduct disorder, and antisocial personality disorder. ODD and conduct disorders are characterized by disruptive behavior such as **negative, disobedient, defiant, destructive, and rule-breaking behaviors.**
8. Enuresis presents with frequent bedwetting and/or wetting of clothes either voluntarily or involuntarily. Many patients with enuresis also complain of constipation or lower intelligence than their peers. Nonpharmacological approaches such as parental re-assurance, Bell and pad method, frequently arousing the child from sleep and making it void, etc. are considered the first choice for the management of enuresis.
9. Encopresis is defined as the failure to achieve fecal continence past the age of toilet training which is a troublesome condition and carries high social stigma and psychological consequences. Treatment of retentive Encopresis involves two stages: fecal disimpaction followed by maintenance therapy with the use of laxatives, adequate water intake, and a high-fiber diet.

BIBLIOGRAPHY

1. Sadock BJ, Sadock VA, Ruiz P. Kaplan and Sadock's synopsis of psychiatry: Behavioral sciences/ clinical psychiatry (11th ed.). 2015. Wolters Kluwer Health
2. Amaral DG. (2017). Examining the Causes of Autism. Cerebrum: the Dana forum on brain science, 2017, cer-01-17.

3. Minshew NJ, & Williams DL. The new neurobiology of autism: cortex, connectivity, and neuronal organization. Archives of Neurology, 2007;64(7):945–50.
4. American Psychiatric Association. Diagnostic and statistical manual of mental disorders. 2013. 5th ed. Arlington, VA: American Psychiatric Association.
5. DeFilippis, M., & Wagner, K. D. Treatment of Autism Spectrum Disorder in Children and Adolescents. Psychopharmacology Bulletin, 2015;46(2):18–41.
6. Sanne te Meerman, Laura Batstra, Hans Grietens & Allen Frances. ADHD: a critical update for educational professionals, International Journal of Qualitative Studies on Health and Well-being, 2017. 12:sup1
7. Thapar A, Cooper M, Jefferies R, Stergiakouli E. What causes attention deficit hyperactivity disorder? Archives of disease in childhood, 2012. 97(3), 260–5.
8. Albrecht B, Uebel-von Sandersleben H, Gevensleben H and Rothenberger A. Pathophysiology of ADHD and associated problems—starting points for NF interventions? Front. Hum. Neurosci. 2015;9:359.
9. Aggarwal A, Marwaha R. Oppositional Defiant Disorder. [Updated 2022 Feb 7]. In: StatPearls [Internet]. Treasure Island (FL): StatPearls Publishing; 2022 Jan.
10. Ghosh A, Ray A, Basu, A. Oppositional defiant disorder: current insight. Psychology research and behavior management, 2017;10:353–67.
11. Mohan L, Yilanli M, Ray S. Conduct Disorder. [Updated 2022 May 2]. In: StatPearls [Internet]. Treasure Island (FL): StatPearls Publishing; 2022 Jan.
12. Matthys, W., Vanderschuren, L., & amp; Schutter, D. The neurobiology of oppositional defiant disorder and conduct disorder: Altered functioning in three mental domains. Development and Psychopathology, 2013;25(1):193–207.

Chapter 17

Mental Retardation

Competency achievement: Students will be able to
1. **PS15.1** Describe the etiology and magnitude of mental retardation
2. **PS15.2** Describe and discuss intelligence quotient and its measurement
3. **PS15.3** Elicit and document a history and clinical examination and choose appropriate investigations in a patient with mental retardation
4. **PS15.4** Describe the psychosocial interventions and treatment used in mental retardation

INTELLECTUAL DISABILITY

Intellectual disability (ID) (previously known as mental retardation) is characterized by a **neurodevelopmental deficit** presenting with limitations in **intellectual functioning and adaptive behavior**. These limitations are because of failure to acquire adequate cognitive and adaptive skills and appear before the age of 18 years. Apart from these limitations, persons with intellectual disabilities may present with **behavioral problems**, depression, anxiety, features of ADHD, and autism. The etymology has undergone several changes over the years from **idiocy** to **mental retardation** and recently the term **intellectual disability** is in widespread use.

The prevalence of ID is around 1% in the general population. 75–90% of all cases of ID fall under the mild category, 10–25% under the moderate category, 5% in severe, and less than 1% in the profound category. There is slight male dominance with male to female ratio of 1.3:1. Around 80% of cases are in developing countries.

Etiology

In many cases and particularly for mild-to-moderate cases of ID, the cause of intellectual disability is not known. In other cases, the causes of ID are mainly divided into **genetic abnormalities** and **environmental factors**. Environmental factors include perinatal and childhood environmental exposures that have adverse effects on the brain development of the child.

1. Genetic Factors

Genetic abnormalities can be due to **single gene mutation**, **copy number variation,** or due to **chromosomal abnormalities**. Genetic abnormalities result in ID by causing neurodevelopmental defects, an inborn error of metabolism, or neurodegeneration.

Following genetic syndromes account for most cases of intellectual disability.
1. Down syndrome
2. Fragile X syndrome

3. Phenylketonuria (PKU)
4. Lesch–Nyhan syndrome
5. Rett syndrome

2. Environmental Factors

Environmental factors include **perinatal and childhood factors** affecting the developing central nervous system. Maternal malnutrition, **TORCH infection**, chronic illnesses like diabetes mellitus, bronchial asthma, and substance abuse (mainly alcohol) adversely affect the developing brain because of the impact on nerve growth due to poor placental oxygen supply. Adverse events during birth like instrumental delivery, **delayed birth cry, hypoxia,** etc. are also significantly associated with the development of ID. Childhood environmental factors include childhood infections like **meningitis and encephalitis**, head trauma, exposure to toxins, asphyxia, malnutrition, and severe abuse. These factors negatively impact the growth of the neural tissue resulting in ID.

Diagnostic Evaluation

According to DSM5 the diagnosis of intellectual disability requires a deficit in intellectual functioning and adaptive functioning with onset before the age of 18 years.

1. Intellectual Functioning

Intellectual functioning includes higher mental functions such as **logical reasoning, problem-solving, verbal skills, and intellectual learning.** These skills are required to understand reality and interact with it appropriately at the full capacity of an individual. These higher mental functions are generally known as intelligence and are **measured by IQ tests**.

2. Adaptive Skill

Adaptive skills involve **competence in social, conceptual, and practical skills.** Social skills include interpersonal skills and social communication, social responsibilities, and the resolution of social problems. Conceptual skills include the ability to understand time, finance, and language. Practical skills refer to the ability to use tools, interact with people, and carry out activities of daily living.

Intelligence Quotient (IQ)

The **IQ test** is widely used to assess the severity of intellectual disability and scores are expressed as "**mental age**" **divided by chronological age multiplied by 100**. Based on the scores attained in IQ tests intellectual disability is categorized as follows:

1. IQ 50 to 70: Mild intellectual disability
2. IQ 35 to 49: Moderate intellectual disability
3. IQ 20 to 34: Severe intellectual disability
4. IQ below 20: Profound intellectual disability

Clinical Presentation

Persons with mild **IDs** find it **difficult to acquire conceptual skills** such as understanding concepts, solving problems, and making decisions. They can communicate almost normally by using proper language but have limitations in social skills. Many can attain academic levels beyond primary school but fail to reach higher secondary schools. These patients can achieve independence in terms of finances by learning basic vocational skills and can live a normal life with minimal support.

Those with **moderate IDs** fail to achieve academic levels beyond primary school. They can independently carry out activities of daily living and can achieve basic skills related to safety and health. However, many cannot manage finances and fail to achieve practical and social skills. They require a good amount of support for living a productive life.

Signs of **severe ID** are evident during childhood as a delay in achieving milestones. They can understand language and can communicate understandably by using minimal language. These patients can independently perform simple daily routines like maintenance of self-care, dressing, eating, etc., but need support in social situations and cannot handle finances. They cannot live independently and need constant supervision in a safe home.

Patients with **profound ID** are unable to live independently and need support from caregivers for carrying out activities of daily living like self-care, dressing, eating, etc. They can only use minimal language for communication and generally are also limited in physical aspects and many fail to attain gross motor milestones. Most cases with profound ID generally have genetic syndromes and other features of these syndromes are clinically evident in these groups of patients.

Comorbidity

The presences of comorbid conditions make the assessment, diagnosis, and management of ID complex and challenging. By far, epilepsy and cerebral palsy are most commonly associated with intellectual disability, especially in severe and profound cases. The presence of epilepsy or cerebral palsy makes a patient with ID less responsive to psychiatric medications and more prone to their side effects.

Behavioral problems such as irritability, aggression, self-harm behavior, etc. are seen in mild to moderate cases of ID. The presence of behavioral problems causes more impairment in day to day functioning of these patients and also adds to the burden of caregivers. Detailed history and assessment are necessary to find out the reasons for these behavioral problems for proper management. Behavioral problems might arise from mood swings, depression, high-level frustration, insecure attachment, etc.

Other childhood psychiatric conditions like **hyperactivity–impulsivity**, features of **autism**, anxiety, and **depression** are also common in patients with ID. Features of ADHD and autism are more common in moderate to severe cases while anxiety, phobia, and depression are more common in mild to moderate cases. Other conditions like sleep disturbances and enuresis are also common.

Another important comorbid condition associated with ID is **pica** which is characterized by the ingestion of non-food materials. The presence of pica makes the patient prone to infections and worm infestations, intoxication, choking, and GI obstructions.

Suggested Investigations

Following investigations may be required in a case of ID to establish cause and assess prognosis and possible treatment options

1. Cytogenetic studies such as subtelomeric studies, fragile X screening, and others to identify chromosomal abnormalities
2. Metabolic investigations to identify inborn errors of metabolism and hormonal ailments
3. Neuroimaging studies such as MRI and CT scans of the brain to identify CNS defects

Treatment

Management should start immediately after diagnosis in a case of ID to prevent further worsening and to improve the quality of daily living. Treatment intervention involves a multifaceted approach involving the following parameters.

1. **Educational support** in special schools provides modified academic approaches and promotes self-sufficiency as the child reaches adulthood. Educational support should involve teaching self-assistance, behavioral skills, social and communication skills, etc.
2. **Behavioral intervention** is needed to promote positive and productive behavior and to discourage negative or problematic behaviors. Using principles of operant conditioning (giving the reward for positive behaviors) promotes productive behavior. CBT is used to teach coping skills to adjust negative thoughts, emotions, and mood swings.
3. **Vocational training** helps these patients to learn necessary earning skills and financial management as they reach adulthood. Acquiring the necessary vocational skills can make these patients live a productive life and reduce dependency on caregivers.
4. **The family intervention** involves psychoeducation of family members regarding the nature of illness and prognosis as they need to understand the incurable nature of the disease and have to limit their expectations. Training of family members is crucial in behavioral activation therapy to promote desirable behaviors and discourage undesirable behaviors.

Psychopharmacological Interventions

Medications are often needed for the management of **behavioral problems and comorbid conditions**. Aggression is the most troublesome behavioral problem and can be treated with low-dose **risperidone** or aripiprazole. Low-dose risperidone is effective in controlling aggression and also has minimal side effects profile.

Other comorbid conditions are treated as per the symptomatic presentation. ADHD symptoms can be controlled with **stimulants**, **atomoxetine**, or clonidine. However, it should be remembered that stimulants are contraindicated in patients with epilepsy or a tic disorder. Symptoms of depression can be adequately managed with low-dose SSRIs such as **fluoxetine**. Fluoxetine can also control repetitive motor movements, impulsive behavior, symptoms of OCD, and anxiety. Sleep problems can be adequately controlled with melatonin. Benzodiazepines should be avoided for fear of excessive sedation, tolerance, and abuse, in some patients they can induce paradoxical reactions leading to aggression and irritability.

SUMMARY

1. Intellectual disability or ID is characterized by a neurodevelopmental deficit presenting with limitations in intellectual functioning and adaptive behavior. These limitations are because of failure to acquire adequate cognitive and adaptive skills and appear before the age of 18 years.
2. Causes ID are mainly divided into **genetic abnormalities** and **environmental factors**. Genetic syndromes commonly account for cases of intellectual disability are Down syndrome, Fragile X syndrome, Phenylketonuria (PKU), Lesch–Nyhan syndrome, and Rett syndrome. Environmental factors include perinatal and childhood environmental exposures that have adverse effects on the brain development of the child.

3. For a diagnosis as per DSM5, intellectual disability requires a deficit in intellectual functioning such as logical reasoning, problem-solving, verbal skills, and intellectual learning and adaptive functioning such as competence in social, conceptual, and practical skills, with onset before the age of 18 years.
4. The IQ test is widely used to assess the severity of intellectual disability and scores are expressed as "mental age" divided by chronological age multiplied by 100. Based on the scores attained in IQ tests intellectual disability is categorized as mild, moderate, severe, and profound.
5. Epilepsy and cerebral palsy are most commonly associated with intellectual disability especially in severe and profound cases while behavioral problems such as irritability, aggression, self-harm behavior, etc. are seen in mild to moderate cases of ID.
6. Management of intellectual disability involves family intervention, behavioral modification, vocational training, and the use of medications to treat behavioral problems and depression, anxiety, psychosis, etc.

BIBLIOGRAPHY

1. Lee K, Cascella M, Marwaha R. Intellectual Disability. [Updated 2022 Feb 7]. In: StatPearls [Internet]. Treasure Island (FL): StatPearls Publishing; 2022 Jan.
2. American Psychiatric Association. Intellectual disability. Diagnostic and statistical manual of mental disorders, 2013. (5th ed.).

Chapter 18

Psychiatric Disorders in the Elderly

Competency achievement: Students should be able to
1. **PS16.1** Enumerate and describe common psychiatric disorders in the elderly including dementia, depression and psychosis
2. **PS16.2** Describe the aetiology and magnitude of psychiatric illness in the elderly
3. **PS16.3** Describe the therapy of psychiatric illness in elderly including psychosocial and behavioural therapy
4. **PS16.4** Demonstrate family education in a patient with psychiatric disorders occurring in the elderly in a simulated environment
5. **PS16.5** Enumerate the appropriate conditions for specialist referral in psychiatric disorders in the elderly

INTRODUCTION

Old age is generally considered to start **after 65 years of age**. Ageing is associated with general deterioration in function, physical appearance, cognitive abilities and increased vulnerability to infection. Regular physical activities and exercise, healthy diet and adequate rest can help retain physical appearance and cognitive abilities to a remarkable degree. Nonetheless, old age is associated with certain psychosocial problems as described below.

1. Social Activity

Maintenance of good social contact and interaction is important to preserve the sense of usefulness and self-esteem. Elderly individuals often find it difficult to remain socially connected because of the death of friends and relatives, due to medical illness and also due to ostracism by the younger generation. Loneliness in these individuals is one of the important factors contributing to the emergence of depression.

2. Ageism

Ageism is the negative attitude displayed by younger generation toward the older persons leading to discrimination against them. Ageism contributes to social isolation, poor self esteem and a feeling of worthlessness.

3. Socioeconomic Aspects

Older individuals, unless getting pension after retirement, are deprived of money and feel poor. This problem is more so in elderly women than in men. Lack of money can deprive them of certain enjoyment (e.g. good food) they dearly want.

4. Retirement

For few elderly individuals retirement may lead to a feeling of loneliness, unproductiveness and associated with poor self esteem. It is also associated with economic hardship for those with no other source of income.

5. Sexual Activity

In older individuals sexual activity largely depends on availability of spouse. In general, sexual activity decreases in frequency in older individuals.

COMMON PSYCHIATRIC DISORDERS IN THE ELDERLY

PREVALENCE AND BURDEN

According to the **World Health Organization**, over 20% of individuals above 60 years of age are suffering from some psychiatric or neuro-psychiatric illnesses. Most common of these are dementia and depression with 5% and 7% of elderly population suffering from them, respectively. Other common psychiatric illnesses in the elderly population are anxiety disorders (3.8%), psychosis and substance abuse disorder (1%). These illnesses account for approximately 17 years lived with disability in these individuals.

DEMENTIA

Dementia is one of the most common causes of disability in the elderly, second only to arthritis. Advancing age is the most important risk factor for development of dementia. Apart from advancing age, other risk factors for dementia in old age are presence of hypertension, diabetes mellitus, poor nutritional status, frequent medical illnesses, alcohol abuse, lack of physical activities, etc. Common types of dementia in the elderly are mentioned below.

1. Alzheimer's disease
2. Vascular dementia
3. Lewi body dementia
4. Dementia with Parkinson's disease
5. Vitamin deficiency dementia
6. Alcohol induced dementia

(Most of these disorders have been described in detail in **Chapter 4** under organic mental illnesses)

Behavioral and psychiatric symptoms (BPSD) are common in patients with dementia. Common presenting features of BPSD are irritability and agitation, aggression, delusions and hallucinations, emotional outburst, depression and anxiety. Common themes of delusions in a case of dementia are delusion of persecution, infidelity, delusion of theft, delusional misidentification, and delusion of parasitosis and other somatic delusions. BPSD is generally managed with behavioral modification, supportive therapy and family psychotherapy (discussed in Chapter 4). Those cases not responding to behavioral therapy may be managed with psychotropic medications. Low dose antipsychotics are frequently prescribed to manage agitation, aggression, delusions and hallucinations. In addition, SSRIs may be prescribed to control emotional outburst, impulsively, depression and anxiety symptoms in dementia. Melatonin is helpful in reversing the altered sleep wake cycle often seen in these patients.

DEPRESSION

Depression is one of the most common psychiatric illnesses in the elderly. The prevalence of depression in geriatric age groups is found to be 15–20% in various studies. Presence of depression negatively impacts the psychological and physical well being of elderly individuals and is associated with significant morbidity and mortality. Suicide is the single most mortality factor associated with depression in these patients.

Age is as such not a risk factor for depression. Followings are some of the important known risk factors for depression in geriatric age groups.

1. **Psychosocial factors** such as loneliness, boredom, lack of friends and lack of family support are important contributing factors in the development of depression in the elderly.
2. **Presence of long standing medical illnesses** especially hypertension and diabetes mellitus significantly contribute to development of depression in elderly individuals. Presence of hypertension and diabetes mellitus leads to microvascular changes leading to cortical atrophy and subcortical white matter changes which contribute to development of depression. Depression arising in this setting is known as **vascular depression** and contributes to more than 50% cases of geriatric depression.
3. **Other long term medical conditions** that make elderly individuals prone to depression are cardiac illnesses, arthritis, inflammatory illnesses, renal impairment, etc.

Long-term use of certain medications also contributes to the development of depression in these individuals.

Clinical Presentation of Geriatric Depression

Geriatric depression does not present with typical symptoms of major depressive disorder as found in young individuals. Common presenting symptoms of geriatric depression are irritable mood, psychomotor agitation or depression, early morning awakening, lack of motivation, somatic symptoms, psychotic symptoms and cognitive symptoms. Cognitive symptoms are a defining feature of geriatric depression and present with poor memory, impaired attention and concentration, impaired judgement and reasoning and disorientation. Depression with cognitive symptoms in elderly individuals may be confused with a case of dementia; hence, the term **pseudodementia** is applied for these cases. Somatic symptoms such as pain over various parts of the body, heaviness of head, burning sensation and stomach upset are also common in elderly patients with depression. Psychotic features such as delusion of guilt, nihilism and persecutory ideas are also common in geriatric depression.

Suicide in Geriatric Depression

Suicide is the most common mortality factor associated with geriatric depression. Risk of suicide is more with geriatric depression than depression in the adults. Risk factors for suicide in geriatric depression are living alone, male gender, agitated depression, lack of insight and presence of psychotic features.

Suggested Investigations

1. Complete blood count
2. Serum electrolyte level
3. FBS and PPBS to rule out diabetes mellitus

4. Thyroid function test
5. Brain imaging studies to rule out dementia

Treatment of Depression in the Elderly

Treatment of geriatric depression should be catered on case to case basis considering many factors: severity of depression, presenting symptoms, presence of comorbidities, drug-drug interaction and tolerability.

Psychotherapy is the treatment of choice for mild to moderate depression. **Cognitive behavioral therapy** is the psychotherapeutic approach of choice for these patients. **Family interventions** in the form of social and emotional support to the patient, being vigilant regarding suicidal tendencies and seeking psychiatric help in case of emergency is also important.

Moderate to severe cases of depression are managed primarily with medications. SSRIs are first choice in these cases because of their better tolerability profile. However, cases of depression with somatic symptoms also need to add on pregabalin or gabapentin along with SSRIs. Similarly, cases of psychotic depression show poor response to SSRIs alone in which cases low dose antipsychotics are added. ECT and other brain stimulation methods are only preserved for severe psychotic depression presenting with stupor, depression with active suicidal tendency and cases with poor medical and nutritional status.

PSYCHOSIS IN THE ELDERLY

1. Schizophrenia

First episode schizophrenia is uncommon in old age. However, there are case reports of first episode schizophrenia in individuals older than 60 years. What is important is that schizophrenia being a lifelong illness, its symptoms persist in old age albeit in lesser severity. There is also ongoing debate regarding the need for treatment of schizophrenic symptoms as they get diminished in the elderly. Furthermore, elderly individuals are also prone to develop EPS, especially Tardive dyskinesia, with typical antipsychotic medications. Elderly schizophrenic patients are also more prone to develop dementia.

2. Delusional Disorders

Delusional disorders are quite common in the elderly and present with well systematised paranoid delusions such as delusion of infidelity, delusion of theft, delusional parasitosis, other somatic delusions and delusion of misidentification. Elderly patients with delusions frequently refuse treatment and medications because of lack of insight, hence, are difficult to manage. These delusional behaviors are more problematic for the family members than the patient himself. Treatment is with low dose second generation antipsychotics such as risperidone.

3. Mood Disorder with Psychosis

Depression is the most common mood disorder in geriatric population. Furthermore, psychotic symptoms are one of the presenting symptoms in geriatric depression. Delusion of guilt, nihilism and persecution are frequently found in geriatric patients with depression. Presence of psychotic symptoms increases the morbidity and mortality by suicide in elderly with depression and also makes the condition non responsive to conventional antidepressants such as SSRIs. It is prudent to add antipsychotics at lower doses to conventional antidepressants in these cases. Manic episodes in the elderly are less common, however, can present with irritable mood, agitation and delusion of persecution and infidelity.

4. Dementia with Psychosis

Alzheimer's disease is the most common cause of dementia in the elderly and around 50% cases of Alzheimer's dementia present with psychotic symptoms. In these cases delusion of persecution, infidelity and delusion of theft are common themes. Other psychotic symptoms associated with Alzheimer's disease are visual and auditory hallucinations, aggression and disorganized behavior. Another common cause of dementia in the elderly is Lewy body dementia or LBD which typically presents with visual hallucinations and other prominent delusions.

5. Substance Induced Psychosis

Alcohol induced psychosis is quite common in the old age group. Another common condition found in elderly alcoholic patients is Korsakoff psychosis presenting with memory impairment and psychosis.

ANXIETY DISORDERS

Anxiety, especially subsyndromal anxiety, is common in the elderly. The most common anxiety disorder seen in geriatric patients are generalized anxiety disorder (7.3%) followed by phobias (3.1%) and the panic disorder (1%). Increased incidences of anxiety disorders in the elderly are mainly due to existential crisis as there is a perception that death is nearing in. Another reason for this is fragility of autonomic nervous individuals in this age group.

Appropriate Conditions for Referral to a Psychiatric Specialist

1. When the general physician is not certain about the diagnosis.
2. Patient having a major psychiatric illness such as advanced stage of dementia or psychotic depression.
3. Patient is showing suicidal tendency.
4. When the patient is confused and disoriented and proper evaluation and investigation is required.
5. Patients showing poor response to initial treatment.
6. Patients requiring family interventions or behavioral therapy.

SUMMARY

1. Old age is associated with certain unique psychosocial problems such as loneliness, ageism, frequent medical illnesses, boredom etc. In old age, it is important to engage in productive activities to get the feelings of purpose in life and to do regular physical activities to stay fit.
2. Dementia is one of the commonest causes of disability in the elderly. Alzheimer's disease is the most common cause of dementia followed by vascular dementia, frontotemporal dementia or FTD, Lewi body dementia etc.
3. Depression is common in old age and presents with low mood, loss of interest, guilt feeling, atypical features, somatic symptoms and psychotic features.

4. Psychosis in elderly individuals can present with aggression, delusions and auditory hallucinations. First episode psychosis in old age points towards some organic cause and must be investigated properly. Common causes of psychosis in old age are dementia, delusional disorder, depression, schizophrenia and substance induced psychotic disorders.
5. Anxiety symptoms are also common in the elderly because of existential crisis and fragility of the autonomic nervous system.

BIBLIOGRAPHY

1. Ghimire K, Dahal R. Geriatric Care Special Needs Assessment. [Updated 2022 Feb 22]. In: StatPearls [Internet]. Treasure Island (FL): StatPearls Publishing; 2022 Jan.
2. Small GW, Liston EH, Jarvik LF. Diagnosis and treatment of dementia in the aged. West J Med. 1981 Dec;135(6):469–81.
3. Fiske A, Wetherell JL, Gatz M. Depression in older adults. Annu Rev Clin Psychol. 2009;5:363–89.
4. Targum SD. Treating Psychotic Symptoms in Elderly Patients. Prim Care Companion J Clin Psychiatry. 2001 Aug;3(4):156–163.
5. Subramanyam AA, Kedare J, Singh OP, Pinto C. Clinical practice guidelines for Geriatric Anxiety Disorders. Indian J Psychiatry. 2018 Feb;60(Suppl 3):S371–82.

Chapter 19

Psychiatric Emergencies

Competency achievement: Students should be able to

1. **PS17.1** Enumerate and describe the recognition and clinical presentation of psychiatric emergencies
2. **PS17.2** Describe the initial stabilization and management of psychiatric emergencies
3. **PS17.3** Enumerate the appropriate conditions for specialist referral in patients with psychiatric emergencies

INTRODUCTION

The two most important psychiatric conditions we encounter in the emergency department are patients with significant aggression and violence and patients with suicidal tendency. Dealing with such patients is quite difficult for internists and junior residents and the skill to manage such patients need to be learned by them. Other psychiatric cases coming to the emergency department are cases of acute psychosis, delirium, panic attack and hyperventilation syndrome.

ACTIVELY SUICIDAL PATIENT

Suicidal risk among psychiatric patients visiting the emergency department (ED) is quite high, even if they are not apparent. So, all psychiatric patients attending ED irrespective of diagnosis should be assessed for suicidal risk. In case a patient is actively suicidal or reveals any plan to do so, proper assessment and evaluation are necessary to prevent suicide.

When an actively suicidal patient or patient with self-harm behavior visits ED, the patient may be shifted to a private room for evaluation. Any harmful objects such as sharp objects and poisonous materials should be removed from the patient's reach to ensure the safety of the patient. The patient is approached with a calm disposition and rapport should be established with empathetic communication. Suicidal risk is assessed by direct questioning in the following areas.

1. **Suicidal intent or ideation:** The patient is enquired about any suicidal idea coming into his mind and why he feels like ending his life. Many patients reveal suicidal thoughts coming into their minds because of hopelessness and helplessness which are signs of depression.
2. **Suicidal plan:** Has the patient made any particular plan to kill himself such as dying by ingestion of poison or shooting himself? He is further enquired regarding any activities he has done to commit suicide such as bringing poison or a firearm to his home.

3. **History of a suicidal attempt:** A person having attempted suicide in the past has already shed the fear of killing themself and is at the greatest risk of committing suicide.
4. **History of psychiatric illness**. It is found that around 80% of patients who commit or attempt suicide has had been suffering from some psychiatric illness, especially depression. History of ongoing major depressive disorder, bipolar depression, schizophrenia with commanding hallucinations, and personality disorders with substance abuse are strong indicators of suicidal risk.
5. **Agitation or restlessness:** An agitated patient in depression (especially found in bipolar depression) is more able to carry out suicidal acts than a severely lethargic patient in depression. Therefore, agitated patients are at greater risk of committing suicide than lethargic patients.

Management of Suicidal Patients in ED

Emergency management of actively suicidal patients involves **patient education, developing coping skills, finding support, and making rapid referrals.** The patient and caregivers are educated about the underlying psychiatric conditions and suicidal risks associated with them. The patient may be given brief counseling on managing emotion with proper coping skills like deep breathing, aerobic exercise, and meditation. A relevant support system must be identified which can be accessed by the patient at the time of crisis. In cases where necessary, proper referral to a psychiatric hospital must be done.

Disposal of the Patient with Suicidal Risk

After careful assessment of suicidal risk, the patient may be admitted to the psychiatric ward if the suicidal risk is high. Most cases are admitted as independent cases but those with severe depression with a lack of insight may be admitted as supported cases after consultation with caregivers. If the suicidal risk is deemed low then the patent may be discharged with proper counseling of caregivers for constant vigilance, removing any lethal weapons or poison from the access of the patient, and proper dosing of medications with supervision. Educating family members about warning signs and proper follow-up visits are planned before discharging the patient.

VIOLENT OR AGITATED PATIENT

Interns and junior residents often find it difficult to examine psychotic patients in the ED because of inexperience and fear of violence. One of the most important aspects to be considered while examining an agitated patient in the ED is the safety of the physician and the patient. It is prudent to follow a standard approach known as the SAFEST approach in such cases as described below.

1. **Spacing:** It means maintaining a safe distance from a psychotic patient while examining him in the ED. The examiner must have access to a door for immediate escape in case of any violent behavior shown by the patient. Do not touch the patient unless necessary.
2. **Appearance:** Most of the history should be taken from an attendant appearing for the patient. Always try to build rapport with an empathetic and nonjudgmental disposition with the attendant by your side. Security staff may be called to handle any violence which may arise. Any harmful object or weapon should be removed from the patient's sight.

3. **Focus:** The examiner should be vigilant about any signs of escalating violence as mentioned below.
   A. Loud talking
   B. Using abusive and sexual language
   C. Accusing clinician of conspiracy
   D. Punching on the wall or bed
   E. Becoming agitated with clenched fists, fiery eyes, etc.
4. **Exchange:** The patient can be calmed with continuous empathetic verbal exchange and establishing good rapport. A non-judgmental approach to a patient's problem can make the patient calm and cooperative.
5. **Stabilization:** The patient can be stabilized using physical or chemical restraint whenever necessary. Chemical restraint can be achieved with parenteral lorazepam along with an injection of haloperidol and promethazine.

Assessment of the Cause of Aggression

Aggression and violence are almost always associated with psychotic disorders. Family members should be enquired about past or present history of any psychiatric illness. The patient should be assessed for symptoms of following psychotic illnesses which are more commonly associated with aggression and violence.

1. Acute mania
2. Paranoid schizophrenia
3. Antisocial personality disorder
4. Substance intoxication such as alcohol intoxication, stimulant intoxication, etc
5. Delirium tremens and
6. Acute psychosis

Management of Aggressive Patients

Restraint methods are applied when a patient becomes violent and pose danger to himself and others. Restraining a mentally ill patient in India is governed by the Mental Healthcare Act, of 2017, and the human rights and dignity of the patient must be maintained while restraining. Some restraining methods (e.g. mechanical restraint) are considered a method of last resort and should be applied when other alternative methods fail and restraint should not be a form of punishment. The nominated representative should be informed about restraining within a period of 24 hours.

A violent or agitated patient can be restrained via the following means.

1. **Chemical restraint** involves the use of medications to calm down the violent patient to prevent him from carrying out any dangerous behavior. Sedatives such as lorazepam or diazepam are most commonly used for chemical restraint. In some cases, neuroleptics such as parenteral haloperidol with promethazine may be required to control the patient.
2. **Physical restraint:** Sometimes force is applied through direct physical contact to restrict the mobility of the patient and to disengage him from a dangerous act.
3. **Mechanical restraint** involves using instruments to restrict mobility. The use of mechanical restraint is quite controversial. Examples of mechanical restraints are using belts to tie the patient to a table, using clothes or chains to tie hands and feet, tying the patient to bed rails to prevent him from getting up from the bed, etc.

OTHER PSYCHIATRIC EMERGENCIES IN THE ED

Delirium

Delirium cases are very common in the emergency department and present with altered sensorium, agitation, and behavioral disturbances. Impairment in consciousness (altered sensorium) is the hallmark feature of delirium. In all cases of delirium, the primary underlying cause should be evaluated for proper management of the case. The primary management approach in a case of delirium is the management of the underlying cause which can vary from case to case. Common causes of delirium are

1. CNS disturbances such as infection, injury, toxicity, or mass occupying lesion.
2. Systemic illnesses causing CNS hypoxia or toxicity such as pneumonia, septicemia, and hepatic or uremic encephalopathy.
3. Substance intoxication or withdrawal (alcohol or opioid intoxication, alcohol withdrawal, etc).

The presence of psychotic features such as fleeting delusions and hallucinations (mostly visual hallucinations) and psychomotor agitation invite psychiatric interventions. Low-dose antipsychotics (low-dose haloperidol or risperidone) are the standard treatment for delirium with psychotic features. Benzodiazepines should be avoided as they add to the confusion and delay recovery.

Acute Psychosis

Patients presenting with acute onset psychotic behavior are quite common in the emergency department. A case of acute psychosis presents with sudden onset behavioral disturbances with agitation, delusions, hallucination, poor self-care, sleep disturbances, crying spells, etc. It is imperative to differentiate a case of functional psychosis from organic psychosis in the emergency department. The presence of the following features points toward a possible organic cause:

1. Presence of confusion or altered sensorium
2. Urinary or fecal incontinence
3. Agitation and irritability
4. Impaired cognitive functions such as memory and orientation

Once any possible organic cause is ruled out, a provisional diagnosis is made considering the presenting symptoms. Causes of acute psychosis include:

1. Acute and transient psychotic disorder
2. Manic episode
3. Psychotic depression
4. Substance-induced psychosis
5. Schizoaffective disorder

Treatment

Antipsychotics are the mainstay of treatment of acute psychosis. Parenteral haloperidol with promethazine is given to control agitation and psychosis in the emergency department in severe cases. Patients presenting with less severe psychosis can be managed with oral antipsychotics such as olanzapine or risperidone in combination with benzodiazepines such as lorazepam. Severe cases may be admitted to the psychiatric ward for proper management.

Hyperventilation Syndrome

A case of hyperventilation syndrome generally presents with sudden onset shortness of breath, chest pain, a feeling of paraesthesia and numbness and sometimes the patient may be gasping. The vast majority of cases are young adolescent patients with poor coping skills who develop these episodes following some acute interpersonal stress. In some cases, it may be the presentation of acute anxiety and panic attacks. Unnecessary investigations may be avoided by careful history and examination. These cases are managed in the ED with reassurance and psychoeducation of family members. Oral or parenteral anxiolytics such as lorazepam and clonazepam may be given to treat acute cases in the ED.

Panic Attack

Panic attacks present with sudden onset excessive fearfulness with a feeling of impending doom or death lasting for 2–5 minutes which may be repeated at intervals. Careful history and examination and necessary investigations are done to rule out organic cases mimicking panic attacks such as mitral valve prolapse, hypoglycemic crisis, and hypertensive emergency.

Once any serious medical condition is ruled out, the case is managed with oral anxiolytics such as etizolam and clonazepam to be taken on SOS (as and when) basis. SSRIs such as paroxetine or escitalopram may be prescribed as prophylaxis to prevent further episodes.

SUMMARY

1. Suicidality among psychiatric patients attending the emergency department is quite high, hence, every psychiatric patient attending ED should be assessed for suicidal risk.
2. After establishing rapport with an empathetic approach, the suicidal risk is assessed in terms of suicidal ideas, planning, and activities, presence of depression, history of suicidal attempts, etc.
3. If a suicidal risk is found then the patient should be shifted to a private room and all harmful objects and substances should be removed from the patient's reach. Proper counseling of the patient and caregivers should be done concerning the need for hospitalization or home-based care.
4. In cases where the suicide risk is very high, the patient should be hospitalized. In low-risk cases, the patient may be sent home with proper counseling from the caregiver regarding safety, vigilance, and dosing of medications.
5. Managing violent patients in the ED is quite difficult and needs skills in communication and assessment. Violence is associated with acute mania, paranoid schizophrenia, ASPD, and substance intoxication and withdrawal.
6. Violent patients in the ED should be managed with the standard SAFEST approach which stands for spacing (maintaining safe distance), Appearance (attendant should appear for the patient), focusing on signs of violence, exchange (empathetic communication to calm down the patient) and stabilization using restraint.
7. Chemical restraint using sedatives and neuroleptics is the method of choice for violent patients. However, in some cases application of physical and mechanical restraint may be necessary.
8. Apart from actively suicidal and violent patients, other psychiatric emergencies are delirium, acute psychosis, acute conversion episodes, and panic attack.
9. One of the most important skills to develop during the evaluation of psychiatric patients in the emergency is to differentiate functional cases from organic cases. Signs of organicity that should be assessed include confusion, disorientation, lowering of consciousness, incontinence, presence of fever, headache, and vomiting.

BIBLIOGRAPHY

1. Betz ME, Boudreaux ED. Managing Suicidal Patients in the Emergency Department. Ann Emerg Med. 2016 Feb;67(2):276–82.
2. Sebastian J, Debnath S. Nursing management of patients with violent behavior. Indian J Cont Nsg Edn 2020;21:129–34
3. Ziaei M, Massoudifar A, Rajabpour-Sanati A, Pourbagher-Shahri AM, Abdolrazaghnejad A. Management of Violence and Aggression in Emergency Environment; a Narrative Review of 200 Related Articles. Adv J Emerg Med. 2018 Nov 29;3(1):e7.
4. Raveesh BN, Lepping P. Restraint guidelines for mental health services in India. Indian J Psychiatry. 2019 Apr;61(Suppl 4): S698–S705.
5. Rosen T, Connors S, Clark S, Halpern A, Stern ME, DeWald J, Lachs MS, Flomenbaum N. Assessment and Management of Delirium in Older Adults in the Emergency Department: Literature Review to Inform Development of a Novel Clinical Protocol. Adv Emerg Nurs J. 2015 Jul-Sep;37(3):183–96; quiz E3.
6. Byrne P. Managing the acute psychotic episode. BMJ. 2007 Mar 31;334(7595):686–92.
7. Mavrogiorgou P, Brüne M, Juckel G. The management of psychiatric emergencies. Dtsch Arztebl Int. 2011 Apr;108(13):222–30.

Chapter 20

Therapeutics

Competency achievement: Students should be able to
1. **PS18.1** Enumerate the indications and describe the pharmacology, dose, and side effects of commonly used drugs in psychiatric disorders
2. **PS18.2** Enumerate the indications for modified electroconvulsive therapy
3. **PS18.3** Enumerate and describe the principles and role of psychosocial interventions in psychiatric illness including psychotherapy, behavioral therapy, and rehabilitation.

INTRODUCTION

Medications are the mainstay of treatment of psychiatric illnesses. Psychotropic medications greatly vary from one another in their mechanism of action, dose, side effects, and indications. It is imperative to understand the basic principles of the pharmacology of these medications for the proper treatment of psychiatric illness. Psychotherapy is often combined with pharmacotherapy, especially in neurotic illnesses, to get the best results. Furthermore, brain stimulation methods such as ECT and transcranial magnetic stimulation (TMS) have their special places in the management of psychiatric illnesses.

PSYCHOPHARMACOLOGY

ANTIPSYCHOTICS

Antipsychotics are the mainstay of treatment of psychotic illnesses such as schizophrenia, acute psychosis, delusional disorders, etc. Since the discovery of the first antipsychotic drug chlorpromazine, a basket of other antipsychotics have been synthesized. These drugs can be classified into two categories such as first-generation antipsychotics and second-generation antipsychotics.

FIRST GENERATION ANTIPSYCHOTICS

These drugs are also known as typical antipsychotics, classical antipsychotics, or major tranquilizers. Because of their mechanism of action, they are also known as dopamine receptor antagonists or DRA. Chlorpromazine, whose antipsychotic effect was discovered in 1951, was the prototypical drug in this category. First-generation antipsychotics are further classified as follows:

1. Phenothiazines
   - With aliphatic side chain such as chlorpromazine

- With piperidine side chain such as thioridazine
- With piperazine side chains such as fluphenazine and trifluoperazine

2. Butyrophenones which include haloperidol and droperidol
3. Thioxanthenes such as flupentixol
4. Heterocyclics such as pimozide and loxapine

Indications

Apart from common psychotic illnesses, typical antipsychotics are also useful in varied psychiatric illnesses as enumerated below:

1. Schizophrenia
2. The manic episode of BPAD
3. Acute and transient psychotic disorder
4. Delusional disorders
5. Organic psychosis
6. Substance-induced psychosis
7. Tic disorder (haloperidol is the drug of choice)

Mechanism of Action

First-generation antipsychotics act as antagonists at dopamine D_2 receptors. As we know that dopamine hyperactivity at the D_2 receptor in the mesolimbic pathway is the basis of psychotic symptoms in functional psychotic illnesses, blocking of the D_2 receptor via these drugs leads to the resolution of psychotic symptoms such as delusions and hallucinations. However, they have no effects on the dopamine D_1 receptors in the mesocortical pathway and hence do not improve negative or cognitive symptoms of schizophrenia.

Side Effects

Apart from acting on D_2 receptors in the mesolimbic pathway, these drugs also act on dopamine D_2 receptors in other dopaminergic pathways which leads to undesirable side effects. The most common of these are extrapyramidal side effects also known as EPS.

Extrapyramidal Side Effects

The action of antipsychotics on D_2 receptors in basal ganglia leads to extrapyramidal side effects (EPS). EPS is more common with high-potency antipsychotics like haloperidol and pimozide due to their strong D_2 blocking action than with low-potency ones such as chlorpromazine. Depending upon the time of onset of symptoms after administration of the drug, EPS can be grouped into the following 3 categories.

Table 20.1: Dose range of typical antipsychotics

Drug	*Minimum effective dose*	*Maximum dose*
Chlorpromazine	100 mg	1000 mg
Thioridazine	100 mg	800 mg
Haloperidol	2 mg	20 mg
Trifluoperazine	5 mg	60 mg
Fluphenazine	2 mg	60 mg

1. Acute Onset EPS such as Acute Dystonia and Oculogyric Crisis

In these cases, symptoms appear within hours of administration of the drug. Acute Dystonia presents with sustained painful contractions of a group of muscles in the head and neck region or limb muscle. Oculogyric crisis presents with sustained and painful involuntary upward rolling of the eyeballs. Both these acute EPS can be managed with promethazine given parenterally. Promethazine, under its anticholinergic action, alleviates the side effects arising from D_2 blockade in the basal ganglia. (D_2 blockades lead to an increase in the acetylcholine activity in the striatum leading to EPS)

2. Subacute Onset EPS such as Pseudoparkinsonism and Akathisia

Pseudoparkinsonism is the most common presentation of D_2 blockade in the basal ganglia by typical antipsychotics. It presents with Parkinsonian features such as akinesia, bradykinesia, rigidity, resting tremor, and drooling of saliva. It occurs due to the blockade of D_2 receptors in the nigrostriatal pathway. Drug-induced Parkinsonian features can be controlled with anticholinergic agents like trihexyphenidyl or benzhexol. Dopamine D_2 receptors blockade in the nigrostriatal pathway leads to excessive cholinergic activity in the basal ganglia such as putamen and caudate nucleus. Blocking of muscarinic cholinergic receptors effectively neutralizes this imbalance of neurotransmitters in the basal ganglia and alleviates symptoms of drug-induced Parkinsonism. Drug-induced Parkinsonian features are bilaterally symmetrical in presentation while those associated with Parkinson's disease tend to be more on one side of the body (for example in Parkinson's disease rigidity on the right or left half of the body will be more than that of the other half).

Akathisia presents with a feeling of inner restlessness, a tendency to move constantly, not finding solace in taking rest, increased heartbeat, sleep difficulties, etc. On observation, these patients are restless, constantly moving around, not able to sit or sleep even for a while, and are visibly distressed. The subjective sensation of inner restlessness and discomfort is so distressing that some patients think of committing suicide. Akathisia is more common with newer agents like aripiprazole and lurasidone but is also common with first-generation antipsychotics. Akathisia can be effectively controlled with anxiolytics like benzodiazepines, propranolol, or low-dose mirtazapine.

3. Chronic Onset EPS such as Tardive Dyskinesia and Tardive Dystonia

Tardive dyskinesia or TD is the most troublesome side effect of long-term treatment with typical antipsychotics. It presents with involuntary, rhythmic contractions of a group of muscles. It typically involves muscles of the head and neck region followed by limb muscles, although truncal muscle can also be involved. Common presentations are the darting movement of the tongue, lip smacking, facial grimacing, head nodding, etc. Symptoms of TD are cosmetically disabling and carry a significant stigma in society and also remain even after discontinuation of the offending agent.

Tardive dystonia is another chronic complication of treatment with typical antipsychotics, but the incidence is rare as compared to TD. It presents with intermittent spasms of muscle groups resulting in painful and distressing muscle contractions such as torticollis and blepharospasm. Injection of botulinum toxin into the muscle is the most efficacious treatment of tardive dystonia.

Mechanism of TD

Chronic blockage of D_2 receptors in basal ganglia with typical antipsychotics leads to receptor hypersensitivity of D_2 receptor and also oxidative damage of dopaminergic neurons in basal ganglia. This leads to compensatory sprouting of dopaminergic pathways in other parts of the basal ganglia via maladaptive neuroplasticity. These maladaptive neuroplastic changes more commonly involve parts of basal ganglia controlling head and neck muscles and limb muscles due to their greater representation in basal ganglia (analogous to a representation of motor homunculus in the precentral gyrus). These abnormal dopaminergic tracts discharge from time to time leading to the abnormal involuntary rhythmic contractions of muscles. These maladaptive neuroplastic changes remain even after the discontinuation of the offending drug which explains the permanent nature of this condition.

Treatment of TD

Treatment involves stopping the offending drug and discontinuing any anticholinergic drugs still being taken by the patient. Clozapine, an antipsychotic which can improve symptoms of TD, may be prescribed to control symptoms of psychosis after withdrawal of the offending antipsychotic medication. Tetrabenazine, a VMAT2 (vesicular monoamine transporter 2) inhibitor is generally prescribed to control TD. Other medications having some efficacy against TD are amantadine, vitamin E, etc. Medications with antioxidant properties such as ginkgo biloba extract and vitamin E have better efficacy in controlling symptoms of TD and should be considered first-line drugs.

Other Side Effects

Blocking dopamine D_2 receptors in the tuberoinfundibular tract leads to an increased level of prolactin in the body. Hyperprolactinemia presents with galactorrhoea, breast engorgement, menstrual irregularities, and secondary infertility in females. In males, increased prolactin level leads to loss of libido, erectile dysfunction, and gynecomastia. These side effects are more common with high-potency antipsychotics like haloperidol and pimozide.

Low-potency antipsychotics like chlorpromazine also block muscarinic cholinergic receptors. They cause anticholinergic side effects presenting with dry mouth, blurring of vision, constipation, urinary retention, etc. These side effects are even made worse by concomitant prescription of anticholinergics like trihexyphenidyl.

Blockade of the H_1 antihistamine receptor leads to sedation (beneficial for patients with sleep problems), increased appetite, and weight gain. Similarly, alpha-1 adrenergic receptor blockade can lead to orthostatic hypotension and pedal edema. However, these side effects are more common with second-generation antipsychotics than first-generation ones.

Neuroleptic Malignant syndrome is a serious side effect associated with typical antipsychotics, especially haloperidol. Risk factors for the development of NMS include higher doses of typical antipsychotics, older age group or young children, manic patients, low body mass, comorbid substance abuse, etc. It presents with hyperthermia, rigidity, autonomic instability, and altered mental status. Complications associated with NMS are electrolyte imbalance, dehydration, muscle breakdown causing myoglobinuria and acute kidney injury (AKI), coma, and death. A prompt diagnosis followed by pragmatic treatment is necessary to save the patient. Treatment involves immediate stopping of the offending drug, cooling with cold sponging, intravenous fluid therapy, securing the airway, etc. Specific antidotes for NMS include dantrolene sodium and bromocriptine.

SECOND GENERATION ANTIPSYCHOTICS

Second-generation antipsychotics are also known as atypical antipsychotics. Under their pharmacodynamic actions, they are also known as serotonin dopamine antagonists or SDAs. Clozapine, marketed in 1970, was the first SDA coming into clinical use for schizophrenia. Clozapine was followed by other SDAs such as risperidone, olanzapine, quetiapine, aripiprazole, ziprasidone, amisulpride, lurasidone and cariprazine (newer agents such as aripiprazole, lurasidone, and cariprazine are both efficacious and metabolically safe and also less prone to develop EPS. These agents are considered as third generation antipsychotics by some authors).

SGAs are known as atypical antipsychotics as they are less prone to develop EPS. However, some SGAs such as risperidone and amisulpride are comparable to typical antipsychotics in terms of proneness to develop EPS and others such as olanzapine can also cause EPS at higher doses. Only clozapine and quetiapine are strictly atypical as they are not associated with the development of EPS. Less risk of development of EPS with SGAs is due to their serotonin antagonistic actions which mitigate the effects of dopamine blockade in the basal ganglia and some such as clozapine and quetiapine do not block dopamine receptors to a significant extent.

Indications

1. Schizophrenia, currently SGAs are the first line of treatment for schizophrenia because of their good efficacy and tolerability.
2. BPAD (SGAs are also indicated in controlling aggression and psychosis in mania and are also indicated in bipolar depression).
3. Acute psychosis
4. Delusional disorders
5. Substance-induced psychosis
6. Behavioral disturbance in ADHD or Autism, low dose risperidone treatment of choice in controlling troublesome behaviors in childhood.
7. To control psychosis associated with organic conditions such as dementia and delirium.

Mechanism of Action

All second-generation antipsychotics have a variable degree of dopamine D_2 antagonistic activity. Some also have actions on other dopamine receptors, e.g. clozapine and

Table 20.2: Dose range of second-generation or atypical antipsychotics

Drug	*Minimum effective dose*	*Maximum dose*
Clozapine*	100 mg	900 mg
Risperidone	2 mg	8 mg
Olanzapine	5 mg	20 mg
Quetiapine	100 mg	400 mg
Aripiprazole	10 mg	30 mg
Amisulpride	50 mg	600–800 mg
Lurasidone	20 mg	80 mg

*Minimum therapeutic dose of clozapine is 100 mg. However, to minimize side effects (sedation and postural hypotension) it is started at a low dose of 12.5 mg, and the dose is gradually increased.

olanzapine have D_4 antagonistic activity and lurasidone and aripiprazole act as D_1 agonists. Apart from action on the dopamine system, all of them also have strong antagonistic action on serotonin 5HT2A/2C receptors which is responsible for a lower probability of EPS with SGAs (detailed discussion of which is beyond the scope of this book). Newer agents such as aripiprazole, lurasidone, and cariprazine also act as agonists on 5HT1 receptors.

Side Effects

Acute side effects of SGAs arise due to their antihistaminic, anticholinergic, and alpha-adrenergic blocking actions. They cause sedation and increased appetite under their H_1 antihistaminic actions. Anticholinergic side effects include dry mouth, blurring of vision, constipation, and urinary retention. Alpha-adrenergic blocking action leads to orthostatic hypotension and lightheadedness. These side effects are mainly seen with pine groups of drugs such as olanzapine, clozapine, and quetiapine. Newer SDAs such as amisulpride, lurasidone, and aripiprazole are less prone to develop these side effects.

Long-term treatment with SGAs can lead to increased cardiovascular risks known as the 'metabolic highway'. It starts with increased appetite ultimately leading to central obesity, insulin resistance, type 2 diabetes mellitus, and hypertension. All these factors increase the risk of adverse cardiovascular events such as MI or stroke. These adverse effects are more common with olanzapine, clozapine, risperidone, and quetiapine but less common with amisulpride, lurasidone, and aripiprazole. Aripiprazole can reverse these risk factors developed after taking other SGAs.

Among SDAs risperidone and amisulpride are significantly more prone to develop EPS and hyperprolactinemia.

General Principles of Antipsychotic Therapy

When a drug-naive psychotic patient comes for treatment, a second-generation antipsychotic is selected depending on patient characteristics, symptomatology, and comorbidities. Patients presenting with prominent positive symptoms (delusions and hallucinations) respond well to strong D_2 blockers like risperidone and amisulpride while those with prominent negative symptoms respond well to olanzapine and lurasidone. A trial of any one antipsychotic is given for a period of 6 weeks and treatment response is evaluated. In case of poor response to the first antipsychotic, it should be stopped and another second-generation antipsychotic or a first-generation antipsychotic should be tried. Efficacy wise both first and second-generation antipsychotics are comparable to one another but first-generation antipsychotics are avoided because of side effects such as EPS and tardive dyskinesia.

In case of poor response to 2 or more antipsychotics given for an adequate period in an adequate dose, the case is diagnosed as resistant psychosis and clozapine should be started. Many cases of resistant schizophrenia respond well to clozapine and improvement in cognition is so much so that it is known as 'cognitive re-awakening '. In the case of the first episode of psychosis, antipsychotics should be given for a period of 1 year and then tapered gradually. In case of relapse, treatment should be continued for life.

ANTIDEPRESSANTS

TRICYCLIC ANTIDEPRESSANT OR TCA

TCAs are antidepressants coming to clinical use in 1959 and imipramine was the first TCA used for the treatment of depression. Subsequently, other TCAs were marketed for the treatment of depression and other neurotic illnesses. Gradually, TCAs were superseded by SSRIs as first-line treatment for depression not because of their superior efficacy but because of better side effects profile and less toxicity on overdose. Despite this, many TCAs are still used for a variety of neurotic illnesses to this date.

TCAs are named as such because of the basic three-ring structure shared by all of them. However, individual agents differ from one another based on side chains attached to the basic three-ring structure. These side chains also determine their receptor binding profile, efficacy, and side effects profile. Following are some of the most commonly used TCAs in psychiatry practice.

1. Imipramine
2. Amitriptyline
3. Nortriptyline
4. Doxepin
5. Dosulepin, formerly known as dothiepin
6. Amoxapine
7. Clomipramine

Another class of antidepressants similar to TCAs is known as tetracyclic antidepressants which include trazodone and nefazodone. Tetracyclines are comparable to tricyclics as per their indications and side effects profile.

Indications

Tricyclic antidepressants are used for several psychiatric illnesses as mentioned below:

1. Depressive disorders including MDD
2. Generalized anxiety disorder
3. Somatic symptom disorders
4. Psychosomatic disorders such as fibromyalgia and irritable bowel syndrome
5. Neuropathic pain disorders
6. OCD (clomipramine is considered a second-line drug)
7. Nocturnal enuresis (imipramine is a second-line drug)

Table 20.3: Dose range of TCAs

Drug	*Dose range*
Imipramine	25–300 mg
Amitriptyline	25–300 mg
Nortriptyline	75–150 mg
Doxepin	25–300 mg
Dosulepin or dothiepin	75–150 mg
Amoxapine	25–500 mg
Clomipramine	25–250 mg

TCAs such as amitriptyline, nortriptyline, and dosulepin are clinically used as first-line medications for functional pain disorders such as somatoform disorder, fibromyalgia, and irritable bowel syndrome. For depressive disorders, they have been replaced by SSRIs and are only used as second-line medications when there is poor response to SSRIs.

Mechanism of Action

TCAs exert their antidepressant actions by increasing the levels of serotonin and noradrenaline in the synaptic clefts by blocking their reuptake back into the presynaptic nerve endings. Individual agents differ in their relative actions on serotonin and noradrenaline reuptake which is responsible for their differential efficacies in various neurotic conditions. For example, clomipramine mainly inhibits serotonin reuptake and is hence better suited for OCD while the action of nortriptyline and doxepin on noradrenergic reuptake is more than serotonin for which they are better suited for functional pain disorders. Apart from this, TCAs also have activities on histamine H_1 receptor, muscarinic cholinergic receptors, and alpha-adrenergic receptors which dictate their side effect profiles.

Side Effects

Because of increased serotonin levels in GI tracts, they can cause gastric discomfort, and sexual side effects are due to increased serotonin levels in the brain. Increased noradrenaline levels in the brain can cause exaggeration of anxiety symptoms at the start of therapy which subsides by itself after some days.

Inhibitory action on the H_1 histamine receptor in the brain and hypothalamus leads to the following symptoms.

1. Sedation, sometimes desirable in patients with depression, GAD, and OCD
2. Increased appetite
3. Weight gain and central obesity

Similarly, anticholinergic symptoms are due to the blockade of muscarinic cholinergic receptors in the body and present with

1. Dry mouth
2. Blurring of vision
3. Urinary retention and
4. Constipation

(These symptoms generally improve on continuing with the drugs for a few weeks) Alpha-adrenergic blockade leads to orthostatic hypotension and light headedness for which they should be prescribed at night and should be prescribed cautiously in older patients because of the risk of falls.

TCA Toxicity

TCAs have a narrow therapeutic index and overdose can lead to life-threatening adverse effects. Overdose generally leads to cardiac toxicity such as heart block and ventricular fibrillations. Because of these life-threatening adverse effects of an overdose of these drugs, TCAs are falling out of favor as treatment of depressive disorders as depression is associated with a significant risk of suicide by consuming prescribed medications in excess amounts. Otherwise, TCAs have good efficacy and desirable effects such as sedation when prescribed for cases of depressive disorders.

SELECTIVE SEROTONIN REUPTAKE INHIBITORS OR SSRIS

Selective serotonin reuptake inhibitors or SSRIs are a group of drugs used for the treatment of several psychiatric conditions ranging from MDD to PTSD.

These drugs are named as such because of their primary mode of action; inhibition of the reuptake of serotonin neurotransmitter from the synaptic cleft after their release from the nerve terminal, thereby increasing their availability to act on the receptors. A lower level of activity of serotonin is implicated in several psychiatric conditions and increasing serotonin level via SSRIs improves these conditions.

There are six principal SSRIs in clinical use which are mentioned below.

1. Fluoxetine
2. Citalopram
3. Escitalopram
4. Sertraline
5. Paroxetine and
6. Fluvoxamine

All SSRIs mentioned above increase serotonin activity in the synaptic cleft as the principal mode of action. However, despite similar principal modes of action, these drugs subtly differ from one another in another minor mode of action (for example fluoxetine has additional 5HT2C receptor antagonist, sertraline has dopaminergic activities via DAT inhibitory action, and paroxetine has additional anticholinergic action). These minor modes of action may be subtle but may be a deciding factor when choosing a drug on a case-to-case basis depending on the presenting symptoms.

Indications

SSRIs are one of the most commonly prescribed psychotropic medications in psychiatric clinics. Their indications range from depression and anxiety in adults to behavioral disturbances in children and during stroke recovery in geriatric patients. A few common indications are mentioned below:

1. Depressive disorders, especially MDD
2. Bipolar depression (along with second-generation antipsychotics)
3. Generalized anxiety disorder
4. Phobic anxiety disorders
5. PTSD

Table 20.4: Dose range of SSRIs

Drug	*Dose range*
Fluoxetine	20–80 mg
Citalopram	20–40 mg
Escitalopram	10–20 mg
Sertraline	50–100 mg
Paroxetine and	10–30 mg
Fluvoxamine	50–300 mg

Higher doses are required in the treatment of OCD.

6. OCD
7. To control stereotypes in autism
8. Borderline personality disorder
9. Eating disorders, e.g. bulimia nervosa
10. Post-stroke depression

Mechanism of Action

Serotonin is synthesized and stored in serotonergic neurons housed in the raphe nuclei situated in the midbrain. Serotonergic neurons from these locations are projected to various other parts of the brain (cerebral cortex, limbic system, etc). Serotonin, once released, acts on various serotonergic receptors ranging from 5HT1 to 5HT7. Once its action is over, it is cleared from the synaptic cleft via reuptake transport (SERT) back into the serotonergic neurons. SSRIs block the reuptake of serotonin from the synaptic cleft back into the serotonergic neurons by blocking the reuptake transporter (SERT) thereby prolonging the availability of serotonin in the synaptic cleft and increasing the activity of serotonin on the receptors. This action of SSRIs helps mitigate conditions arising due to low serotonin activity in the brain.

Side Effects

Apart from increasing serotonin in the CNS, SSRIs also increase serotonin levels in other parts of the body such as in the GI tract, which is responsible for most of the side effects of SSRIs as mentioned below.

1. Gastric discomfort, nausea, vomiting, and diarrhea due to increased serotonin in the GI tract.
2. Sexual dysfunction such as decreased libido, erectile dysfunction, and delayed ejaculation due to an increase in the level of serotonin in the brain.
3. Increased risk of bleeding due to impaired platelet aggregation.
4. Increased suicidal ideation in young patients
5. Manic switch, when SSRIs are prescribed alone for bipolar depression, the patient may switch from a depressive episode to a manic episode.
6. Serotonin syndrome is a rare but dreadful adverse effect of SSSIs. It is characterized by confusion, vasomotor instability, increased temperature, and rigidity. The risk of developing serotonin syndrome is more with the co-prescription of serotonergic agents such as one SSRI along with another SSRI, SNRI, or TCA. Because of this, co-prescription of serotonergic agents should be avoided.

Discontinuation Syndrome

Sudden stoppage of ongoing therapy with an SSRI leads to discontinuation syndrome characterized by low mood, subjective discomfort, irritability, tingling and numbness of limbs, and an electric shock-like sensation inside the brain (known as brain zaps). These symptoms are more common with paroxetine and escitalopram and are less common with fluoxetine because of its longer washout period (half-life is 8–12 days). Discontinuation symptoms can be avoided or at least minimized by stopping an SSRI in tapering doses or replacing other SSRIs with fluoxetine at the time of stopping. Once developed, discontinuation symptoms can be managed by re-introducing the earlier SSRI or by giving another SSRI such as fluoxetine.

SELECTIVE SEROTONIN AND NOR-EPINEPHRINE REUPTAKE INHIBITORS OR SNRIS

These are a group of drugs that selectively block the reuptake of both serotonin and nor-adrenaline. These two principal amine neurotransmitters are implicated in several neuroses such as anxiety disorders, somatic symptom disorders, and depressive disorders. These are mainly preserved as second-line medications and are prescribed when the response to SSRIs is poor. The drugs in this class are

1. Duloxetine
2. Venlafaxine
3. Desvenlafaxine and
4. Milnacipran

Mechanism of Action

SNRIs selectively block the reuptake of serotonin and noradrenaline neurotransmitters from the synaptic cleft leading to their continued availability for their action on respective receptors. In this regard, SNRIs differ from TCAs (which also inhibit serotonin and noradrenaline reuptake from synaptic cleft) as TCAs are nonselective and also possess other properties such as antihistamine and anticholinergic properties. SNRIs are devoid of these undesired actions and hence impart fewer side effects than TCAs. At the same time, being selective both for serotonin and noradrenaline, they have a greater range of therapeutic actions than SSRIs which have only serotonin reuptake inhibitor properties.

Indications of SNRIs

SNRIs have a wide range of indications encompassing all psychiatric diagnoses where SSRIs and TCAs can be prescribed. However, they are generally preserved as second-line medications and are indicated only when the response to an SSRI is unsatisfactory. Under their noradrenergic action, SNRIs are a good choice for any neurotic condition presenting with associated somatic symptoms. Few indications where they can be given even as first-line medications are

1. Major depressive disorder
2. Premenstrual dysphoric disorder or PMDD
3. Anxiety disorders
4. Somatic symptom disorders and
5. Fibromyalgia

Side Effects

All the side effects associated with SSRIs are also seen with SNRIs. Furthermore, due to noradrenergic action, few additional side effects may be seen with these drugs. Common side effects are:

1. Gastric discomfort with nausea, vomiting, and diarrhea
2. Increased anxiety and restlessness for the first few days to weeks
3. Sleep disturbances, especially when taken at night
4. Increased blood pressure, should be prescribed cautiously in patients with HTN
5. Suicidal ideation in young children
6. Manic switch in bipolar depression cases
7. Sexual dysfunctions are less common with SNRIs under their noradrenergic actions
8. Serotonin syndrome especially when co-prescribed with other serotonergic drugs

9. Discontinuation syndrome is seen when SNRIs are stopped suddenly. Symptoms are similar to that of SSRI discontinuation syndrome.

MONOAMINE OXIDASE INHIBITORS OR MAOIs

Monoamine oxidases or MAOs are enzymes involved in clearing off monoamines from the synaptic cleft. Inhibiting these enzymes leads to an increase in the level of monoamines such as serotonin and noradrenaline in the synaptic cleft. There are two types of MAOs such as MAO-A and MAO-B. MAO-A is principally involved in metabolizing serotonin and noradrenaline while MAO-B targets dopamine. MAO inhibitors can be selective for MAO-A or MAO-B or may be non-selective as mentioned below:

1. Nonselective MAO inhibitors
   - Isocarboxazid
   - Phenelzine
   - Tranylcypromine
2. Reversible inhibitors of MAO-A or RIMAs
   - Moclobemide
   - Lazabemide
3. MAO-B inhibitors
   - Selegiline
   - Rasagiline

Indications

1. MAO inhibitors are one of the most efficacious drugs for major depressive disorder. However, because of unwanted side effects, they are reserved for resistant cases of depression.
2. Bipolar depression, there is good efficacy in bipolar depression.
3. Anxiety disorders, especially agoraphobia and social anxiety disorder.
4. OCD, as second-line therapy in resistant cases of OCD
5. MAO-B inhibitors are used for the treatment of Parkinson's disease

Side Effects

MAO inhibitors increase the levels of serotonin and norepinephrine in the brain and also in other parts of the body which explain their side effects profile.

1. Gastric discomfort
2. Increased anxiety for a few days after starting therapy
3. Sexual side effects
4. Insomnia especially when taken at night
5. Manic switch in cases of BPAD

Tyramine Reaction

Tyramine is a monoamine present in some food sources like aged cheese, wine, etc, and is cleared from the body via degradation by MAO enzymes. When these foods are consumed by a person taking MAO inhibitors, tyramine is not able to be degraded leading to an increased level of nor-adrenaline (tyramine triggers nerve cells to release noradrenaline). This can lead to hypertensive crises and death. Therefore, tyramine-containing foods are contraindicated in persons taking MAOIs.

Reversible inhibitors of MAO or RIMAs such as moclobemide are not associated with tyramine reaction as being reversible they can be replaced from their binding sites by increased levels of tyramine. However, RIMAs are somewhat less efficacious than nonselective MAOIs such as tranylcypromine.

MISCELLANEOUS ANTIDEPRESSANTS

Mirtazapine

Mirtazapine is an atypical antidepressant with a unique mode of action that is different from classical antidepressants such as TCAs and SSRIs. It is classified as NaSSA or noradrenergic and selective serotonin antidepressant which means it blocks the reuptake of noradrenaline and acts as an antagonist at serotonin receptors. It is an efficacious antidepressant with additional sedating, anxiolytic and antiemetic properties under its antihistaminic action. Because of its good sedative properties, mirtazapine is particularly suitable for agitated depression with suicidal tendencies. Mirtazapine is indicated in the following cases mostly as add-on therapy with other primary agents.

1. Major depressive disorder
2. Bipolar depression
3. Generalized anxiety disorder
4. Anxiety associated with some stressful events
5. Primary insomnia

Side effects of mirtazapine include excessive sedation, postural hypotension, lethargy, etc.

Bupropion

Bupropion is an atypical antidepressant whose primary targets are noradrenaline and dopamine neurotransmitters. It is classified as NDRI or noradrenaline and dopamine reuptake inhibitor. It blocks the NET (noradrenaline transporter) in the cerebral cortex which is responsible for the reuptake of both noradrenaline and dopamine. Increased activity of noradrenaline and dopamine in the cerebral cortex relieves depressive symptoms and improves cognition and attention. Indications of bupropion are:

1. Major depressive disorder
2. Bipolar depression
3. Seasonal affective disorder
4. Smoking cessation
5. SSRI-induced sexual dysfunction
6. Adult ADHD

Bupropion therapy can increase anxiety (should not be given in depression with prominent anxiety symptoms) and is associated with insomnia when given at night, poor appetite, and agitation. Bupropion is safe in bipolar depression as there is less chance of manic switch when compared with SSRIs and SNRIs.

MOOD STABILIZERS

Mood stabilizers have antimanic, antidepressant, and prophylactic properties and are the mainstay of treatment for bipolar disorder. Lithium, the first mood stabilizer used clinically, is the gold standard mood stabilizer. Subsequently, carbamazepine (and oxcarbazepine), sodium valproate, and lamotrigine also came into clinical use as mood stabilizers. The most important clinical aspect is to select a specific agent for a patient with BPAD, considering various patient-specific factors. Some mood stabilizers such as lithium and sodium valproate have good antimanic properties while others, especially lamotrigine, have good antidepressant properties. Recently, second-generation antipsychotics are widely used as mood stabilizers either in combination with other mood stabilizers or as monotherapy.

LITHIUM AS A MOOD STABILIZER

The mood-stabilizing property of lithium was discovered serendipitously in 1948. In those days it was in rampant use for gouty arthritis and was available as 'bear lithia water'. Subsequently, it was used as an antimanic and prophylactic agent in patients with BPAD. Until the late 1980s, it was the sole mood-stabilizing agent available in the market. In the 1980s anti suicidal action of lithium was discovered further bolstering its use as a mood stabilizer.

Mechanism of Action

Lithium is handled by the body as it handles sodium. Hence, hyperactive nerve cells (in patients of BPAD) intake lithium in place of sodium to some extent resulting in depleted levels of sodium ions inside these cells. As a consequence, the sodium-dependent intracellular cascade involving the IP3-DAG pathway fails to get activated as the required level of sodium ion is not achieved. This leads to the failure of the nerve cells in achieving hyperactivity. This is how lithium exerts its antimanic and mood-stabilizing actions.

However, just a slight increase in the level of lithium further replaces intracellular sodium ions and these cells cannot get activated normally leading to lithium toxicity. This explains the narrow therapeutic index of lithium.

Lithium is available as lithium carbonate which is to be taken orally. It is indicated in the following conditions.

1. In the manic episode of BPAD, lithium is indicated in clear-cut cases of BPAD presenting with euphoric mania, with good interepisode functioning, and in patients with a family history of mood disorder. It usually takes 1–3 weeks to exert its antimanic action.
2. Prophylaxis of BPAD (is quite effective in preventing manic episodes in cases of BPAD and somewhat less effective in preventing depressive episodes).
3. As an augmenting agent in resistant depression.
4. Cyclothymia
5. In borderline personality disorder with frequent self-harm behaviors. Lithium has proven efficacy in controlling self-harm and suicidal behavior.

Side Effects

The use of lithium is limited by its side effects which are described below.

1. Fine tremor
2. Bradycardia
3. Polydipsia and polyuria
4. Sialorrhea
5. Diarrhea

6. Hyper- or hypothyroidism
7. Teratogenic effects, when given in an early period of pregnancy can cause a cardiac defect known as Abstein anomaly.

Lithium Toxicity

Lithium has a very narrow therapeutic index and just a slight increase in the dose can lead to devastating toxic effects. A therapeutic blood level of lithium ranges from 0.8 to 1.2 mEq/L. Toxic effects start just above the blood level of 1.5 mEq/L. Because of the narrow therapeutic index, blood level monitoring is advised in all cases of lithium therapy. Because of the toxic effects on the heart, kidney, and thyroid gland, kidney and thyroid function tests and ECG should be done in all cases before lithium therapy. Symptoms of lithium toxicity are:

1. Confusion with coarse tremors and ataxia
2. Seizure
3. Sick sinus syndrome and heart block
4. Diarrhea and vomiting
5. Acute renal failure

Lithium toxicity is treated with adequate hydration and hemodialysis to eliminate the excess amount of lithium ions present in the body.

ANTIEPILEPTICS AS MOOD STABILIZER

SODIUM VALPROATE

Sodium valproate is an antiepileptic agent used as an antimanic drug in cases of BPAD. It is a sodium salt of valproic acid which in turn is derived from valeric acid. Another sodium salt of valproic acid is known as divalproex sodium, which is a mixture of sodium valproate and valproic acid. Sodium valproate is not effective in the depressive phase of BPAD.

Mechanism of Action

Sodium valproate is a broad-spectrum antiepileptic agent with varied mechanisms of action. It acts as a sodium channel blocker, calcium channel blocker, and GABA mimetic. Its sodium channel-blocking action is primarily responsible for its antimanic and prophylactic properties in cases of BPAD.

Indications

Sodium valproate is a commonly used antiepileptic medication and is also frequently prescribed in psychiatric clinics. Some of the major indications of sodium valproate are:

1. Manic episodes of BPAD (it is particularly useful for dysphoric mania and BPAD with comorbid substance abuse).
2. Prophylactic treatment of BPAD is effective in controlling manic episodes but less effective in controlling depressive episodes.
3. Sodium valproate is the drug of choice for rapid-cycling bipolar disorder.
4. In controlling aggression associated with any psychiatric conditions.
5. Migraine prophylaxis and
6. In generalized seizure disorders such as GTCS, absence seizure, etc.

Side Effects of Sodium Valproate

Sodium valproate is generally well tolerated. However, it is associated with the following side effects

1. Gastric discomfort with nausea and vomiting as sodium valproate is acidic in nature.
2. Dry mouth and sedation
3. Weight gain on long-term use
4. Alopecia which is quite troublesome for young patients
5. For PCOS, sodium valproate is not preferred in women of childbearing age groups because of the development of PCOS.
6. Fine tremor
7. Teratogenicity (sodium valproate is contraindicated in the first trimester of pregnancy as it is associated with neural tube defects. If sodium valproate cannot be avoided then concomitant folic acid administration is necessary to reduce the risk).

Adverse Toxic Effects of Sodium Valproate

Treatment with sodium valproate can lead to some life-threatening toxic effects although such adverse effects are rare. Some of these such as fulminant hepatic failure and acute pancreatitis are idiosyncratic while others are dose-dependent. A psychiatrist must be vigilant regarding the possible emergence of these life-threatening adverse effects and warn the patient regarding such possibility. These adverse effects are enumerated below:

1. Acute fulminant hepatitis
2. Acute hemorrhaging pancreatic
3. Steven–Johnson syndrome (SJS)
4. Hyperammonemia
5. Acute encephalopathy presenting with confusion, tremor, and ataxia

Sodium valproate is safe and effective in the manic state of bipolar disorder. However, while prescribing sodium valproate proper patient selection and monitoring for the possible emergence of side effects must be considered.

CARBAMAZEPINE AND OXCARBAZEPINE

Carbamazepine is an antiepileptic medication frequently used as an antimanic agent and also for prophylactic therapy in BPAD. Carbamazepine is quite effective but carries black box warnings for the development of SJS and agranulocytosis. Its congener, oxcarbazepine, is associated with far fewer incidences of SJS and agranulocytosis. However, there is less evidence in support of its efficacy in bipolar disorder.

Indications of Carbamazepine

1. The manic episode of BPAD
2. prophylactic therapy in bipolar disorder
3. Seizure disorders, especially partial seizures, and also some generalized seizures.
4. Trigeminal neuralgia, it is drug of choice for prophylaxis of trigeminal neuralgia
5. Alcohol withdrawal, especially uncomplicated alcohol withdrawal state
6. Neuropathic pain disorders

Mechanism of Action

Carbamazepine (and oxcarbazepine) inhibits voltage-gated sodium channels, thereby inhibiting excessive activation of the cerebral cortex. As we know that hyperactivity of the frontal cortex is associated with manic symptoms, inhibition of cortical tissue leads to the gradual resolution of manic symptoms. Continuing treatment with carbamazepine also prevents further excessive activation of cortical tissue which explains its prophylactic efficacy in cases of BPAD.

Side Effects of Carbamazepine

1. Sedation
2. Gastric discomfort with nausea and vomiting
3. Ataxia
4. Diplopia or double vision
5. Confusion

Treatment with carbamazepine can results in some life-threatening adverse effects most of which are idiosyncratic (non-dose dependent) as follows

1. Bone marrow suppression leading to agranulocytosis and aplastic anemia
2. Hepatotoxicity
3. Steven–Johnson syndrome and toxic epidermal necrolysis, more common with carbamazepine than oxcarbazepine
4. Hyponatremia is especially associated with oxcarbazepine

Carbamazepine may be used as a mood stabilizer in cases where sodium valproate is not considered safe. However, the therapist must be vigilant about the possible emergence of serious adverse effects such as SJS and agranulocytosis.

LAMOTRIGINE

Lamotrigine is an antiepileptic drug used as a mood stabilizer in cases of bipolar disorder. Lamotrigine is primarily indicated for depressive episodes of bipolar I and bipolar II disorders. It is especially efficacious in preventing depressive episodes and somewhat less effective against manic episodes.

Mechanism of Action

Lamotrigine exerts its antiepileptic effects probably by blocking voltage-gated sodium channels and voltage-gated calcium channels. Its inhibitory action on sodium and calcium channels explains its effectiveness in bipolar disorders.

Indications of Lamotrigine

1. The depressive episode of bipolar disorder. It is used as second-line medication for this indication.
2. Prophylactic therapy in bipolar disorders. Lamotrigine is especially effective in preventing depressive episodes than manic episodes. As bipolar II disorder is associated with frequent depressive episodes, lamotrigine is best suited for this category of bipolar disorder.
3. Generalized seizure disorders such as GTCS, is a first-line drug for generalized seizure disorders

4. Focal onset seizure disorders, it is usually used as adjunctive therapy in resistant cases of focal onset seizures
5. Lamotrigine is also used off-label for neuropathic pain disorders, trigeminal neuralgia, migraine prophylaxis, etc.

Side Effects of Lamotrigine

Treatment with lamotrigine is associated with the following side effects.

1. Sedation and lethargy
2. Gastric discomfort with nausea and vomiting
3. Headache
4. Dizziness
5. Tingling of extremities

Adverse Effects of Lamotrigine

Lamotrigine is associated with serious skin rash often leading to the development of SJS and toxic epidermal necrolysis (TEN). The incidence of serious allergic reactions with lamotrigine is 1 in 100. Any history of allergic reaction to other food products or history of allergic rhinitis or dermatitis should be enquired about before starting lamotrigine. Skin rash with lamotrigine is idiosyncratic in nature and generally occurs within a few days to weeks after treatment and is rare after months of treatment. The patient and family members must be made aware of the possible emergence of skin allergies. In case of rash or other severe skin reactions, the medicine must be stopped and the patient should be immediately brought to the casualty department. Treatment is with intravenous injection of hydrocortisone and antihistamines such as promethazine or diphenhydramine. In case of the development of SJS and TEN, the patient must be hospitalized and homeostasis should be maintained.

Second-generation Antipsychotics as Mood Stabilizers

There is a new trend in the treatment of bipolar disorder with second-generation antipsychotics replacing conventional mood stabilizers in the treatment of acute episodes (both manic and depressive episodes). Olanzapine is the first SGA approved for the treatment of acute manic episodes. Subsequently, a few other SGAs were also approved for this indication. Currently, the following 6 SGAs are in clinical use for acute episodes of BPAD

1. Olanzapine
2. Quetiapine
3. Aripiprazole

Table 20.5: Dose range of mood stabilizers in bipolar disorder

Drug	*Starting dose*	*Maximum daily dose*	*Plasma level*
Lithium	300 mg	900–1800 mg	0.6–1.2 mEq/L
Sodium valproate	500 mg	1500 mg	50–125 μg/mL
Carbamazepine	400 mg	1500–1800 mg	4–12 μg/mL
*Lamotrigine	12.5–25 mg	400 mg	—

*Therapeutic dose range of lamotrigine is 200–400 mg per day. However, it is started at low doses for fear of the emergence of an allergic reaction.

4. Ziprasidone
5. Lurasidone and
6. Cariprazine

Olanzapine is primarily indicated for acute manic episodes either as monotherapy or in combination with other mood stabilizers. Olanzapine in combination with fluoxetine is also first-line therapy for bipolar depressive episodes. Quetiapine is also mentioned as a first-line drug for bipolar depression. Both olanzapine and quetiapine can also be used in the maintenance therapy of BPAD either as monotherapy or in combination with conventional mood stabilizers. However, long-term treatment with these drugs can lead to weight gain, obesity, insulin resistance, and dyslipidemia. Therefore, they are of limited use in patients with metabolic syndrome.

Newer SGAs such as aripiprazole, lurasidone, and cariprazine have potent antidepressant efficacy and are approved for the treatment of bipolar depression. These medications are suitable for patients where pines are not considered safe. Aripiprazole, lurasidone, and cariprazine can be used either alone or in combination with other conventional mood stabilizers for the maintenance therapy of BPAD.

Overall, second-generation antipsychotics are both safe and effective alternatives for the treatment of acute episodes of BPAD and also for prophylaxis. However, specific agents should be selected according to patient characteristics.

SEDATIVES AND HYPNOTICS

Sedatives are drugs that induce calmness in a person while hypnotics are drugs that induce arousable sleep. Many drugs used for sedation also have hypnotic potential and vice-versa. General anesthetics are drugs that induce complete loss of consciousness with loss of bodily sensations, while vital functions remaining unimpaired. Sedatives and hypnotics often act as anesthetic agents at relatively higher doses.

Gamma-aminobutyric acid (GABA) is the primary inhibitory neurotransmitter in the brain which induces calmness and sleep. The action of GABA on the GABA-A receptor is primarily responsible for these actions. GABA-A receptor is a pentamer having five structural subunits: 2 alpha, 2 beta and 1 delta subunits. These subunits span across the cell membrane and are arranged circularly, forming an anion channel at the center which functions as a chloride (Cl^-) channel. In the extracellular part, these subunits form binding sites for various ligands: two GABA binding sites and one BDZ (benzodiazepines) binding site. GABA is the primary endogenous ligand at the GABA binding site leading to the opening of the Cl- channel at the center. This results in increased activity of Chloride inside the cell and subsequent inhibition of the cell resulting in CNS sedation and induction of sleep.

Classification of Sedatives and Hypnotics

1. Barbiturates
2. Benzodiazepines
3. Z-drugs
4. Miscellaneous
   - Antihistamines
   - Buspirone
   - Second-generation antipsychotics

- Doxepin
- Trazodone

BARBITURATES

Barbiturates are sedative-hypnotics drugs derived from barbituric acid. Apart from being used as sedative and hypnotic drugs, they are also widely in use as antiseizure drugs and as general anesthetic agents. Currently, barbiturates are largely replaced by benzodiazepines as sedatives and hypnotics. This is mainly because of the higher abuse potential of barbiturates and increased fatality at toxic doses with no antidote available to treat barbiturate toxicity.

Barbiturates are classified into 4 groups depending on their onset and duration of action

- Long-acting (6 hours) such as phenobarbitone
- Intermediate-acting (3–6 hours) such as amobarbital
- Short-acting (2–3 hours) such as pentobarbital and secobarbital
- Ultra-short acting (duration is less than 30 minutes) such as thiopentone sodium and methohexital sodium)

Mechanism of Action

Barbiturates are GABA mimetics. They bind to the alpha-beta subunits of GABA-A receptors and increase the duration of the opening of the chloride channel thereby increasing the level of chloride ions inside the cell. Increased chloride ions inside the cell result in subsequent deactivation of the nerve cell. This explains the sedative, hypnotic, anxiolytic, anticonvulsant, and anesthetic actions of barbiturates.

Indications

Barbiturates are among the first sedatives and hypnotics used clinically for inducing sleep in cases of insomnia. They were also used for treating anxiety disorders. However, benzodiazepines have largely replaced barbiturates for this use because of their better safety profile and less risk of abuse and dependence. Currently, barbiturates are used for the following conditions:

1. Neonatal seizure, phenobarbital is the drug of choice for neonatal seizures.
2. Status epilepticus
3. Thiopentone sodium and methohexital sodium are used for induction of anesthesia, especially in short procedures such as ECT and dental procedures.

Barbiturates are contraindicated in status asthmaticus, acute intermittent porphyria, and in cases of previous allergic reactions to barbiturates.

Abuse and Dependence

Barbiturates carry high risks of abuse and dependence. Prescribing barbiturates for more than 2–4 weeks for insomnia and anxiety is likely associated with the development of tolerance and dependence. Once dependence has been established, suddenly stopping the drug can lead to severe withdrawal symptoms such as tremors, anxiety, irritability, insomnia, withdrawal seizure, and delirium. The use of barbiturates for insomnia and anxiety is largely limited by the development of tolerance and risk of dependence.

Barbiturate Toxicity

Barbiturates have a narrow therapeutic index and slightly higher doses can lead to toxicity presenting with a lowering of consciousness and labored breathing. The patient may go into a deep coma and can die of respiratory failure. There is no specific antidote for barbiturates overdose. Haemodialysis can help remove the drug from the bloodstream and can prove lifesaving.

BENZODIAZEPINES

Benzodiazepines are a class of sedatives and hypnotic drugs and have largely superseded barbiturates for these indications. The first benzodiazepine, chlordiazepoxide, came into clinical use in 1960. All of them share the same basic chemical structure: fusion of a benzene ring with a diazepine ring. Benzodiazepines are the most commonly prescribed psychotropic medication and are prescribed by both psychiatrists and general physicians alike.

Benzodiazepines are classified according to their predominant clinical role into the following categories:

- Hypnotics (diazepam, lorazepam, nitrazepam, alprazolam, triazolam)
- Anxiolytics (clonazepam, alprazolam, chlordiazepoxide, oxazepam)
- Anticonvulsants (lorazepam, midazolam, clobazam) and
- Muscle relaxants (diazepam, lorazepam)

Although the above classification is more practical and clinically relevant, benzodiazepines are also classified by many authors based on their duration of action: long-acting (chlordiazepoxide), intermediate-acting (lorazepam), short-acting (triazolam) and ultra short-acting (midazolam).

Mechanism of Action Benzodiazepines

Similar to barbiturates, benzodiazepines also enhance the action of GABA by acting on GABA-A receptors. However, in contrast to barbiturates, benzodiazepines increase the frequency of opening of chloride channels. This increase in the frequency of opening of the chloride channel leads to increased activity of chloride ions inside the nerve cells with its subsequent inhibition. This mechanism explains the anxiolytic, sedative, and anticonvulsant actions of benzodiazepines.

Indications of Benzodiazepines

1. Insomnia, benzodiazepines are frequently used both for primary and secondary insomnia. They help in reducing sleep latency time and prevent frequent nighttime awakenings.

Table 20.6: Dose range of commonly used benzodiazepines

Drug	*Dose range*
Diazepam	2–20 mg
Lorazepam	2–10 mg
Clonazepam	0.5–4 mg
Alprazolam	0.25–4 mg
Chlordiazepoxide	25–100 mg

2. For anxiety disorders, short-course benzodiazepines help reduce anxiety symptoms till other anxiolytics such as SSRIs start exerting their action.
3. Aggression and violence, benzodiazepines can effectively calm down an aggressive and violent patient.
4. For seizure disorders, parenteral benzodiazepines are frequently used in emergency departments to control active seizures.
5. Status Epilepticus, intravenous midazolam can control resistant status epilepticus.
6. For alcohol withdrawal symptoms, benzodiazepines such as chlordiazepoxide and lorazepam effectively control alcohol withdrawal symptoms.

Contraindications

Benzodiazepines are contraindicated in angle closure glaucoma and for those who are sensitive to benzodiazepines. Relative contraindications include a history of COPD, sleep apnoea, and head injury, in younger and older patients and pregnancy. There is little evidence that benzodiazepines induce fetal defects but when given in the later stages of pregnancy they can cause respiratory depression and withdrawal in the newborn.

Side Effects

Benzodiazepines are frequently associated with the following side effects:

1. Daytime drowsiness, more common with long-acting benzodiazepines such as chlordiazepoxide
2. Unsteady gait and slurred speech
3. Frequent fall which in older individuals can cause limb fractures and head injuries. Because of the risk of falls, benzodiazepines should be given with caution in older patients.
4. Paradoxical reactions. The paradoxical reaction is more common in the elderly, children, patients with a head injury, cerebral defects, and patients with personality disorders and substance abuse.
5. Cognitive impairment such as impairment in attention, concentration, and judgment.
6. Impairment in motor performance, because of these benzodiazepines should be prescribed with caution in drivers and heavy machinery workers.
7. For impaired memory, benzodiazepines should be avoided in patients with dementia.

Risk of Abuse and Dependence

Benzodiazepines are highly addictive drugs that can cause physical dependence on long-term use. For this reason, benzodiazepines should never be prescribed for more than 1 month and should be tapered and stopped within a period of 2–3 weeks.

Benzodiazepines cause a sense of well-being by activating the pleasure circuit and causing relaxation. This acts as positive reinforcement which compels the person to use the drug again and again. Continued use leads to tolerance and dependence and withdrawal reaction on suddenly stopping the drug. Withdrawal reactions act as negative reinforcement for which the person continued abusing benzodiazepines. Benzodiazepines withdrawal is akin to alcohol withdrawal and presents with

1. Tremor and restlessness
2. Insomnia
3. Irritability and dysphoria

4. Withdrawal seizure
5. Delirium

Treatment of benzodiazepine withdrawal and dependence is similar to that of alcohol withdrawal and dependence (Chapter 5).

Toxicity

Benzodiazepine overdose can lead to respiratory suppression, coma, and death. Toxicity happens more commonly when benzodiazepines are consumed with other CNS depressants such as alcohol and opioids. Benzodiazepine toxicity is treated with supportive measures such as maintenance of airway and circulation and intubation in case of respiratory failure. Flumazenil is a specific antidote that effectively neutralizes the toxic effects of benzodiazepines. Flumazenil, which is given as an intramuscular injection, should be started at a low dose and is given frequently till the patient gains adequate respiratory control and regain consciousness. Sudden administration of flumazenil at high doses can precipitate severe withdrawal reactions such as withdrawal seizure and delirium.

Z-DRUGS

A group of drugs primarily developed for the treatment of primary insomnia in the 1990s are colloquially known as non-benzodiazepines. These are also known as Z-drugs as their names start with the letter Z and include:

1. Zaleplon
2. Zolpidem
3. Zopiclone and
4. Eszopiclone

These drugs are more or less similar to benzodiazepines in their mechanism of action, side effects, toxicity, and abuse potential but differ from them in selectivity under their distinct chemical structure.

Mechanism of Action

These drugs selectively act on GABA-A1 subtypes of GABA-A receptors. They act as positive allosteric modulators by binding at the BZD site of the GABA-A1 receptor thereby increasing the frequency of opening of the centrally located Cl^- channel. This explains their sedative action. However, because of their selective actions on GABA-A1 receptors, these drugs more or less lack anxiolytic, anticonvulsant, and muscle relaxation actions.

Indications

Z-drugs are primarily indicted for primary insomnia. They improve sleep latency, sleep quality, and total duration of sleep. Unlike benzodiazepines, they can be given for a prolonged time, e.g. 3–5 months for this indication. They are quite useful in patients requiring tapering of their benzodiazepine doses. However, they are not devoid of the risk of addiction and dependence and should be given with caution. Currently, other medications such as melatonin or low-dose doxepin and maintenance of sleep hygiene are considered first-line therapy for primary insomnia. Z-drugs are prescribed when these measures fail.

Side Effects

1. They can cause significant memory impairment and impairment in other cognitive functions and motor performance.
2. Cases of angioedema with a risk of airway obstruction have been reported, especially with zolpidem.
3. They can precipitate abnormal behaviors during sleep such as somnambulism, sleep eating, and sleep driving which can be dangerous. Sleep-deprived persons are at the highest risk when these drugs are taken.
4. They can provoke aggression, irritability, and strange behaviors in patients with brain defects, cluster B personality disorders, and with history of polysubstance abuse.
5. When given to elderly patients they increase the risk of falls and fractures.

Overdose of these drugs can lead to toxicity with respiratory suppression, coma, and death. Flumazenil can be used as an antidote similar to that benzodiazepine toxicity. They are also associated with the risk of abuse, addiction, and dependence. Sudden stoppage of these drugs in dependent individuals can precipitate withdrawal reactions with tremors, autonomic hyperactivity, and seizure.

Buspirone

Buspirone is an azapirone initially developed as an antipsychotic but was discontinued for this purpose due to poor efficacy and later re-introduced as an anxiolytic medication. It is generally prescribed as a second-line medication for generalized anxiety disorder. It is especially important as an augmenting agent with SSRIs and helps ameliorate sexual side effects associated with them.

It acts as a partial agonist at the 5HT1A serotonin receptor which is thought to be responsible for its anxiolytic potency. It does not affect GABA receptors and hence does not cause addiction and dependence. However, actions of buspirone take 2–3 weeks to emerge and it also has no rapid anxiolytic effects as that of benzodiazepines.

STIMULANT MEDICATIONS

Introduction

Stimulants are naturally obtained or synthetically prepared substances which increase the activity of the central nervous system. Some stimulants are widely used for various psychiatric conditions which are mentioned below.

1. Dextroamphetamine
2. Combination of amphetamine and dextroamphetamine
3. Methylphenidate
4. Pseudoephedrine
5. Modafinil and armodafinil

Mechanism of Action of Stimulants

Stimulants increase the activity of CNS by increasing the activity of dopamine or noradrenaline or both. This is achieved by blocking the DAT (dopamine transporter) or NAT (noradrenaline) transporters or both.

Indications of Stimulants

Some common indications of stimulants are:

1. ADHD (dextroamphetamine and methylphenidate are first-line drugs)
2. Narcolepsy and other hypersonic disorders (modafinil and armodafinil are a treatment of choice)
3. Obesity as an appetite suppressant
4. In nasal or sinus congestion a decongestant

Side Effects of Stimulants

Treatment with stimulants may give rise to the following side effects:
1. Poor appetite which may lead to growth retardation in children
2. Stomach ache
3. Insomnia, especially when taken at night
4. Headache
5. Anxiety and tremor

Stimulant Overdose

Stimulant overdose presents with anxiety with panicky feelings, tremors, perspiration, and tachycardia. Severe cases of overdose may present with psychosis and cardiovascular instability. Death may occur due to ventricular arrhythmia and malignant hypertension. Cases of stimulant overdose are managed with benzodiazepines (help in sedation and alleviate anxiety), and beta-blockers (decrease heart rate, hypertension, and perspiration). The presence of ventricular arrhythmia may require treatment with anti-arrhythmic drugs.

BRAIN STIMULATION METHODS

Electroconvulsive Therapy

Electroconvulsive therapy (ECT) is one of the most widely used and effective non-pharmacological interventions available for serious psychiatric illnesses. ECT is both safe and effective and commonly indicated for mental illnesses presenting in severe conditions or those not amenable to medications. It employs electrical current to induce seizure which is necessary and sufficient for its therapeutic effect. In the past, direct ECT was in widespread use but these days in many countries including India, direct ECT is legally banned, hence modified ECT under general anesthesia is currently available for use.

History

The camphor-induced seizure had been a modality of treatment for psychotic illnesses since the seventeenth century. At first, Belgian neurologist Ladislas Von Meduna observed that the density of glial cells in the brain of schizophrenic patients is diminished while in that of epileptic patients, glial cell density is increased. From this observation, he concluded that if a seizure is induced by any means in psychotic patients, it may induce glial cell proliferation leading to improvement in psychotic symptoms. His team successfully treated a schizophrenic patient presenting with a catatonic stupor by a camphor-induced seizure in 1934. Ugo Cerlleti and Lucio Bini proposed the use of electricity to induce seizure as a treatment modality for psychotic illnesses. They successfully induced seizure in a psychotic patient by application of electrical impulses in 1938. Subsequently, necessary improvement in the ECT delivery system (e.g. brief pulse therapy) was introduced to make the procedure both safe and effective. To reduce the stigma associated with the ECT procedure (which is aesthetically unconvincing), modified ECT under general anesthesia was introduced.

Indications

Currently, ECT as a treatment modality in psychiatry is useful for severe or acute cases needing urgent improvement or those cases not responding to medications as mentioned below.

1. Severe depression with active suicidal tendency
2. Patients with severe psychotic depression refusing medications
3. Treatment-resistant depression (cases not responding to at least 2 antidepressants given for adequate time)
4. Catatonic schizophrenia
5. Psychotic patients presenting with poor nutritional status
6. Manic patients presenting in a delirious state with electrolyte imbalance (manic delirium)

Contraindications

ECT is quite safe and has very few relative contraindications as mentioned below.

1. Patients with raised intracranial pressure (due to space-occupying lesion or mass effect). Seizures in these patients can lead to cerebral herniation and death.
2. Another important contraindication is pheochromocytoma as ECT in these patients can result in a hypertensive crisis.
3. Patients with cardiac conduction defects.
4. Patients with poor cardiovascular function
5. Cerebral aneurysm or AV malformation (ECT may trigger a rupture event)

In older patients and pregnancy, ECT is the safest modality of treatment available in the psychiatric realm.

Set-up and Procedure

ECT is delivered by a team consisting of a psychiatrist, an anesthetist, and a psychiatric nurse. Prior work-ups to rule out any cardiac defects or raised intracranial pressure are mandatory. The primary setup involves a delivery room with an available oxygen delivery system, EEG monitor, ECG monitor, and suction apparatus and with instruments needed for putting the patient under general anesthesia.

As ECT is given under GA, the patient must remain orally nil for at least 6 hours before the commencement of the procedure. After inducing GA, an electrical pulse is delivered across the skull with electrodes placed over the temples via an ECT delivery machine. The occurrence of seizure can be either evaluated electronically using the EEG monitor or visually by observing the twitching of fingers of a hand (which is deprived of muscle relaxant by raising the pressure cuff above systolic pressure before giving muscle relaxant)

Mechanism of Action

The occurrence of seizure is necessary and sufficient for therapeutic response with ECT. The mechanism underlying the ECT-induced antipsychotic effect is largely unknown. Many authors have formulated various hypotheses such as the neurotransmitter hypothesis (ECT normalizes neurotransmitter imbalance in psychotic patients), neurotrophic factors hypothesis (ECT induces production of neurotrophic factors such as BDNF to bring structural changes which resolve the psychotic symptoms), anticonvulsant hypothesis, etc.

The anticonvulsant hypothesis suggests that electrically induced seizure raised the threshold of neural activation. As we know that both mania and depression occur due to abnormal overactivation of cortical neurons, and raising thresholds to prevent this abnormal overactivation lead to the resolution of symptoms. Recent studies have suggested that ECT decreases the connectivity within the brain default mode network causing reduced activity of this network which is thought to be hyperactive both in depression and schizophrenia.

Side Effects

ECT is generally safe and has few side effects. Common side effects of modified ECT are-

1. Amnesia. This is the most troublesome of all side effects. The patient can not remember anything that happened a few hours to days before the procedure (retrograde amnesia) and in rare cases, retrograde amnesia can be extensive spanning months to years before the procedure. It may take a few days to months to gain the memory back.
2. Disorientation and confusion following the procedure are common (post-ictal confusion).
3. Nausea and vomiting due to raised ICP after the procedure.
4. Death is rare and is mostly due to complications of GA

TRANSCRANIAL MAGNETIC STIMULATION

Transcranial magnetic stimulation (TMS) is a novel noninvasive therapeutic modality for psychiatric illnesses. It is based on the concept of electromagnetic induction and employs rapidly changing electric fields to alter the activities of the neural tissue. In TMS, an alternating current is passed through a coil placed over the scalp which induces current flow in the neural tissue lying underneath, known as eddy current. This can change the excitability of the neural tissue and improve symptoms of any psychiatric illness arising due to abnormal neural activity.

The clinical response of a single application of TMS is short lasting, hence for long-lasting recovery, TMS is applied repeatedly and the process is known as repetitive TMS or rTMS. rTMS is indicated for resistant depression, OCD, anxiety disorder, etc. For an effective response, the magnetic coil must be placed over the brain area thought to be responsible for the specific illness e.g. dorsolateral prefrontal cortex in depression.

rTMS is both effective and safe and is devoid of serious side effects. Few patients complain of headache, lightheadedness, localized scalp pain, transitory twitching of facial muscles, etc. The presence of magnetic devices such as pacemakers is an absolute contraindication for rTMS while raised ICT and cardiac ailments are relative contraindications.

VAGUS NERVE STIMULATION (VNS)

The Vagus nerve is the 10th cranial nerve arising from the brainstem. About 80% of nerve fibers contained within it are afferent (going into the brainstem from the periphery). Vagus nerve stimulation (VNS) of the can activate these up-going afferent nerves which in turn modulate the activities of the brainstem nuclei such as locus coeruleus and raphe nuclei.

As we know that these brain stem nuclei are the seat of monoaminergic neurotransmitters such as serotonin and norepinephrine, and activation of the vagus nerve can alter the level of these chemicals in the brain. VNS is primarily indicated for recurrent resistant depression not responding to antidepressants and ECT.

VNS involves stimulation of the left vagus nerve with an electric pulse generator embedded in the chest wall. This procedure is invasive and can cause neck pain, voice change, local infection, and in rare cases vocal cord paralysis and cardiac arrest. Hence, VNS is only reserved for resistant recurrent depression.

PRINCIPLES OF PSYCHOTHERAPY

Introduction

Psychotherapy is an alternative therapeutic approach and is as important as a psychopharmacological approach in the treatment of psychiatric illnesses. As a modality of treatment, psychotherapy is especially important in the treatment of neurotic illnesses such as mild depression, anxiety neurosis, OCD, dissociative and conversion disorders, personality disorders, eating disorders, etc. Psychoanalytic psychotherapy, based on principles of Freudian psychology, was the treatment of choice for neurotic illnesses in the early part of the 20th century and is known as **first-wave psychotherapy.** Later, behavioral and cognitive approaches came to the forefront and superseded the psychoanalytic approach in the middle part of the 20th century. Behavioral and cognitive therapies such as CBT are known as **second-wave psychotherapy.** Recently, therapies based on humanistic principles such as client-centered therapy and mindfulness-based psychotherapy are taking over along with cognitive behavioral approaches. Therapies based on humanistic principles are known as **third-wave psychotherapy.**

PSYCHOANALYTIC PSYCHOTHERAPY

Psychoanalytic psychotherapy is based on the principles of ego psychology, defense mechanisms, and topological theory of mind (see Chapter 13). Psychoanalysis involves following basic steps:

1. Therapeutic alliance
2. Recollection
3. Working through and
4. Conflict resolution

1. Therapeutic Alliance

The therapist and the client come together willingly for the evaluation of the problem and its resolution by forming a mutually understanding relationship known as a therapeutic alliance. It is a time-bound contract between the two and the therapist must show an empathetic approach toward the client and listen to his/her problems in a nonjudgmental way for the smooth evaluation and resolution of the illness.

2. Recollection

It is the procedure to get access to the unconscious to evaluate the repressed memories and desires which are responsible for the present problem. This can be achieved by any of the three procedures: dream analysis, hypnosis, or free association.

a. ***Dream analysis:*** According to Freud, repressed unconscious memories and wishes are important components of a dream and one can know about these repressed materials by analyzing the dream of the patient.
b. ***Hypnosis:*** Hypnosis is the process of inducing a hypnotic trance by suggestion. In the hypnotic trance state, the boundaries between conscious, preconscious, and unconscious compartments are broken and the therapist can easily access the conflict buried in the unconscious compartment by bringing it to the conscious compartment. Hypnosis is used as the first procedure in psychoanalytic psychotherapy to evaluate the unconscious conflict responsible for the neurotic state the patient is suffering. Another procedure developed by Freud himself to gain access to the unconscious compartment is known as 'free association'.
c. ***Free association:*** Free association is a procedure during which the patient is asked to tell the therapist every thought coming into his/her mind. As the patient goes on speaking her mind, gradually the repressed memories and conflictual themes buried inside the unconscious compartment make their way into the consciousness from time to time and are revealed by the patient to the therapist which is known as the 'slip of the tongue' phenomenon.

3. Working Through

During the process of psychoanalysis, the therapist makes the patient relive the phallic phase by posing himself as the parental figure. The client gradually develops romantic attraction toward the therapist assuming him as the father (in cases of female patients) which is known as transference. Sometimes, the client may hesitate to get involved with the therapy procedure known as resistance. However, the therapist must persist in his endeavor to know about the real incident causing the intrapsychic conflict ultimately leading to the illness which is known as working through.

4. Conflict Resolution

The conflict is gradually resolved by bringing the painful memories to the consciousness and making them acceptable to the ego. Acceptance of the memory of the traumatic event causes the abolition of the defense mechanisms employed by the ego and the neurotic condition vanishes.

Indications of Psychoanalytic Psychotherapy

Currently, this therapeutic approach is becoming less and less popular because of its complexity and lack of objectivity; however, it is still in use in some parts of the world for the following conditions.

- Dissociative disorders
- Conversion disorders
- Somatic symptoms disorders
- Paraphilic disorders
- Substance deaddiction

BEHAVIORAL THERAPY

The concepts of behavioral therapy have been derived from theories of behaviorism developed during the early part of the 20th century. Behavioral therapy was a drastic change from the classical approaches such as psychoanalytic psychotherapy and shapes the psychotherapeutic approach during the mid-20th century. Behavioral therapy is still widely used even today, although in modified forms and combined with cognitive therapy.

Behavioral therapies are based on principles of learning theories developed by Ivan Pavlov, Watson, and BF Skinner such as classical conditioning and operant conditioning (Chapter 2).

Behavioral Therapies: Application of Learning Theories

1. Aversion therapy employs the principles of operant conditioning to discourage undesirable behavior. Aversion therapy involves presenting the patient with some unpleasant stimulus when he performs an undesirable behavior.
   The use of disulfiram in cases of alcohol dependence is a beautiful example of aversion therapy. Disulfiram is an aldehyde dehydrogenase inhibitor and blocks the conversion of acetaldehyde into acetic acid leading to the accumulation of acetaldehyde in the body. Therefore, when a person on disulfiram drinks alcohol, there is an accumulation of acetaldehyde in the body leading to dysphoria, headache, abdominal cramps, vomiting, etc. (disulfiram reaction) which are highly unpleasant for the patient. After experiencing a disulfiram reaction 2–3 times the person develops an aversion to alcohol intake and ultimately stops drinking alcohol altogether.
2. Systematic desensitization employs the principles of classical conditioning to treat an illness. It is regularly employed to treat phobic anxiety disorders. A phobia is defined as an excessive and irrational fear of harmless objects or situations which occurs due to the pairing of these harmless stimuli with some harmful stimulus. In systematic desensitization, a patient suffering from a phobia is first relaxed (by taking benzodiazepines or by performing relaxation exercises) and gradually exposed to the phobic stimulus in a stepwise manner. Now, due to the pairing of relaxation with phobic stimulus, the conditioned fear response is gradually unlearned and when the session is complete, the patient is no more fearful of the harmless stimulus anymore (resolution of symptoms).
3. Flooding is another desensitization technique based on principles of classical conditioning, developed for phobias. It differs from systematic desensitisation by the fact that exposure to flooding is sudden and not in a stepwise manner. The basic principle is that when a patient with a phobic anxiety disorder is suddenly exposed to a phobic stimulus, there is a sudden onset of excessive fear with a panicky feeling, but on continuing with the exposure, the patient gradually realizes the harmlessness of the stimulus and becomes relaxed after some time. Patients are also taught to practice relaxation exercises during the exposure to make the fear go at the earliest. Desensitization occurs on repeated exposure and the patient no more feels fearful of the phobic stimulus.
4. Applied behavior analysis is a technique based on principles of operant conditioning to encourage desirable behavior in children with autism, ADHD, and disruptive disorders. It usually involves giving a reward in the form of verbal praise, candy, toys or token economy when the child successfully performs a desirable behavior e.g. making a step toward socialization in case of autism. Punishment is seldom used in ABA to discourage undesirable behaviors. ABA is highly effective in developing social skills, language skills, and communication skills and minimizing self-harm

behavior in autism. Similarly, it is effective in promoting attention and concentration and minimizing hyperactivity in ADHD.

5. Contingency management employs the principles of operant conditioning to help patients of substance addiction in maintaining abstinence from drug abuse. It employs money, prizes, and lottery tickets as a reward for these patients on submission of drug-negative urine samples as evidence of abstinence. There is considerable evidence in support of contingency management in the treatment of substance abuse disorders although not frequently used.

COGNITIVE BEHAVIORAL THERAPY

Cognitive Theory

The cognitive theory was developed by the American psychiatrist Aron T Beck in the early 1960s. While examining patients of depression in his clinic, he observed that patients with depression harboured mental frameworks and attitudes about themselves and about the world which are invalid and irrational. As per his observation, patients with depression have negative views regarding themselves, their environment, and their future leading to feelings of worthlessness, helplessness, and hopelessness. However, these views are irrational and invalid arising out of their faulty thought processes. Based on these observations, Beck put forward his famous cognitive model of depression which was later extrapolated to develop a general cognitive theory of personality.

According to cognitive theory, early childhood experiences such as trauma, abuse, neglect or praise, love, affection, etc. lead to the development of mental frameworks about self and the objects and situations in the environment which are enduring and last for life. These mental frameworks about self and the environment are known as 'core beliefs' which shape our views about ourselves and our surrounding environment. Core Beliefs can be positive such as 'I am confident, I am loveable', or can be negative such as 'I am ugly; I am incompetent 'etc. Core beliefs are further strengthened by subsequent experiences wrapped over it layer after layer to form the 'schemas'. These schemas are like filters which shape our perspectives about our external world. These perspectives may match or mismatch with the true nature of objects or situations in reality.

As the individual grows, these core beliefs or schemas formed in childhood are retained throughout life. When the individual is exposed to a stressful life event, various aspects of the stressful situation are perceived through the lenses of core beliefs and schemas. If the core beliefs of the person are negative then during stress they lead to the development of negative automatic thoughts such as 'I am sinful and destined to suffer, no one can help me out of this misery', etc. Similarly, negative schemas can act as filters and give a distorted picture of the environment which is known as a cognitive distortion. Some of the important cognitive distortions are:

1. Mind reading (assuming that people are thinking negatively of you)
2. Catastrophizing (expecting a disaster after hearing about a problem)
3. Dichotomous thinking (also known as all or none thinking, thinking only about the extremes without giving importance to any possibilities in between)
4. Emotional reasoning (assuming the emotional reaction to a situation as the ultimate truth and behaving accordingly)
5. Mental filtering (extracting only the negative aspects of a situation by filtering out all the positive aspects)

6. Overgeneralizations (making a sweeping general conclusion from a single piece of evidence)
7. Personalization (entirely blaming oneself for the negative outcome of a situation without taking into account other possibilities)
8. Should statement (thinking only about how things should have been in the past without giving importance to the practical aspects of a situation)
9. Minimization (downplaying the positive aspects of self or of a situation)

Negative automatic thoughts and cognitive distortions lead to negative emotions (sadness, anxiety, and guilt) which ultimately shape our behavior (social withdrawal, lack of interest, self-harm behavior) which are characteristics of depressive psychopathology.

Example: Let us analyze a case of paranoid personality disorder. Negative life events such as abuse by parents in childhood might lead to the development of negative core beliefs such as 'I am vulnerable' and negative schema about people as malevolent and deceitful. In adulthood, in every stressful situation, the person tends to view it through the lens of these core beliefs leading to negative automatic thoughts such as 'people are trying to harm me, people are conspiring against me', etc. The cognitive distortion of overgeneralizations can make all people deceitful and malevolent for the patient. These automatic thoughts and cognitive distortions ultimately lead to negative emotions such as 'fear and insecurity' which lead to paranoid behaviors of social isolation, sensitivity, and quarreling behavior which are characteristic features of paranoid personality disorder.

Application of Cognitive Theory

1. Cognitive behavioral therapy
2. Dialectical behavioral therapy
3. Rational emotive behavior therapy (REBT)

Techniques of CBT

1. ***Identifying negative automatic thoughts:*** It is the first and most difficult step in CBT. The therapist and client sit together and try to evaluate the thought process of the client through Socratic questioning (rationality and logicality of the thought). With this, those thoughts that are irrational and invalid (negative automatic thoughts) come to the forefront.
2. ***Challenging 'core beliefs:*** After identifying negative automatic thoughts, the core beliefs giving rise to these automatic thoughts are identified. These core beliefs are challenged via questioning (Socratic questioning).
3. ***Cognitive restructuring and practicing new skills:*** After identifying negative automatic thoughts, the next step is developing new real-world perspectives of self and the environment and handling real world problems in a practical way. This requires the acquisition of new practical skills (relaxation, mindfulness, aerobic exercise, etc) that helps positively handle stress.
4. ***Goal setting:*** The therapist must teach the client how to set short and long-term goals which help in recovering from current mental illness. These goals must be SMART (specific, measurable, attainable, relevant, and time-bound).

5. ***Problem-solving:*** Practical problem-solving skills help the client deal with stressors rationally and practically. Problem-solving involves identifying a problem, listing possible solutions, evaluating the pros and cons of each solution, choosing a rational solution, and implementing the solution.
6. ***Self-monitoring:*** This is the most important part of CBT. The client must maintain a diary to track all stressful situations, her emotional and behavioral reactions to them, and how he/she is implementing the techniques of CBT to deal with them.

Indications

CBT is effective in a wide variety of psychiatric illnesses. A few common indications are:

1. Depressive disorders
2. Obsessive–compulsive disorder
3. Anxiety disorders and PTSD
4. Personality disorders
5. Eating disorders
6. Substance use disorders
7. Delusional disorders

Dialectical Behavioral Therapy (DBT)

DBT was developed by Marsha M Linehan specifically for the treatment of borderline personality disorder and especially to manage self-harm behavior in these patients. DBT aims to improve self-harm behavior and disruptive behavior in patients of BPD by learning distress tolerance and emotional regulation with mindfulness, healthy coping skills and interpersonal effectiveness. DBT is a program involving a team of therapists to deal with each component of the program and is considered the most effective therapeutic modality for the treatment of borderline personality disorder.

HUMANISTIC THERAPIES

These are based on the principles of humanistic psychology developed by Carl Roger and Abraham Maslow. Client-centered therapy, logotherapy, gestalt therapy, and mindfulness-based psychotherapies are included in this approach.

Client-centered Therapy

It was developed by Carl Roger, the founder of humanistic psychology, who believed that much of the psychological problems can be resolved by the patients (also known as the client) himself/herself via self awareness and self acceptance, the therapist only playing an active supporting role. It is based on the principle of unconditional positive regard which means the therapist must encourage the client to share his/her problems with the therapist who listens to them with empathy, warmth, and consideration. This leads to the development of a secure and trustworthy relationship between the two and the client gradually starts sharing all his/her feelings and distress with the therapist. The therapist must understand and clarify all these problems in a non-judgemental manner and make them acceptable to the client in a positive way. This therapy helps in self-awareness and self-acceptance of the ongoing problems with the therapist only working as a warm empathetic guide.

OTHER PSYCHOTHERAPY APPROACHES

Family Therapy

Family members are the most important part of the social support system, so it is prudent to involve family members in the therapeutic process of a mentally ill person. Most of the time family members lack information on various aspects of a psychiatric illness and how to handle them. Furthermore, a distorted family dynamic due to miscommunication between family members can be the reason for perpetuation, poor therapeutic response, and relapse of a psychiatric illness.

Family therapy is aimed at reducing stress and conflict within a family by improving communication between family members. Various components of family therapy are:

1. Exploring the internal dynamics within a family and its contribution toward mental illness.
2. Restructuring the internal dynamics within a family by improving communication between family members.
3. Improving the problem-solving capabilities of a family by teaching new coping skills.

Indications

1. Marital conflicts
2. Parent–child conflict
3. Problem between siblings
4. Psychoeducation about an index case within the family
5. Handling expressed emotions
6. Adjustment problems between family members

Group Psychotherapy

Group psychotherapy involves the treatment of a group of patients with some commonality at once by a therapist. Group therapy is aimed at inducing behavioral correction, development of social and interpersonal skills, development of new coping skills, and the eventual return of the patient to society.

Stages of Group Development

1. ***Forming stage:*** In the forming stage, the patients experience nervousness and uncertainty and are mostly dependent on the therapist for group functioning.
2. ***Storming stage:*** In this stage patients start to open up and start sharing their personal experiences with other members. But, the therapist should be aware that conflict may develop between some members at this stage and he should resolve it accordingly.
3. ***Norming stage:*** After the successful resolution of conflict, the cohesiveness among the group members improves and there is greater sharing of experiences in this stage. Now, the therapist intervenes less and less and the group members generally take the therapy forward.
4. ***Performing stage:*** At this stage, the group has already gained maturity and all the members understand each other and their strengths and weaknesses better than before. The therapist is just a mere supervisor as the group almost functions independently.

5. ***Adjourning stage:*** When the therapy sessions come to the end, the group members may feel sad and anxious. The therapist should help members manage their feelings about the closing of the session and counsel them about ways forward in life outside the group.

Indications

Group psychotherapy is indicated in the following conditions.
1. Emotional trauma
2. Grief or loss
3. Anxiety disorders
4. Depression
5. Relationship problems
6. Low self-esteem

PSYCHIATRIC REHABILITATION

Individuals with psychiatric disabilities often face problems in carrying out self-care, managing tasks of daily living, socialization, and working productively. Psychosocial rehabilitation programs are aimed at improving social-communication skills and vocational skills to make the life of a psychiatric patient purposeful and productive.

Strategies of Psychosocial Rehabilitation

The two basic strategies of psychosocial rehabilitation are:
1. Interventions that enhance the functioning of psychiatric patients with disability by the acquisition of social and instrumental skills through training or retraining.
2. Interventions that modify the patient's social and physical environment to compensate for disabilities.

Skill development interventions attempt to change the patient's behavior by improving self-care (grooming and personal hygiene), management of the tasks of daily living, communication, vocational and employment roles, coping with residual symptoms, and ameliorating cognitive deficits through remediation. Three basic components of skill development interventions are:
1. Social skills training
2. Vocational rehabilitation and
3. Cognitive remediation

Social Skills Training

Social skills tainting aims to improve social interaction to further integrate the patient back into society. It is achieved via videotapes of other psychiatric patients and of the patient himself, role-playing therapy, and homework assignments for the specific skills to be practiced.

Vocational Rehabilitation

Vocational rehabilitation programs include proactive measures that enable the psychiatrically disabled individual to function to his or her optimal capacity, either in a competitive environment or in a sheltered but stimulating setting, depending on the preference.

Cognitive Remediation

It is a fairly recent approach that aims at improving the cognitive skills of the patients, which in turn improves social, communication, and vocational skills. It employs computational approaches such as computer-generated exercises, neural networks, virtual reality, etc. to improve cognition, working memory, spontaneity, and working capacity.

Interventions to Reduce the Family Burden

In the Indian context, family members are the primary caregivers, therefore attempting to assist family members is likely to enhance the care they can provide to the disabled individual. These could be in the form of emotional support to the primary caregivers, offering daycare facilities to the severely disabled, and assisting the economically deprived disabled individual or a member of his or her family to obtain gainful employment.

SUMMARY

1. Antipsychotics are the mainstay of treatment of psychotic disorders such as schizophrenia, mania, ATPD, delusional disorders, etc. Currently, atypical antipsychotics such as olanzapine and risperidone are in widespread use replacing typical antipsychotics such as chlorpromazine and haloperidol. Antipsychotics act by blocking dopamine and serotonin receptors and are associated with side effects such as pseudo-parkinsonism, akathisia, tardive dyskinesia, metabolic syndrome, etc.
2. Antidepressant medications such as SSRIs, TCAs, and SNRIs are the mainstays of treatment of depressive disorders, anxiety disorders, and OCD. They act by inhibiting the reuptake of serotonin from the synaptic cleft and are associated with gastric discomfort, sexual side effects, and increased risk of bleeding and discontinuation syndrome when stopped abruptly.
3. Mood stabilizers are drugs used in the prophylactic treatment of bipolar disorders. Lithium is the classical mood stabilizer while anti-epileptic drugs such as sodium valproate, carbamazepine, and lamotrigine can also be used as mood stabilizers. They act by inhibiting abnormal activation of neural tissue by blocking ion channels or by inhibiting intracellular activation cascade.
4. Sedatives and hypnotics such as benzodiazepines and Z-drugs have widespread use, especially in controlling aggression, anxiety, and insomnia. They act by activating GABA-A receptors in the CNS and are associated with significant abuse and dependence potential when prescribed for a longer period.
5. Brain stimulation methods such as ECT and rTMS are reserved for special cases such as depression with active suicidal tendencies, resistant depression, resistant schizophrenia, and psychotic patients with poor health conditions. ECT is highly efficacious and response is rapid, although short lasting.
6. Psychotherapy such as psychoanalytic psychotherapy, behavioral therapy, and cognitive therapy are alternative treatment approaches mainly indicated for neurotic illnesses such as dissociative and conversion disorders, anxiety disorders, mild depression, and OCD.

BIBLIOGRAPHY

1. Chokhawala K, Stevens L. Antipsychotic Medications. [Updated 2022 Mar 8]. In: StatPearls [Internet]. Treasure Island (FL): StatPearls Publishing; 2022 Jan.
2. Taylor DM, Barnes TRE, Young AH. The Maudsley prescribing guidelines in psychiatry, 2018. (13th ed.)
3. Teo JT, Edwards MJ, Bhatia K. Tardive dyskinesia is caused by maladaptive synaptic plasticity: a hypothesis. Mov Disord. 2012;27:1205–15.
4. Mailman RB, Murthy V. Third generation antipsychotic drugs: partial agonism or receptor functional selectivity? Current pharmaceutical design, 2010. 16(5), 488–501.

5. Moraczewski J, Aedma KK. Tricyclic Antidepressants. [Updated 2022 May 2]. In: StatPearls [Internet]. Treasure Island (FL): StatPearls Publishing; 2022 Jan.
6. Chu A, Wadhwa R. Selective Serotonin Reuptake Inhibitors. [Updated 2022 May 8]. In: StatPearls [Internet]. Treasure Island (FL): StatPearls Publishing; 2022 Jan.
7. Sansone RA, Sansone LA. Serotonin-norepinephrine reuptake inhibitors: a pharmacological comparison. Innovations in clinical neuroscience, 2014;11(3-4):37–42.
8. Fiedorowicz JG, Swartz KL. The role of monoamine oxidase inhibitors in current psychiatric practice. Journal of psychiatric practice, 2004;10(4):239–48.
9. Gould TD, Chen G, Manji HK. Mood stabilizer psychopharmacology. Clinical neuroscience research, 2002;2(3-4):193–212.
10. Jameson JL, Loscalzo J. Harrison's Principles of Internal Medicine, 2015. (19th edition.). New York: McGraw Hill Education.
11. Tripathi KD. Essentials of Medical Pharmacology, 2018. (8th ed.).
12. Brandt, Jaden, and Christine Leong. "Benzodiazepines and Z-Drugs: An Updated Review of Major Adverse Outcomes Reported on in Epidemiologic Research." Drugs in R&D vol. 17,4 (2017): 493-507.
13. Farzam K, Faizy RM, Saadabadi A. Stimulants. [Updated 2022 Jun 16]. In: StatPearls [Internet]. Treasure Island (FL): StatPearls Publishing; 2022 Jan.
14. Salik I, Marwaha R. Electroconvulsive Therapy. [Updated 2022 May 8]. In: StatPearls [Internet]. Treasure Island (FL): StatPearls Publishing; 2022 Jan.
15. Mann SK, Malhi NK. Repetitive Transcranial Magnetic Stimulation. [Updated 2022 Mar 9]. In: StatPearls [Internet]. Treasure Island (FL): StatPearls Publishing; 2022 Jan.
16. Pycroft L, Stein J, Aziz T. Deep brain stimulation: An overview of history, methods, and future developments. Brain Neurosci Adv. 2018 Dec 12;2:2398212818816017.
17. Marks S. Psychotherapy in historical perspective. Hist Human Sci. 2017 Apr;30(2):3–16. doi 10.1177/0952695117703243. Epub 2017 Apr 20.
18. Chand SP, Kuckel DP, Huecker MR. Cognitive Behavior Therapy. [Updated 2022 May 29]. In: StatPearls [Internet]. Treasure Island (FL): StatPearls Publishing; 2022 Jan.
19. Varghese M, Kirpekar V, Loganathan S. Family Interventions: Basic Principles and Techniques. Indian J Psychiatry. 2020 Jan;62(Suppl 2):S192-S200.
20. Ezhumalai S, Muralidhar D, Dhanasekarapandian R, Nikketha BS. Group interventions. Indian J Psychiatry. 2018 Feb;60(Suppl 4):S514–S521.
21. M Sarada Menon. Psychosocial Rehabilitation: Current Trends. NIMHANS Journal Volume: 14 Issue: 04 October 1996 Page: 295–305.
22. DeBattista C, Schatzberg AF. The Black Book of Psychotropic Dosing and Monitoring. Psychopharmacol Bull. 2021 Jan 12;51(1):8-58.
23. Indian Pharmacopoeia Commission, Ministry of Health and Family Welfare, Government of India. NFI National Formulary of India, 4th Edition 2011.

Chapter 21

Miscellaneous

Competency achievement: Students should be able to

1. **PS19.1** Describe the relevance, role, and status of community psychiatry
2. **PS19.2** Describe the objectives strategies and contents of the National Mental Health Programme
3. **PS19.3** Describe and discuss the basiç legal and ethical issues in psychiatry
4. **PS19.4** Enumerate and describe the salient features of the prevalent mental health laws in India
5. **PS19 5** Describe the concept and principles of preventive psychiatry
6. **PS19.6** Enumerate and describe the identifying features and the principles of participatory management of mental illness occurring during and after disasters

COMMUNITY PSYCHIATRY

Definition

Community psychiatry is a relatively new concept in India. It was started in Amritsar Mental Hospital in the 1950s on an experimental basis when the hospital started involving family members in the care of mentally ill patients. The scope of community psychiatry expanded greatly with the implementation of the **National Mental Health Programme in 1982** and further with the implementation of the **District Mental Health Programme in 1996**.

Purpose

The purpose of community psychiatry is to deliver affordable basic mental healthcare at the community level using community resources and through the primary healthcare system. Community mental health in India includes the following components.

1. **Treatment** of mental disorders at the community level as far as possible.
2. **Promotion** of Mental health and prevention of mental illnesses at the community level.
3. **Inclusion of community groups** (religious groups, self-help groups, local bodies) in the mental healthcare delivery system.
4. **Rehabilitation** of chronically ill psychiatric patients with disability in the community itself.
5. **Prevention of substance abuse** behavior such as alcohol abuse in the community.
6. **Plans for removal of stigma** associated with mental illnesses in the community.

District Mental Health Programme

The National Mental Health Programme was started in India in 1982 to decentralize mental health care and to deliver basic mental health care at the community level by integrating mental health care with the primary healthcare system. District mental health programme was started in 1996 under NMHP to further strengthen the mental healthcare delivery process at the community level. Objectives of DMHP are:

1. To deliver minimum affordable mental healthcare to the underprivileged and vulnerable sections of society.
2. Early detection and treatment of mental illnesses at the community level.
3. To reduce the stigma associated with mental illnesses through various awareness programs.
4. To rehabilitate patients with chronic mental illnesses within the community.

DMHP had adopted the following core approaches to achieve the above objectives

1. **Human resource support:** For proper implementation of the DMHP agenda, the involvement of a psychiatrist, clinical psychologist, psychosocial worker, psychiatric nurse, and case registry assistant are necessary. At least one from each of the above-mentioned resource personnel should be posted at the district level for the smooth running of the system.
2. **Training programs:** Training programs are carried out from time to time to train primary physicians, nurses, pharmacists, community health workers, and ASHAs regarding the identification of prevalent mental illnesses, basic treatment approaches, and timely referral to higher centers. These training programs are carried out by psychiatrists at PHC and CHC levels.
3. **Community awareness camps:** These are organized at the village and community levels to make the general public aware of the identification of mental health issues, seeking medical treatment for mental health illnesses, removal of stigma associated with mental illnesses in the community, etc.
4. **Community participation:** Community participation by linkage with self-help groups, family and caregiver groups, and NGOs working in the field of mental health.
5. **Running of daycare centers:** Under the DMHP program daycare centers are run to provide rehabilitation services to the mentally ill and to continue with the treatment initially provided under DMHP for relapse prevention. It also aims at enhancing the skills of family members and caregivers in taking better care of mentally ill patients.
6. **Intersectoral linkage**: It involves outreach services such as school mental health services, workplace stress management services, satellite clinics, etc. These outreach services are specifically targeted towards at-risk groups or especially vulnerable groups.

Outreach Components under DMHP

1. **Satellite clinics**, at least 4 satellite clinics should be carried out at CHC and PHC levels by the DMHP team every month.
2. **Targeted interventions** such as workplace stress management services, jail visits, suicide prevention services, and school and college intervention services are to be carried out from time to time. The school mental health program developed by NIMHANS, Bengaluru has the following components:

a. **Teacher's orientation** program in which teachers are trained on how to identify mental health problems among students and how to seek proper mental health care for needy students.
b. **Skills training** for teachers involves training programs that improve the counseling skills of teachers to reduce stress among students.
c. **Student enrichment programs** are aimed at training students how to handle stress, prepare for exams effectively, improve interpersonal relations and student-teacher relations, etc.
d. **Life skills education** programs for students aimed at acquiring practical skills in planning their future.

PREVENTIVE PSYCHIATRY

Introduction

The global burden of psychiatric illnesses is rising at an alarming rate. The majority of the common psychiatric illnesses such as depression, bipolar disorder, schizophrenia, OCD, dementia, etc, are associated with significant disability and loss of productivity. There is a need to push for preventive strategies in the field of mental health to reduce this burden in near future by lowering the incidence and prevalence of psychiatric illness.

The concept of prevention in psychiatry has been largely borrowed from preventive medicine. However, the most difficult aspect of employing these strategies in psychiatry is the lack of clear-cut causal factors for psychiatric illnesses, although some probable risk factors have been identified. Furthermore, there is a huge treatment gap in the field of mental health due to a lack of manpower and resources making early detection and treatment difficult. DMHP has addressed this problem to some extent in India.

Phases of Prevention

As we have studied in preventive medicine, prevention can be of three types depending upon the timing at which preventive strategies have been applied.

1. **Primary prevention** means applying preventive strategies before the onset of an illness to reduce the incidence and prevalence of the disease. Although primary prevention is the most attractive one, it is also the most difficult one in terms of execution.
2. **Secondary prevention** involves early detection and treatment of psychiatric illnesses to reduce disability and/or death. Currently, the entire task force in the field of psychiatry is focused on this aspect of prevention.
3. **Tertiary prevention** involves the rehabilitation of psychiatric patients having some disability arising from psychiatric illnesses.

Primary Prevention in Psychiatry

Primary prevention is defined as the application of preventive strategies before the onset of a psychiatric illness to reduce its incidence and prevalence. There are various modes and methods of primary prevention in psychiatry. Based on the target population, primary prevention can be of the following types.

1. **Universal prevention strategies** are **targeted at the entire population**. The concept of universal prevention in psychiatry is in its nascent stage and will take some time to meet its objectives. At the present scope of universal prevention is limited to **improving maternal health, decreasing birth complications and neonatal**

infection, promoting nutrition of school-going children, etc. All these measures can significantly reduce neurodevelopmental diseases such as autism, ADHD, and schizophrenia.

2. **Selective prevention** strategies are **targeted at individuals at risk** of developing a psychiatric illness such as family members of an index case. Coping skill training, adequate nutrition, regular physical exercise, mindfulness, and intermittent CBT are a few interventional methods included in this strategy. Marital counseling and genetic counseling also fall within the purview of selective prevention strategies.
3. **Indicated prevention** strategies are targeted **at individuals who have already developed some prodromal symptoms** of a psychiatric illness. Management of schizophrenia prodrome may fall in this category and persons with prodromal psychosis are usually treated with CBT and nutritional supplements such as alpha-lipoic acid (neuroprotective supplement). Antipsychotic medications are usually not indicated in these patients. Another example of indicated prevention is preventing the development of PTSD in individuals exposed to extreme stress with psychological support, CBT, and by giving prazosin for a few days to weeks in especially vulnerable cases.

Mental Health Promotion

Mental health promotion has gained considerable traction in recent times, especially in the post-COVID-19 period. Urban middle-class people are becoming more and more conscious about their mental health and well-being. There are a few strategies that can be adopted to promote good mental health and well-being.

1. Improving coping skills
2. Adopting principles of positive psychology such as positive emotion (love, compassion, joy), positive experiences (achievements, hobbies, traveling), and positive institutions (family and friendship)
3. Regular physical exercise and healthy diet and
4. Mindfulness meditation

Both primary prevention and health promotion strategies are still in their infancy in psychiatry. However, already the time has come; we should seriously pay attention to psychiatric prevention strategies to decrease the burden of psychiatric illnesses in the community.

FORENSIC PSYCHIATRY

Introduction

Forensic psychiatry deals with the application of knowledge in psychiatry in the administration of law. Many times, a medical officer may be asked by the court of law to give an opinion on the state of mind of an accused at the time of committing a crime or the present state of mind of a person awaiting trial. In these cases, the medical officer must be aware of the implications of his opinion and its social, moral, and legal ramifications.

As per the Indian Lunacy Act 1912, a 'lunatic' is defined as an idiot or a person of unsound mind. Insanity is a legal term that implies unsoundness of mind and is frequently used in a court of law. Mental illness has a broader concept and is clearly defined in the Mental Healthcare Act 2017.

Criminal Responsibility of the Insane

The criminal responsibility of the insane is the assessment of the legal responsibility of an insane or mentally ill person who has committed a crime, for his crime.

In India, IPC 84, which is solely based on the M'Naghten rule, deals with the criminal responsibility of the insane. As we look into history, on one fine day in 1843 England, a young man named M'Naghten, shot Edward Drummond (personal secretary of British PM) dead after mistaking him for the UK Prime Minister Sir Robert Peel. Subsequently, he was acquitted by a panel of judges on the ground of insanity, and on that day a groundbreaking rule was formulated which is famously known as the M'Naughten rule.

Section 84 of IPC, which is based on the M'Naghten rule states that "nothing is an offense which is done by a person who, at the time of doing it, because of unsoundness of mind, is incapable of knowing the nature of the act, or that he is doing what is either wrong or contrary to law."

Civil Responsibilities

1. Management of Properties

The insanity of a sufficient degree can make a person incapable of managing his properties. In case of any relative filling such an application on the ground of insanity, the onus is on the court to enquire into the matter. If it is found that the person in question is indeed incapable of managing his/her properties then the court may appoint and empower a person to manage his properties. In case of a report of the person being cleared of insanity, a repeat inquiry may be ordered by the court to ascertain whether the person has cleared of insanity or not and the managing power of his properties may be returned to him.

2. Marriage and Divorce

As per Hindu Marriage Act 1955 (with 1976 amendment in force) a marriage contract is considered invalid if, at the time of marriage, either party is

a. Incapable of giving valid consent to marriage in consequence of unsoundness of mind or
b. Though capable of giving valid consent, has been suffering from a mental disorder of such a kind or to such an extent as to be deemed unfit for marriage and procreation of children or
c. Has been subject to recurring episodes of insanity

In case of violation of any of the conditions mentioned in the act, the marriage will be considered null and void.

3. Testamentary Capacity

Before trying to understand testamentary capacity, we have to understand what a Will is. A Will is a legal document regarding a person's wish to dispose of his/her movable or immovable properties and material wealth after his/her death. So, a Will is made by a person to dispose of his wealth and properties to the persons of his liking after his death. Testamentary capacity is the capacity of a person to make a valid Will. Indian Succession Act, of 1935 (based on the Banks Vs Goodfellow criteria) makes the following observations.

a. Any person of sound mind can make a Will.
b. Persons, who are ordinarily insane, may make a Will during an interval when they are of sound mind (lucid interval)

c. No person can make a Will while he is in such a state of mind, whether arising from intoxication or illness or any other cause so he does not know what he is doing.

Banks vs Goodfellow criteria for testamentary capacity
1. Understanding of the nature of the will making and its effects
2. Knowledge of the nature and extent of one's assets
3. Knowledge of persons who have a reasonable claim to be beneficiaries
4. Understanding of the impacts of the distribution of the assets of the estate
5. A confirmation that the testator is free of any delusion that influences the disposition of the assets
6. Ability to express wishes clearly and consistently in an orderly plan of disposition)

MENTAL HEALTH ACTS IN INDIA

1. The Lunacy (Supreme Courts) Act, 1858
2. The Lunacy (District Courts) Acts, 1858
3. The Indian Lunatic Asylum Act, 1858
4. The Indian Lunacy Act, of 1912
5. The Mental Health Act, of 1987 and
6. The Mental Healthcare Act, 2017

Salient Features of Mental Healthcare Act, 2017

1. Definition of Mental Illness

"Mental illness means a substantial disorder of thinking, mood, perception, orientation or memory, that grossly impairs judgment, behavior, capacity to recognize reality or ability to meet the ordinary demands of life, mental conditions associated with abuse of alcohol or drugs, but does not include mental retardation which is a condition of arrested or incomplete development of mind of a person, especially characterized by sub-normality of intelligence." This act also clearly defines mental health professionals, mental health institutes, mental health review boards, etc.

2. Advance Directive

An advance directive is a newly introduced concept in this act according to which a person can make a wish in writing in advance regarding the way he wants to be treated and who will be his nominated representative in case he will develop any mental illness in the future. As per the law, an advance directive can be vetted by a medical health professional.

3. Nominated Representative

The nominated representative is a person empowered by a mentally ill person (while still symptom-free) to make treatment decisions and get access to his medical document in case he develops any mental illness. The nominated representative must not be a minor and should be a person who can understand basic ethics, morality, and conduct.

4. Decriminalization of Suicidal Attempt

The suicidal attempt was a criminal offense punishable by law under section 309 of IPC. The Mental Health Care Act has decriminalized suicidal attempts and states that "any person who attempts to commit suicide shall be presumed, unless proved otherwise, to have under severe stress and shall not be tried and punished under the said code."

5. Rights of the Person with Mental Illness

The Mental Healthcare Act recognizes the following rights of a person with mental: illness

a. Right to community living with dignity
b. Right to access treatment equal to that of other physical illnesses
c. Protection from inhuman and degrading treatment
d. Right to access medical records and information regarding treatment
e. Right to confidentiality
f. Right to contact and communicate with persons or organizations of their liking

6. Admission of Mentally Ill Patients

a. 'Independent admission' means an admission of a patient with mental illness who retains the capacity to make mental health care and treatment decisions. According to provisions in this bill, all admission should be independent admission unless conditions make supported admission unavoidable.
b. Supported admission means an admission of patients who have attempted bodily harm to themselves or have behaved violently toward others. Treatment decisions in such cases are made after a thorough examination of the patient by a psychiatrist and a mental health professional or a general practitioner. The duration of supported admission should not exceed 30 days initially, after which the need for continued admission is reviewed.
c. Admission of minor

A mentally ill minor patient can be admitted to a mental health establishment after due application by the nominated representative to the in-charge and after thorough examination by 2 psychiatrists or 1 psychiatrist, and a mental health professional or one psychiatrist and one general medical practitioner. The in charge of the institute must inform about admission of the minor to the medical board within 72 hours. The nominated representative or a female attendant appointed by the NP (in case a minor is a female) should stay with the minor patient throughout the admission period.

7. Discharge of Mentally Ill Patient

In the case of an independently admitted patient, the discharge can be done at the request of the patient. But, in case of supported admission, while discharging the patient the nominated representative, family members, and caregivers should be consulted before discharging the patient.

8. Modified ECT

The Mental Healthcare Act 2017 has banned direct ECT (ECT without Anaesthesia) and also **restricts its use in minors**. ECT can be administered in mental health establishments under general anesthesia only, which is known as modified ECT. In the case of minors, the decision to give ECT can be taken by a mental health review board along with the guardians.

9. Rehabilitation of Mentally Ill

The Mental Healthcare Act has tasked each state government to rehabilitate mentally ill persons back into the community or in safe homes or ashrams in collaboration with NGOs. The local authority and police establishment also must rescue vagrant and wandering mentally ill patients and bring them to mental health establishments for treatment.

NARCOTIC DRUGS AND PSYCHOTROPIC SUBSTANCES ACT (NDPSA)

NDPS Act, which was enacted in the year 1985, prohibits the cultivation, production, trafficking, and possession of narcotic drugs and psychoactive substances except for medical or research purposes that are also under license. This Act has the following features.

1. **The criminalization of drug use and possession:** Possession and use of certain drugs is illegal under this act and invites penalty which depends upon whether the drug was meant for selling or personal use.
2. Possession of **small quantities** (which varies from drugs to drugs as mentioned in Table 21.1) is assumed as for personal use while possession of commercial quantity is presumed as for selling purposes and invites different penalty terms.
3. The penalty for possession of small quantities is imprisonment for 6 months or a fine up to Rs 10,000 or both while that for commercial quantity is imprisonment of 10–20 years and a fine of rupees 1–2 lakh or both.

Treatment Provisions under the NDPS Act

1. An 'addict' is defined as a person dependent on any narcotic drugs or psychoactive substances
2. If addicts are convicted of consumption or offenses involving small quantities then instead of imprisonment they can be admitted to a rehab center for de-addiction treatment.
3. Those convicted addicts who volunteer for treatment are given immunity against conviction.

Table 21.1: Small and commercial quantities of psychoactive substances and prescribed punishment as per the NDPS Act revised, 2001

Drug	*Small quantity*	*Punishment*	*commercial quantity*	*Punishment*
Heroin	5 g	Maximum of 6 months of rigorous imprisonment or a fine up to Rs. 10,000 or both	250 g	Rigorous imprisonment of 10 years (min) to 20 years (max.) and a fine from Rs. 1 lakh to 2 lakh
Opium	25 g		2.5 kg	
Morphine	5 g		250 g	
Ganja	1 kg		20 kg	
Charas	100 g		1 kg	
Cocaine	2 g		100 g	
Methadone	2 g		50 g	
Methadone	2 g		50 g	
LSD	0.002 g		0.1 g	

Ethics in Psychiatry

Indian Psychiatric Society (IPS), in the year 1989, formulated the following codes of ethics for psychiatrists in this country. Every psychiatrist practicing in India should follow some basic ethical principles as follows:

1. **Responsibility,** a psychiatrist should have basic responsibility toward his patients and the society at large and should provide mental health services through observation, investigation, experimentation, and research.

2. **Competence**, he should update his knowledge through continued education and should understand that for this regard, lifetime, learning is necessary.
3. **Benevolence**, the patient's interest, and his health should be given primary importance above all.
4. **Moral standards**, a psychiatrist should follow all moral standards and expectations from society and should not indulge in any kind of activity that brings a bad reputation to the profession.
5. **Patient's welfare**, a psychiatrist should refrain from treating a case that does not fall within his competencies.
6. **Confidentiality**, it is mandatory for a psychiatrist to maintain the confidentiality of the patient's information while teaching or doing research work.

DISASTER PSYCHIATRY

Definition

The term disaster means bad star (*dis-astro*). Oxford Dictionary defines a disaster as a sudden accident or a natural catastrophe that causes great damage or loss of life. WHO in 1998 came up with the following definition of disaster: "a serious disruption of the functioning of a community or a society causing widespread human, material, economic or environmental losses that exceed the ability of the affected community or society to cope using its resources." In India the Disaster Management Act comes into force in the year 2005 which defines a disaster as: "a catastrophe, mishap, calamity, or grave occurrence in any area, arising from natural or manmade causes, or by accident or negligence which results in substantial loss of life or human suffering or damage to, and destruction of property, or damage to, or degradation of, environment and is of such a nature or magnitude as to be beyond the coping capacity of the community of the affected area". This is by far the most complete and wholesome definition of disaster although a complex one.

Types of Disasters

Natural and Man-made

Disasters can be natural or man-made. Natural disasters are generally considered by common folks as the wrath of god against their wrongdoings and their impact on psychological well-being is minimal. Man-made disasters can be accidental or deliberate. Fukushima nuclear fallout is an example of an accidental man-made disaster while the 9/11 terrorist attack is a well-known deliberate man-made disaster. The impact of the man-made disaster on psychological well-being is considerably high and even more so when it is due to deliberate acts.

Mental Health Conditions Associated with Disaster

Some of the most common psychiatric conditions associated with the disaster are mentioned below.

1. Relapse of previous psychiatric illness
2. Dissociative disorders
3. PTSD
4. Acute stress reaction
5. Grief, depression, anxiety neuroses
6. Substance abuse disorder
7. Somatoform disorder

Role of Mental Health Professional

Disasters are associated with an array of psychological problems and psychiatric illnesses which need to be taken care of by mental health care professionals. Mental health professionals have the following duties and responsibilities following a disaster.

Training of Resource Personnel

One of the first steps toward providing psychiatric care during a disaster is the training of resource personnel as they are the foot shoulders involved in identifying persons in need of psychiatric care. Training of resource persons includes teaching basic expertise in identifying mental health problems associated with the disaster, giving basic counseling, and referring those in need of specialized psychiatric evaluation and care. They are also trained in employing triage to assort people needing mental health care at different levels.

Psychological Rehabilitation

In the post-disaster period, many require psychiatric treatment in the form of counseling, reassurance, and emotional support. Resource personnel may be trained in providing basic psychological counseling and emotional support. Brief session psychotherapy and group psychotherapy are of great value in providing emotional support and reassurance in the immediate post-disaster period.

Specialized Care

Only a few cases need specialized care by trained psychiatrists. Cases in need of specialized care are those having PTSD, severe depression, prolonged grief, suicidal tendencies, etc. These patients need to be evaluated by experts and appropriate treatment with psychotherapy or pharmacotherapy should be given. Cognitive behavioral therapy is an evidence-based psychotherapeutic approach that can mitigate symptoms of many of the conditions requiring specialized care. Institutionalized treatment in a psychiatric hospital may be needed in some cases, especially for those with severe depression with active suicidal tendencies.

Prescribing Psychotropic Medications

Prescription of psychotropic medications should be discouraged in the post-disaster psychiatric management approach. However, few medications such as prazosin and propranolol are efficacious in preventing the development of PTSD in vulnerable cases. Similarly, those with severe depression and suicidal tendencies may be prescribed antidepressant medications. However, it is advisable to give medications only when necessary and for a short duration of time.

SUMMARY

1. The purpose of community psychiatry is to deliver affordable basic mental healthcare at the community level using community resources and through the primary healthcare system.
2. The National Mental health program was started in India in 1982 to decentralize mental health care and to deliver basic mental healthcare at the community level by integrating mental health care with the primary healthcare system. The district mental health program was started in 1996 under NMHP to further strengthen the mental healthcare delivery process at the community level.

3. Forensic psychiatry deals with the application of psychiatric knowledge in the administration of law. Many a time psychiatrists are summoned by the court of law to give their expert opinion on civil and criminal matters about a mentally ill patient.
4. The criminal responsibility of a mentally ill person is assessed in India based on 84 IPC which is based on M'Naghten's rule. According to this law, nothing is considered an offense done by a mentally ill person if he is incapable of knowing the nature of his act and its consequences.
5. Civil responsibilities of a mentally ill person involve management of personal property, marriage and divorce, and testamentary capacity. These aspects are dealt with by various laws of the Indian judicial system.
6. Currently in India, the Mental Healthcare Act, of 2017 is in force superseding all previous Mental Health Acts. New provisions in this Act are a concept of advance directive, nominated representative, rights of persons with mental illness, decriminalization of suicidal attempts, and banning of direct ECT.
7. NDPS Act, which was enacted in the year 1985, prohibits the cultivation, production, trafficking, and possession of narcotic drugs and psychoactive substances except for medical or research purposes that are also under license.
8. Practicing psychiatrists are advised to follow some ethical obligations such as responsibility, benevolence, competence, moral standards, and confidentiality.
9. Disaster is associated with various psychological problems such as acute stress reaction and PTSD, depression and suicide, grief, survivor's guilt, anxiety neurosis, etc.
10. The role of mental healthcare professionals during a disaster is to train resource personnel in identifying and managing psychological disaster-associated problems and providing psychological rehabilitation and specialized care to the affected.

BIBLIOGRAPHY

1. Wig NN, Murthy SR. The birth of a national mental health program for India. Indian J Psychiatry. 2015 Jul-Sep;57(3):315–9.
2. Pandya A, Shah K, Chauhan A, Saha S. Innovative mental health initiatives in India: A scope for strengthening primary healthcare services. J Family Med Prim Care. 2020 Feb 28;9(2):502–7.
3. Sood M, Krishnan V. Preventive psychiatry in clinical practice. Indian J Soc Psychiatry 2017;33:79–85.
4. Kobau R, Seligman ME, Peterson C, Diener E, Zack MM, Chapman D, Thompson W. Mental health promotion in public health: perspectives and strategies from positive psychology. Am J Public Health. 2011 Aug;101(8):e1–9.
5. Tirpude BH, Sheikh Nishat A, Chaudhary BL. Psychiatry and Civil Law. Vol. 6, No. 4 (2006-10-2006-12)
6. Kamath RM. Psychiatry and law: past, present and future. Mens Sana Monogr. 2015 Jan-Dec;13(1):105–13.
7. Math SB, Basavaraju V, Harihara SN, Gowda GS, Manjunatha N, Kumar CN, Gowda M. Mental Healthcare Act 2017 - Aspiration to action. Indian J Psychiatry. 2019 Apr;61(Suppl 4): S660–6.
8. Gundugurti Prasad Rao, Bhattacharyya Ranjan, Kondepi Sandeep, Chakraborty Kaustav, Mukherjee Abir. Ethics and Law. Indian Journal of Psychiatry: March 2022 - Volume 64 - Issue Suppl 1 - p S7–S15.
9. Math SB, Nirmala MC, Moirangthem S, Kumar NC. Disaster Management: Mental Health Perspective. Indian J Psychol Med. 2015 Jul-Sep;37(3):261–71.

Chapter 22

Integration

Competency achievement: Students should be able to

1. **PY10.7** Describe and discuss functions of cerebral cortex, basal ganglia, thalamus, hypothalamus, cerebellum and limbic system and their abnormalities
2. **PY10.8** Describe and discuss behavioural and EEG characteristics during sleep and mechanism responsible for its production
3. **PY10.12** Identify normal EEG forms
4. **FM5.4** Differentiate between true insanity from feigned insanity (facticious disorder and malingering)
5. **FM3.17** Describe and discuss the sexual perversions fetishism, transvestism, voyeurism, sadism, necrophagia, masochism, exhibitionism, frotteurism, and necrophilia

NEURODEVELOPMENT

A mammalian zygote, just after its formation, is divided many a time to give rise to a mass of cells known as a **morula**. Soon, a fluid-filled cavity, known as **blastocoel, is formed** inside the cell mass and now it is known as a **blastula**. Further growth and differentiation of the blastula give rise to a three-layered structure called a **germ plate**. A germ plate consists of **outer ectoderm, middle mesoderm,** and **inner endoderm**. The nervous system (both CNS and PNS) is derived entirely from the dorsal ectoderm of the germ plate. This process of development of the nervous system from the ectoderm is known as neurodevelopment.

Neurodevelopment starts with the formation of a ridge-like structure on the specially differentiated part of the dorsal ectoderm (**neuroectoderm**), along the rostrocaudal axis (head-tail axis) of the germ plate, known as the **neural plate**. This process of differentiation of the dorsal ectoderm to form a neural plate is called **neural induction**. Subsequently, the edges of the neural plate get elevated as neural crests form a neural groove. Neural crests grow curving medially and meet at the midline closing the neural groove to form a neural **tube**. The process of formation of the neural tube from the ectoderm is known as **neurulation**.

The neural tube is a fluid-filled structure lined with **neuroepithelial cells** which give rise to all the structures of the CNS. The rostral (head end) part of the neural tube forms **three distinctive dilatations** known as **primary brain vesicles**, from head to tail direction. These primary vesicles are the **prosencephalon (forebrain)** lying at the head end, the **mesencephalon (midbrain**) in the middle, and the **rhombencephalon (hindbrain)** lying at the tail end. These primary dilatations further give rise to **secondary dilatations**. Prosencephalon is further divided into **telencephalon** and **diencephalon, mesencephalon** remains undivided while rhombencephalon further gives rise to **metencephalon** and **myelencephalon**.

Cerebral hemispheres and basal ganglia are derived from the telencephalon and the diencephalon gives rise to the thalamus, hypothalamus, and other associated diencephalic structures. The midbrain structures and colliculi are derived from the mesencephalon. Metencephalon gives rise to pons and cerebellum while medulla oblongata is derived from myelencephalon.

Neural Migration

Neurons and neural glial cells are derived from the totipotent neuroepithelial cells lining the neural tube by a process known as **neurogenesis**. Neurons are post-mitotic; they will not divide again throughout their lifetime after their generation. After neurogenesis, these cells migrate toward the place of their destination through a process called **neural migration**. Neural migration is a complex process involving various homing chemicals or chemotactic factors, neurotrophic factors, and the expression of a slew of genes. Neuronal migration to their destined location from their place of origin can occur radially or tangentially. Depending upon the paths of migration, neuronal migration can be **radial or tangential**.

1. Radial Migration

The **pyramidal cells** of the cerebral cortex are derived and **deposited in a layered manner** by this process. The neural progenitor cells lining the primitive ventricles of the forebrain are known as neural glial cells. These totipotent cells proliferate and give rise to the first batch of neural cells which migrate toward the surface and form a layer just below the pia mater known as pre-plate consisting of **Cajal–Retzius cells**. A network of elongated glial cells now occupies the space between the neural glial cells and pre-plate forming a supportive scaffolding for the migration of neurons. The subsequent neural cells derived from the neural glial cells are guided by these scaffolding glial cells and the cell migration occurs toward the surface (pia mater) along their axons. These migrating cells also have one of their ends attached to the pia and their cell body or soma is gradually pushed toward the surface with the help of microtubules. Ultimately these cells reach near the surface and form a layer (Fig. 22.1). The subsequent batch of neural cells migrates similarly and cross passes the previous layers and is laid above them. By this process, all the layers of the cerebral cortex are laid one above the other in an **inside-out** manner meaning younger cells are laid above the older cells.

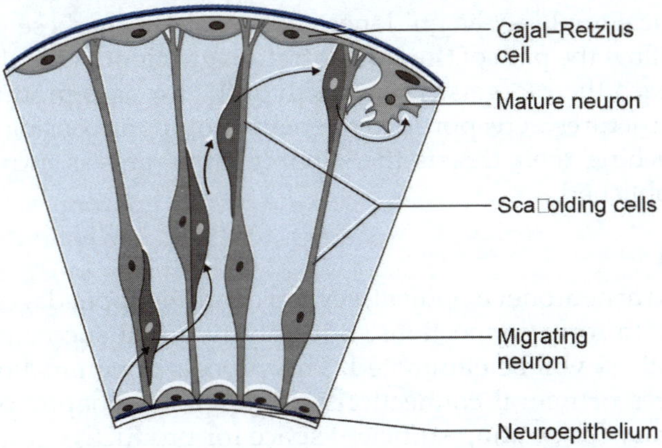

Fig. 22.1: Radial migration of pyramidal neurons.

2. Tangential Migration

The **interneurons** of the cerebral cortex are derived from the **ganglionic eminence** (GE) and subsequently **follow a tangential path** to reach the cerebral cortex. The ganglionic eminence is a structure consisting of totipotent cells and is situated between the telencephalon and diencephalon of the embryonic brain (between the thalamus and caudate nucleus). These totipotent cells of GE proliferate and give rise to neurons destined to be interneurons of the cerebral cortex. These newly generated cells follow a path parallel to the preplate and perpendicular to the neural glial cells to reach the space between the migrating pyramidal cells. This process of migration of interneurons perpendicular (tangential) to the neural glial cells is known as tangential migration (Fig. 22.2).

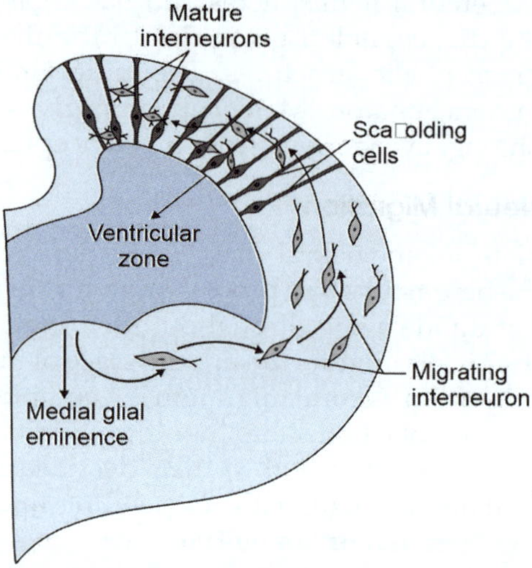

Fig. 22.2: Tangential migration of interneurons.

Neural Differentiation

The migrated nerve cells (both pyramidal cells and interneurons) are immature and devoid of any appendages. Soon after reaching their place of destination, they start developing **outgrowths** forming **axons and dendrites**. To establish connections between one another synaptic apparatus are developed at the ends of these appendages known as dendritic filopodia. Through these processes, these cells start appearing matured and well connected.

Axon Guidance

The process by which neurons of the CNS send out their growing axons to their correct targets is known as axon guidance. It starts with the formation of a specialized structure at the point of axon growth known as the **growth cone**. Growth cones express certain receptors which are stimulated by chemotactic signals coming from the target organ. These **chemotactic signals** act as guidance cues. Assisted by these guidance cues the growing axons follow the path of **the concentration gradient** of the chemotactic factors and ultimately reach their targets. The growth of the axons is promoted and directed by cytoskeletal structures in response to the neurotrophic actions of these chemotactic signals. After reaching their targets the synaptic apparatus is formed and a proper connection is established.

Synaptic Pruning

During the process of neurodevelopment, several dendritic appendages **fiercely compete** with one another to form connections. But only two will succeed to form a secure connection and others will be eliminated. This process of elimination of unnecessary neural appendages or neural connections is known as synaptic pruning. Synaptic pruning is necessary for creating sufficient space for productive connections between neurons for their optimal functioning.

Activity-dependent Plasticity

Neurogenesis, neural migration, subsequent differentiation, dendritic and axonal outgrowth, and axon guidance are activity-independent processes and are hard-wired in the genetic blueprint of the individual.

A growing child gains experiences through interaction with his surroundings. Through these experiences, a child acquires language skills, and motor skills and develops learning, and forms memories. These skills are acquired and mastered by processes occurring at the neuronal level known as activity-dependent neuroplasticity. The mechanisms responsible for activity-dependent plasticity are **long-term potentiation (LTP),** synaptogenesis, synaptic pruning, and adult neurogenesis.

Long-term potentiation or LTP is a process by which existing synaptic connections are further strengthened. LTP is the underlying neural mechanism responsible for memory formation and learning. Active LTP has been demonstrated in the hippocampus (brain region responsible for memory formation) and in the cerebellum (responsible for acquiring motor skills).

Synaptogenesis is the process by which new synapses are formed. The brain-derived neurotrophic factor (BDNF) and nerve growth factor are secreted at specific areas in response to certain experience-driven stimuli and stimulate the sprouting of new neuronal outgrowths and establishing connections between them. Contrary to this, those connections which are deprived of growth factors (BDNF or NGF) are subsequently eliminated by the processing of pruning.

Adult neurogenesis has been detected in the hippocampus and some other areas of the brain. The formation of newer neurons in the hippocampus is necessary for memory formation and its consolidation into long-term memory.

BRAINSTEM

The brainstem is an elongated structure consisting mainly of white fiber tracts with embedded nuclei (collections of gray matter inside the CNS), connecting the cerebral hemispheres with the spinal cord. The brainstem is divided from top to bottom into **four parts**: **diencephalon, midbrain, pons, and medulla oblongata.**

Diencephalon is a part of the forebrain (along with cerebral hemispheres) and consists of a collection of nuclei surrounding the third ventricle. Diencephalon has four distinct parts **thalamus, hypothalamus, epithalamus, and subthalamus.**

Thalami (plural for thalamus) are bilateral wedge-shaped gray matter structures situated **lateral to the walls** of the third ventricle and lie medial to the posterior limbs of internal capsules. Thalamus is further divided into **four regions**: **anterior, posterior, medial, and lateral** with each region containing several nuclei. Thalami act as the primary **relay station** for all incoming sensory inputs and send them to the cerebral cortices via thalamic radiations. The anterior nucleus of the thalamus which is connected to the mammillary bodies via the mammillothalamic tract is also a part of the limbic system and **Papez circuit** (*See* Fig. 22.7).

Hypothalamus is a collection of grey matter surrounding the third ventricle and lying below the thalami, somewhat anteriorly. Apart from consisting of a large number of nuclei it also contains several prominent structures like **mammillary bodies, infundibulum, and hypophysis**. Functional aspects of the hypothalamus have been discussed in the limbic system section.

The **epithalamus** is the uppermost part of the diencephalon and consists of the **pineal gland, habenular nuclei, habenular commissure, and posterior commissure**. Habenular nuclei are involved in the regulation of motivation and behavior while the **pineal gland** is important for the secretion of **melatonin** that regulates the sleep-wake cycle.

Subthalamus is the portion of the diencephalon extending into the midbrain. It contains the **nucleus basalis of Meynert** which serves as the seat of **cholinergic neurons** and projects to the cerebral cortex.

Midbrain

Midbrain is the part of the brainstem lying below the diencephalon. The **aqueduct of Sylvius** which connects the third ventricle with the fourth ventricle lies within the midbrain. The aqueduct is surrounded by a mass of gray matter known as **periaqueductal grey (PAG).** PAG is a **part of the reticular activating system (RAS)** and is involved in arousal and pain modulation. Other important nuclei present within the midbrain are the substantia nigra, raphe nuclei, and ventral tegmental area (VTA).

1. **Substantia nigra** harbors **dopaminergic neurons** which project to the striatum (**nigrostriatal pathway**). This pathway is involved in **Parkinson's disease** and **antipsychotics-induced EPS** (extrapyramidal symptoms).
2. **Raphe nuclei** (dorsal and median raphe nuclei) are the principal **serotonergic nuclei** and project to various areas of the brain which are involved in the regulation of mood and emotions.
3. **The ventral tegmental area (VTA)** also harbors **dopaminergic neurons** which project to the nucleus accumbens. This pathway is involved in **reward and motivation**, **substance addiction,** and also in producing **positive symptoms** of schizophrenia.

Pons

The pons is somewhat swollen anteriorly and hollowed out posteriorly. The posterior part of the pons forms the floor of the fourth ventricle.

The most important structure lying within the pons is the **locus coeruleus**. It is a collection of **noradrenergic neurons** and is situated bilaterally at the **roof of the fourth ventricle**. Locus coeruleus is the principal nucleus containing noradrenergic neurons and sends afferents to various parts of the brain. It is involved in **arousal, attention, and the sympathetic response of emotions**.

A group of scattered nuclei present within the pons are known as **pontine nuclei**. The **pedunculopontine tegmental nuclei** and **lateral dorsal pontine nuclei** are **cholinergic** in nature and involved in reward and motivation. Other important pontine nuclei are **parabrachial nuclei** and **lateral tegmental nuclei** which are parts of the RAS and are involved in arousal.

Medulla Oblongata

It is the lowermost part of the brainstem and continues below the spinal cord at the foramen magnum. Medulla oblongata harbors the vasomotor center which regulates cardiovascular functions and reflexes. It also contains the dorsal and ventral respiratory nuclei which regulate respiratory functions.

Reticular-activating System (RAS)

The RAS is a **part of the reticular formation** and consists of a network of nuclei distributed at the anterior part of the brain stems across its length. This network of nuclei is divided into 4 major groups (Fig. 22.3).

1. **Locus coeruleus** (seat of noradrenergic neurons)
2. **Pedunculopontine tegmentum** (seat of glutaminergic neurons)
3. **Raphe nuclei** (seat of serotonergic neurons) and
4. **Posterior tuberomammillary hypothalamus** (seat of histaminergic neurons)

Each of these nuclei groups contains **monoaminergic neurons** and projects widely throughout the brain.

The primary function of RAS is the **maintenance of wakefulness, arousal, and attention**. Activation of RAS starts with the secretion of **orexin A and B** from the **lateral hypothalamus** in response to external light stimulus. Orexins act primarily on locus coeruleus leading to **bursts of noradrenergic activity** which make the animal awake and alert. Other components of the RAS release monoamines such as **histamine and glutamine** which complement noradrenaline in maintaining wakefulness, arousal, and attention.

BASAL GANGLIA AND CEREBELLUM

Basal ganglia are the collections of gray matters lying underneath the cerebral hemispheres which are involved in **initiation of motor movement** and maintenance of body posture. The functional components of basal ganglia are the striatum (**caudate and putamen**), globus pallidus, substantia nigra and subthalamic nuclei, **caudate** being the most important part of the basal ganglia complex. The primary task of the caudate nucleus is to **filter out the signals** for un-necessary movements coming from the cerebral cortex. Excessive activation of caudate nucleus filters out motor signals excessively leading to akinesia and bradykinesia as seen in **Parkinson's disease** and **drug induced EPS**. On the other hand, poor activation of caudate nucleus leads to ineffective filtering of motor signals resulting in un-necessary movements such as tic, stereotype and mannerism as seen in **Tourette syndrome,** autism and schizophrenia. Cerebellum is also involved in fine coordination of motor movements. The importance of cerebellum in psychiatry is limited.

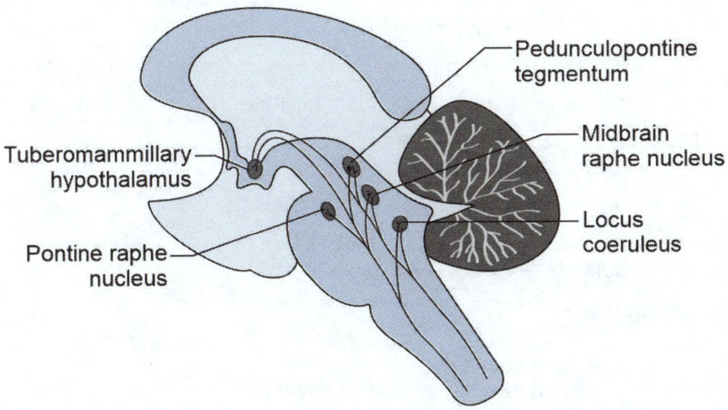

Fig. 22.3: Components of the reticular-activating system.

LIMBIC SYSTEM

The Limbic System consists of several structures surrounding the brain stem and lying underneath the cerebral hemispheres. The term **limbus (border)** signifies their position at the bordering area between the brainstem and cerebral hemispheres. It contains brain structures derived both from the telencephalon and diencephalon and is the primary center for emotional regulation, behavior, and memory formation.

Depending upon their location, the limbic structures can be grouped into the following three regions (Fig. 22.4).

1. **Cortical structures or the limbic cortex**
   - **Orbitofrontal cortex** associated with subjective sensation of emotion
   - **Anterior cingulate cortex** is the center for reward processing, ethics, and morality
   - **Hippocampus** is the primary brain area responsible for memory consolidation
   - **Parahippocampal gyrus**
2. **Subcortical structures**
   - **Septal area**
   - **Amygdala** is involved in the processing of emotions and emotional learning
   - **Nucleus accumbens** is associated with reward and pleasure (pleasure center)
3. **Diencephalic structures**
   - **Hypothalamus** is involved in the autonomic response of emotions
   - **Mammillary bodies**
   - An **anterior nucleus of the thalamus**

Lateral Ventricles of the Brain

Understanding the anatomy of the lateral ventricle is necessary to develop a clear idea about the anatomical position of structures of the limbic system. The cerebral hemispheres are **hollow structures** and each of them contains one elongated **fluid-filled cavity** known as the lateral ventricle. Each lateral ventricle has **a body** and three appendages known as **horns**. The **anterior horn** extends forward into the frontal lobe, the **posterior horn** extends into the occipital lobe and the inferior horn lies within the temporal lobe. Limbic system structures are found around the **inferior horn** of the lateral ventricle (Fig. 22.5).

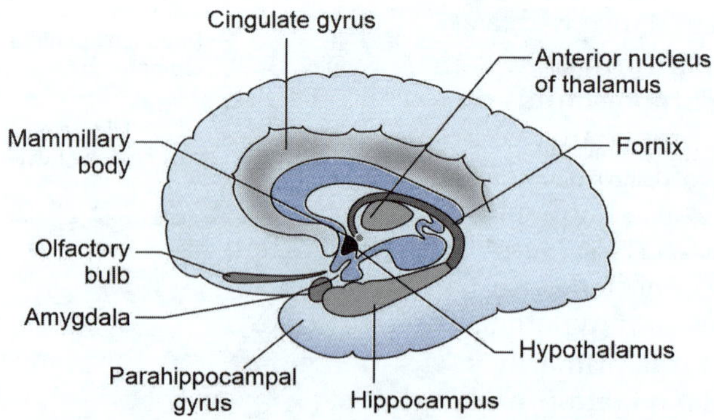

Fig. 22.4: Major components of limbic system.

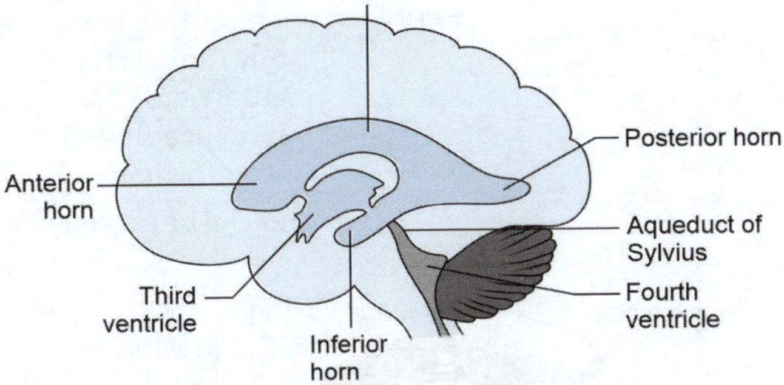

Fig. 22.5: Ventricular system of the brain.

LIMBIC CORTEX

Orbitofrontal Cortex

The orbitofrontal cortex (OFC) is a part of the frontal lobe and is situated on its ventral surface sitting on the **orbital plate**. Functionally, it is considered a part of the prefrontal **cortex** and synonymous with the **ventromedial prefrontal cortex (VMPFC)**. It is the center for cognitive **appraisal of emotion** (the subjective sensation of emotion), **cognitive modulation of emotions, empathy, and impulsivity**.

Anterior Cingulate Cortex

The cingulate cortex is a part of the frontal lobe on its medial surface lying **above the corpus callosum**. The part of the cingulate cortex lying anteriorly and inferiorly to the **genu of the corpus callosum** is called the anterior cingulate cortex which is a part of the limbic system. It is involved in **reward processing, pleasure sensation** in response to good experiences and memory, and also regulates **fear and aggression**.

Hippocampus

To find the hippocampus we have to trace the surface of the temporal lobe first downward and then medically along its outer surface till we reach the brainstem. The medial most of the temporal lobe is known as the medial temporal cortex and medially further lies the parahippocampal gyrus. Just above the parahippocampal gyrus, there is an elongated structure along the upper surface of the **inferior horn of the lateral ventricle.** This elongated structure is known as the hippocampus. It gets its name due to its uncanny resemblance with **a seahorse (hippocampus)**.

The hippocampal formation is a structure consisting of three distinct parts, the **dentate gyrus, the hippocampus proper, and the subiculum** (Fig. 22.6). Dentate gyrus and hippocampus proper are two interlocked C-shaped structures. The hippocampus proper or simply hippocampus is a C-shaped structure that resembles the sea horse or a **ram's horn** and is also known as cornua ammonis **(CA)**. Histologically, it is divided into **4 zones CA1, CA2, CA3,** and CA4 each containing special types of neurons. The Hippocampus is connected with the parahippocampal gyrus, amygdala, thalamus, mammillary bodies, and hypothalamus.

The hippocampus is primarily associated with **memory consolidation, emotional regulation, spatial navigation, and cognitive processing**. Memory consolidation is the process by which short-term memory is converted into long-term memory. This process

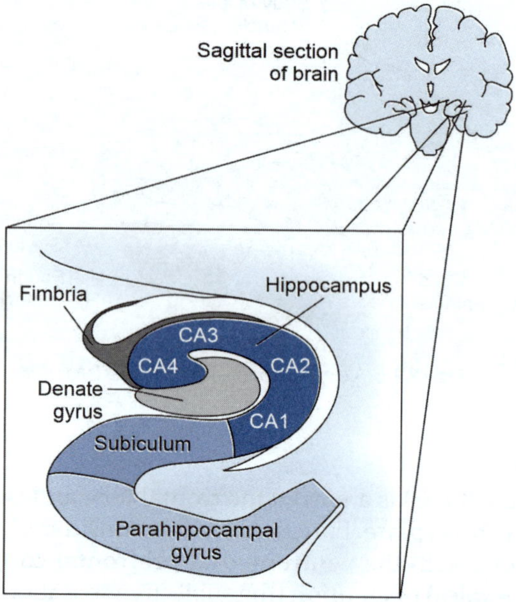

Fig. 22.6: Structures of the hippocampal formation.

involves the hippocampus-assisted strengthening of synapses and the formation of new synapses in the frontal cortex via a process known as **long-term potentiation (LTP).** Memories are stored permanently in the form of new synapses and also as strengthening of already existing synapses.

Amygdala

Amygdala is the primary brain center for the **regulation of emotions, aggression, emotional memory, and social cognition.**

The amygdala is an **almond-shaped structure** lying at the anterior end of the hippocampus underneath the medial most of the temporal lobe (known as uncus). Amygdala gets its name from its resemblance to an almond. The amygdala is a collection of large numbers of nuclei grouped into five functional groups: basolateral nuclei, central nuclei, cortical-like nuclei, other amygdaloid nuclei, and extended amygdala.

Amygdala gets inputs primarily from the sensory association cortex (parietal-temporal-occipital cortex). It sends output signals via two output tracts: **the dorsal tract and the ventral tract**. It sends signals to the **orbitofrontal and anterior cingulate cortices** which are responsible for the **subjective sensation of emotions and their cognitive modulations**. Amygdala also activates the hypothalamus and other brain stem nuclei associated with sympathetic activities in response to emotion. These connections mediate the hormonal response and bodily symptoms of emotions. Amygdalar connections with the hippocampus are responsible for emotional memory formation for emotionally charged stimuli.

Hypothalamus

Hypothalamus is a center for extensive sensory integration and motor output and is involved in controlling **autonomic, endocrine, and somatic behavior.**

Hypothalamus is a bilateral collection of several nuclei surrounding the third ventricle. It is situated at the center of the brain just above the midbrain somewhat anteriorly and below the thalami. Hypothalamus is divided into three zones: **periventricular zone, middle zone, and outer zone**. The periventricular zone regulates endocrine functions while medial and lateral zones are involved in the regulation of autonomic and somatic functions.

Hypothalamus is extensively connected with the cerebral cortex, hippocampus, amygdala, brain stem, and other parts of the brain.

From a psychiatric point of view, hypothalamus-mediated **regulation of sleep, appetite, and regulation of the HPA axis** is important. **The feeding center** lies in the **ventromedial nucleus** of the hypothalamus and is regulated by certain chemicals such as ghrelin, leptin, orexin, and neuropeptide. Activation of the **anterior hypothalamus induces sleep** while the posterior hypothalamus promotes wakefulness. This flip-flop is regulated by various sleep and wakefulness-promoting chemicals such as GABA, adenosine, histamine, norepinephrine, etc. It is the **ventrolateral preoptic nucleus** of the hypothalamus that secretes GABA in response to adenosine and inhibits the wakefulness-promoting brainstem apparatus known as **RAS.**

Nucleus Accumbens

The nucleus accumbens is a small rounded structure situated at the basal forebrain between the caudate nucleus and putamen, anterior-inferior to the head of the caudate nucleus. Each cerebral hemisphere has its nucleus accumbens. Along with the olfactory tubercle, it forms the **ventral striatum** which is a part of the basal ganglia (caudate nucleus and putamen form the dorsal striatum). The Nucleus Accumbens consists of a core and a shell and the shell contains medium-spiny neurons bearing **dopamine D_1 and D_2 receptors**.

Nucleus accumbens is known as the **pleasure center of the brain** and is involved in **reward and motivation**. The pleasure circuit projects from the **ventral tegmental area (VTA)** in the brainstem to nucleus accumbens and is activated by such stimuli as good food, personal achievements, and sexual intercourse. Activation of the pleasure circuit leads to the secretion of dopamine in NAc which gives the sensation of pleasure. Nucleus accumbens is involved in drug addiction and also in **psychosis**.

Papez Circuit

Papez circuit was discovered by **James Papez** via his ingenious experiment in which he injected **live rabies virus** into the hippocampus and traced the path it traversed through the various structures of the brain and found a circuit loop. Initially, he thought that this circuit is involved in the **regulation of emotions.** However, subsequently, it was discovered that it is involved in memory formation.

The circuit starts with the hippocampus. From the posterior end of **hippocampi** arise the white fiber tracts and meet at the midline to form the **fornix**. Fornix curves upward and anteriorly and enters the hypothalamus and again splits into two tracts. These tracts enter the **mammillary bodies** (which lie below the hypothalamus) of respective sides. Now the **mammillothalamic tract** arises from the mammillary body and goes upward into the anterior **nucleus of the thalamus**. Next, the circuit projects from the anterior nucleus of the thalamus as a part of thalamic radiation and goes to the cingulate **cortex**. The white fiber tracts from the cingulate cortex arise at the posterior end as the

cingulum and go to the **parahippocampal gyrus**. At last, the parahippocampal gyrus sends the output again to the hippocampus completing the circuit (Fig. 22.7).

Papez circuit is primarily involved in **memory formation** and consolidation of short-term memory into long-term memory. Damage to any structure of the **Papez circuit** can hamper this process and presents with **anterograde amnesia**. In Korsakoff syndrome there is free radical damage to mammillary bodies and the anterior nucleus of the thalamus due to thiamine deficiency. That's why anterograde amnesia is the hallmark sign of **Korsakoff syndrome**.

CEREBRAL CORTEX

Below the bony skull lie the **three-layered meninges** covering the brain. The folded cerebral cortex, the outer layer of the cerebrum lies below the innermost meningeal layer (the pia mater). The cerebral cortex is the grey matter part of the cerebrum and it appears grey as it is devoid of myelination. Cerebrum is divided into two **cerebral hemispheres**: the **right cerebral hemisphere and the left cerebral hemisphere**. At the bottom, these two cerebral hemispheres are connected by a bundle of white fiber tracts known as the **corpus callosum**. Each cerebral hemisphere is further divided into **four lobes: frontal lobe, parietal lobe, temporal lobe, and occipital lobe.** Each of these lobes has been assigned special functions known as higher mental functions or cognitive functions.

Concept of Cerebral Dominance

There is a widely held **misconception** that cerebral dominance is determined by a **person's handedness,** e.g. right-handed persons have left dominance and vice-versa. But it should be remembered that cerebral dominance has nothing to do with a person's handedness and about 70% of left-handed persons have left the dominant hemisphere. Another widely held misconception is that the dominant hemisphere is superior in terms of functions. But as far as function is concerned both hemispheres are equivalent to each other.

So, what determines cerebral dominance in a person? It is the **location of language functions** that determines cerebral dominance. The language function is lateralized in all human beings. If the language function is located in the left cerebral hemisphere

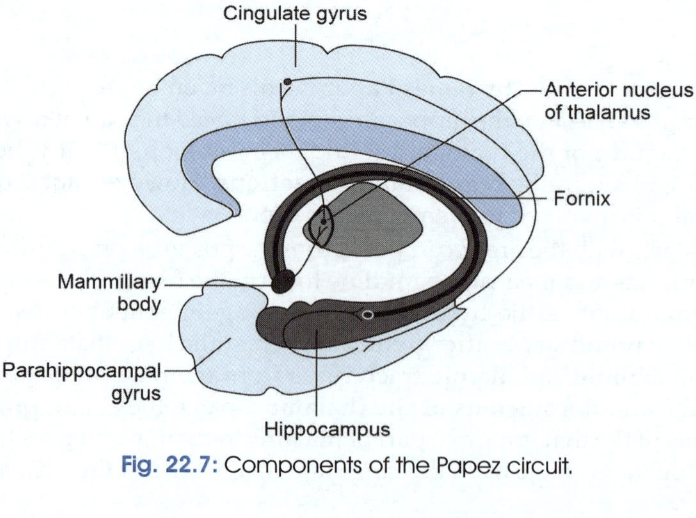

Fig. 22.7: Components of the Papez circuit.

then the person is left dominant and vice-versa. Left dominance does not mean that the left hemisphere is superior in function but it is just the location of language function on the left cerebral cortex and nothing else.

FRONTAL LOBE

The frontal lobe is the **largest part** of the cerebrum. Anatomically, the frontal lobe is the **anterior-most** of the cerebral hemisphere located anterior to the **central sulcus**. It is separated from the parietal lobe by the central sulcus and from the temporal lobe by the **Sylvian fissure**. The frontal cortex has **three surfaces**: dorsolateral surface, medial surface, and orbital surface. Its dorsolateral surface bears the **precentral gyrus** which lies just anterior to the central sulcus and runs vertically and is the **primary motor cortex.** Anterior to the precentral gyrus lies **three horizontal gyri:** superior, middle, and inferior frontal gyri. The medial surface of the frontal lobe contains the superior medial frontal gyrus and cingulate gyrus. The orbital surface is divided by an **H-shaped** sulcus into four parts.

Prefrontal Cortex (PFC)

(Much of our early understanding of functions of the prefrontal cortex came from the **case of Phineas Gage**. He was **an American railroad construction worker** and met with an accident in 1848 in which an iron rod got penetrated his skull injuring his left anterior frontal lobe. Surprisingly Gage survived the accident and lived for another 12 years. But once a loving father and caring husband with a calm and friendly personality, Gage became irritable, sulky, and careless, short-tempered with sudden aggression at times after the accident. This subsequent **change in Gage's personality** was famously termed by his friends as **'no longer Gage'**. This incident changed our understanding of the relationship between the brain and mind forever).

PFC is a functionally distinct part of the frontal cortex lying at the anterior part. It is the **most advanced** part of the brain and is highly developed in humans. It is the center of all the higher mental functions which make us distinctly human: **planning, judgment and reasoning, abstract thinking, and personality.**

The anatomical demarcation of the prefrontal cortex is **diffused and indistinct**. As per consensus, any part of the frontal cortex whose stimulation does not evoke a motor response is a part of the prefrontal cortex. It is also known as 'the **granular frontal cortex' or the 'frontal association cortex'**. The prefrontal cortex is divided into the following parts.

1. Lateral prefrontal cortex
2. Ventromedial prefrontal cortex

The dorsolateral prefrontal cortex **(dlPFC)** and ventrolateral prefrontal cortex **(vlPFC)** are two functionally distinct parts of the lateral **prefrontal cortex**. dlPFC lies anterior to the premotor and motor association cortices and contains the **frontal eye field**. It is part of the brain which is **involved in executive functions** (judgment, reasoning, planning, working memory, etc.), sustained attention, motivation, intelligence, and personality. **Ventrolateral PFC** is the part around **Broca's area** and involved in abstract mediation of the **verbal expression of language.**

Ventromedial PFC is further divided into **ventral PFC and medial PFC**. Ventral PFC is also known as the **orbitofrontal cortex (OFC)** and is involved in the regulation of mood and emotions, impulsivity, and subjective sensation of emotions via its extensive and reciprocal connections with **the limbic system**. **Medial PFC** consists of the **anterior cingulate cortex (ACC)** and regulates attention, reward, aggression, and cognitive modulation of emotions.

MAJOR NEUROTRANSMITTER SYSTEMS

Neurotransmitters are chemicals that **carry messages between neurons** and are essential for information processing in the CNS. Abnormal activities of neurotransmitters are implicated in almost all psychiatric illnesses.

From chemical aspects, neurotransmitters can be grouped as **amino acids** (glutamate, GABA), **peptides** (neuropeptide Y, endorphins), **lipids** (acetylcholine), **amines** (dopamine, serotonin, norepinephrine, etc), **steroids,** etc. But, when the functional aspect is considered they can be **either absolute or relative**. Absolute neurotransmitters are either excitatory or inhibitory. Glutamate is the absolute excitatory and GABA is the absolute inhibitory neurotransmitter. On the other hand, relative neurotransmitters impart either excitatory or inhibitory action depending upon the receptors they act on. This category includes dopamine, serotonin, noradrenaline, etc. as they can be either excitatory or inhibitory depending on the receptors they act.

MECHANISM OF ACTION

Neurotransmitters are **chemical messengers** which transmit messages across the synaptic junction. They are stored in **specialized vesicles** in the presynaptic terminal. When excitation of the presynaptic neuron reaches the axon terminal it results in an opening of the **calcium channels**. Calcium influx into this terminal leads to the docking of neurotransmitters containing vesicles with the presynaptic membrane and its **subsequent release** into the synaptic cleft. After their release, they act on the **specialized receptors** on the postsynaptic terminals and result in the opening of either excitatory (Na^+, Ca^{2+}) or inhibitory (Cl^-, K^+) channels and respectively either excite or inhibit the postsynaptic neuron.

AMINO ACID NEUROTRANSMITTERS

Glutamate

Glutamate is the principal **excitatory neurotransmitter** in the brain. It is a **non-essential amino acid** synthesized by the body itself. Glutamate is involved in **memory consolidation and learning**.

Glutamate acts on glutamate receptors such as **NMDA** (N-methyl-D-aspartate), **AMPA** (α-amino-3-hydroxy-5-methyl-4-isoxazole propionic acid), **kainate receptor, and metabotropic** glutamate receptors. NMDA, AMPA, and kainate receptors are ion channels (Na^+ or Ca^{2+} ion channels) while metabotropic receptors are coupled with stimulatory G-protein (Gs).

Actions of glutamate-mediated via **NMDA receptors** are essential for **memory formation and learning**. The neural mechanisms underlying memory and learning (i.e. **long-term potentiation**) occur through NMDA receptor-mediated glutamate activity. LTP, which requires the repetitive firing of glutaminergic neurons, is the underlying mechanism for memory consolidation in the hippocampus and learning in cerebral and cerebellar cortices.

GABA

Gamma-amino-butyric acid (GABA) is the principal **inhibitory neurotransmitter** in the mammalian brain. GABA is **derived from glutamate** by the process of decarboxylation. GABA acts on various GABA receptors such as **GABAa, GABAb, and GABAc**, all of which are inhibitory. GABAa and GABAc are chloride (Cl^-) ion channels while GABAb is an inhibitory G-protein (Gi) coupled metabotropic receptor.

Functions of GABA include induction of **sleep, regulation of emotions** and feedback, and feeding forward inhibitions of neural cells via GABAergic interneurons.

MONOAMINE NEUROTRANSMITTERS

Dopamine

Dopamine is synthesized from the amino acid **tyrosine**. Dopamine is involved in **motivation, reward, motor control,** etc. the major dopaminergic pathways in the brain are:

1. **Mesolimbic pathway**—projecting from VTA (ventral tegmental area) to NAc (nucleus accumbens), involved in reward and positive symptoms of schizophrenia
2. **Mesocortical pathway**—projecting from VTA to the prefrontal cortex, involved in motivation and negative symptoms **of schizophrenia**
3. **Nigrostriatal pathway**—projecting from substantia nigra to the putamen. Involved in motor planning and processing. Degeneration of dopaminergic neurons of these tracts leads to Parkinson's disease.
4. **Infundibular pathway**—projecting from mammillary bodies to pituitary. Involved in the inhibition of prolactin secretion
5. **Thalamocortical** and **corticothalamic pathways**

Dopamine acts on dopamine receptors which are grouped as **D_1 type** which includes D_1 and D_5 receptors and **D_2 type** which includes D_2, D_3 and D_4 receptors. D_1 type receptors are coupled with **stimulatory G protein**, excitatory in action, and are involved in motivation and reward. In contrast, D_2 receptors are coupled with **inhibitory G protein**, inhibitory in action, and mediate motor control and inhibition of prolactin secretion.

Serotonin

Serotonin or **5-hydroxy tryptamine** is synthesized from the amino acid tryptophan via hydroxylation. Serotonin is involved in the **regulation of mood, emotions, and behavior.**

The principal **serotonergic neuronal** masses in CNS are located in the **pons** and are known as **raphe nuclei.** Serotonergic neurons from raphe nuclei are projected to other parts of the brain such as the limbic system, midbrain, cerebral cortex, etc.

There are seven classes of serotonin receptors ranging from **5HT1 to 5HT7.** Among these, 5HT1 and 5HT5 are inhibitory (coupled with Gi) while others are excitatory. After its action on various receptors, serotonin is cleared off the synaptic cleft either by re-uptake into the presynaptic terminal via SERT (serotonin reuptake transporter) or transformed into the end product 5HIAA (5 hydroxy indoles acetic acid) via the enzyme **MAO (monoamine oxidase).**

Noradrenaline

Norepinephrine in the brain is involved in arousal and **wakefulness, attention, sympathetic activation** (fights or flight response), regulation of emotions, sensory gating, etc. It is synthesized from dopamine via the process of beta-hydroxylation. Noradrenergic neurons are principally found in the **locus coeruleus** located in the pons at the **roof of the fourth ventricle** and project to other areas of the brain.

Noradrenergic receptors are categorized as α and β **receptor** families. α receptors are further divided into α-1 which is coupled with Gs and is excitatory in nature and α-2 which is coupled with Gi and is inhibitory in nature. β adrenergic receptors are further divided into β-1, β-2, and β-3 receptors all of which are excitatory in nature.

Acetylcholine

Acetylcholine is a lipid consisting of an acetyl group attached to a choline group and derived from phospholipids. In the CNS, it is involved in **cognition** (memory, executive functions, etc.), **arousal, reward, and motivation.**

Cholinergic neurons in the brain stem are concentrated in the pedunculopontine **nucleus** and **dorsolateral tegmental nuclei** from where they project mainly to other parts of the brainstem and limbic system. Cholinergic activity in these pathways is involved in arousal, alertness, reward, and motivation. Cholinergic neurons in cerebral hemispheres are concentrated in the basal **forebrain nucleus of Meynert** and septal nucleus and project to other areas of the cerebral cortex. Cholinergic activities in these pathways are involved in **memory and cognition.**

Acetylcholine receptors are grouped as Muscarinic and nicotinic receptors. Muscarinic receptors are further divided into 5 types ranging from M_1 to M_5. The action of acetylcholine in CNS is mainly mediated through M_1 muscarinic receptors, which is a G-proteins (Gq) coupled metabotropic receptor. After its action, acetylcholine is cleared off the synaptic cleft by the action of the enzyme acetylcholinesterase which cleaves it into acetyl and choline parts.

Histamine

Histamine is an amine derived from the **amino acid, histidine**. The major brain histaminergic pathway projects from the **tuberomammillary nucleus** in the posterior hypothalamus to various parts of the brain. A major role of histamine is the regulation of the sleep-**wake cycle, appetite regulation, and promoting arousal**.

Histamine receptors are of four types **H_1–H_4**. The H_1 histamine receptor is involved in the regulation of the sleep-wake cycle and suppresses appetite while the H_3 histamine receptor regulates the activities of other amine neurotransmitters (dopamine, serotonin, and noradrenaline). Because of its involvement in the sleep-wake cycle, molecules with H_1 antagonistic activity (first-generation antihistamines, second-generation antipsychotics, and TCAs) induce sleep and increase appetite leading to weight gain.

Melatonin

Melatonin or 5 methoxy-N-acetyl tryptamine is the main hormone secreted by the **pineal gland**. **Pinealocytes** in the pineal gland synthesize melatonin from the **amino acid tryptophan** and release it into circulation.

Melatonin secretion is enhanced by darkness and is **inhibited by light** which is controlled by the light signals coming from the eyes via the **suprachiasmatic nucleus**.

Melatonin acts on melatonin receptors **ML_1 and ML_2.** The action of melatonin via ML_1 receptors in a **suprachiasmatic nucleus** is responsible for the regulation of **circadian rhythm** and **sleep-wake cycle.**

BASICS OF EEG

The pyramidal neurons in the human cerebral cortex are arranged in an orderly fashion perpendicular to the scalp surface and discharge synchronously. This synchronous electrical activity of the pyramidal neurons can be measured using voltage sensors placed over the scalp. This technique of measuring the electrical activity of pyramidal cells by placing electrical leads on the scalp is known as EEG. EEG in humans was first performed by German Psychiatrist Hans Berger in 1924.

Techniques of EEG

EEG is performed by following the universal 10–20 system in which scalp electrodes are placed at regular intervals (at 10% or 20% of scalp distance) over the scalp. Electrodes placed on the right side of the scalp are noted with an even number while those placed over the left side are noted with an odd number. Similarly, electrodes are also denoted with a letter depending on their area of placement, pF for prefrontal, F for frontal, P for parietal, T for temporal, and O for occipital. So, F1 lead represents the first electrode placed over the left-sided frontal cortex.

Concept of Montage

EEG leads measure the potential differences between cortical regions of the brain they are placed over. The montage means this measurement of potential differences between various cortical regions using electrodes by placing them in an orderly fashion. Commonly, **bipolar and referential montages** are used during routine EEG recordings.

Provocative Techniques

During the performance of EEG, various provocative maneuvers are used to elicit epileptiform discharges in cases where epileptiform discharges are not coming on normal awake EEG, however, epilepsy is strongly suspected. Commonly employed **provocative techniques are hyperventilation, photic stimulation, and sleep deprivation**. These maneuvers irritate cortical pyramidal cells located in seizure focus inducing epileptiform discharges on EEG.

Basic Waveforms in EEG

EEG waveforms are characterized by their location, frequency, amplitude, morphology, continuity, and synchronicity. The most important aspect of EEG waves is their frequency and based on the frequency EEG waves are named as follows.

1. **Delta waves** have a frequency of 0.5–4 Hz. They are prominently found over the frontocentral part of the head in persons in deep sleep (N3 stage of sleep). Generalized delta frequency is also found in patients with deep coma and severe encephalopathy.
2. **Theta waves** (4–7 Hz) come into the picture during the N1 and N2 phases of sleep and are more prominent in the frontal cortical region. Theta waves in the awake state indicate the onset of cerebral dysfunction such as encephalopathy.
3. **Alpha waves** (8–13 Hz) are seen in a normal awake person over the occipital region of the skull. Alpha waves are the defining background feature of normal EEG recording

in healthy adults. Slowing of background alpha rhythm in awakened adults indicates the onset of cerebral dysfunction.

4. **Sigma waves** or sleep spindles are characteristic features of N2 sleep. They may appear as slow waves (12–14 Hz) or as fast waves (14–16 Hz).
5. **Beta waves** range from 13 to 30 Hz on the frequency and are the most prominent waveform in the EEG of healthy adults and children.

Indications of EEG

1. Seizure disorders such as epilepsy, to classify types of seizure (focal or generalized) and to locate the seizure focus
2. Brain dysfunction arising from any cause to identify the degree of dysfunction, e.g. encephalopathy
3. To distinguish encephalopathy from catatonia
4. To ascertain Brain death
5. Sleep studies and sleep disorders
6. Some psychiatric illnesses such as ADHD, Autism, Dementia, etc
7. To ascertain the depth of anesthesia during surgery

ABNORMAL WAVEFORMS IN EEG

Triphasic Wave

Triphasic waves are distinctive waveforms consisting of three phases (1st positive sharp deflection, 2nd negative deflection, and 3rd slow positive recovery) and are easily recognizable in routine EEG. Triphasic waves are pathognomonic of encephalopathy, more so for hepatic encephalopathy.

Interictal Epileptiform discharges (IED)

Interictal epileptiform discharges are synchronous discharges arising from an epileptic focus. They represent the hyper-excitable state of neurons constituting an epileptic focus in the antiepileptic period. The probability of getting an IED in a patient with idiopathic epilepsy with a regular 30 minutes EEG recording is almost 40% and this probability increases with repeated EEG. IEDs can present in the EEG as following patterns:

1. Spike and wave pattern, spikes are pointed waves of short duration (20–70 ms) and are usually followed by a wave component that represents the compensatory action of GABAergic interneurons. One of the most known examples of a spike-wave pattern is the 3 Hz spike-wave pattern found in the absence of seizure. Generalized spike and wave patterns are seen in generalized epilepsy.
2. Sharps are also pointed waves but are of longer duration (70–200 ms)

Nonepileptiform Abnormalities

1. Slowing

Slowing in the EEG is seen in cases of cerebral dysfunction such as encephalopathy of any cause, in a person under general anesthesia, and deep sleep. Slowing presents in the EEG as generalized delta waves. Slowing can be diffuse or focal.

Diffuse slowing presents with delta waves in the EEG throughout the scalp. It represents generalized cerebral dysfunction such as deep sedation, encephalopathy of any cause, and diffuse cerebral infection.

Focal slowing presents with delta finding over a specific area of the scalp. Continuous focal slowing indicates underlying cerebral defects such as brain tumors, cerebral hemorrhage, brain abscess, etc.

2. Electrocerebral Inactivity

In ECI no EEG activity is noted and is indicative of brain death. However, to be certain the EEG should be of good quality and should be performed for at least 30 minutes using a complete set of scalp electrodes.

3. Burst Suppression Pattern

It is characterized by intermittent bursts of high-amplitude EEG activity of short duration followed by isoelectric EEG patterns (suppression). Burst suppression patterns are seen in a coma, general anesthesia, and hypothermia.

SLEEP PHYSIOLOGY AND EEG CHANGES

INTRODUCTION

Sleep is a behavioral state characterized by lowering of consciousness with diminished response to external stimuli and decreased motor activities. Adequate sleep is necessary for the proper functioning of higher mental activities like memory, judgments, reasoning, perception, and motor activities. Sleep has been divided into two distinct phases, e.g. **NREM** (nor rapid eye movement) **s**leep and **REM (**Rapid eye movement) sleep. However, recent research suggests the behavioral state of human beings can be divided into **three states,** e.g. **awakened state, NREM sleep, and REM sleep**.

In an awakened state, both the brain and motor system are active and can be voluntarily controlled. In NREM sleep, the brain is inactive while the skeletal system is somewhat active. REM sleep is considered a distinct behavioral state characterized by increased brain activity while the body is virtually paralyzed.

Non-REM Sleep

Non-REM sleep, also known as **slow-wave sleep**, starts as soon as a person falls asleep. The period between going to sleep and the onset of sleep is known as **sleep latency** and the duration varies from person to person. The first phase of sleep, the **N1 phase** (lasting for the first 1–7 minutes) is characterized by a relaxed mind and body with diminished brain activity; however, the person can be awakened with minimal stimulation. Then the person enters into the second **phase (N2 phase)** which is characteristically deeper than the first phase but still, the person can be awaked with stronger stimuli but is not confused after getting out of sleep. In EEG, the second phase can be identified by **characteristic k-complexes** during polysomnography. The person enters into a **deep sleep** (phase 3 and phase 4 or **N3 phase**) after remaining in the second phase for 40–50 minutes. Deep sleep is characterized by a slow **delta wave pattern in the EEG** (hence the name slow wave sleep). Brain activity is minimal during these phases and it is quite difficult to wake the person from a deep sleep and the person is visibly confused when forcefully awakened during these phases. The person remains in deep sleep for 25–30 minutes and then enters REM sleep.

REM Sleep

This sleep phase is considered **a distinct behavioral state** characterized by an active brain and a virtually paralyzed body. It starts after getting out of deep sleep (N3), about

Table 22.1: EEG changes during sleep	
Behavioral stage	***EEG changes***
Wakefulness	Mixed frequency background rhythm dominated by alpha activity.
N1 sleep (stage 1)	Mixed frequency background dominated by theta activity
N2 sleep (stage 2)	Appearance of characteristic sleep spindles and K-complex
N3 sleep (stages 3 and 4)	Background is dominated by high voltage low frequency delta waves
REM sleep	Mixed frequency background rhythm with saw tooth waves

90 minutes after the onset of sleep. Brain activity in this phase is even more robust than in the awakened state and this state is associated with vivid dreaming. The highly active cerebral cortex sends inhibitory signals to the brainstem **RAS, paralyzing the skeletal system** so that we do not act out our dreams. However, these inhibitory signals spare the nerves controlling eye movement as their nuclei are above the reticular activating system (RAS). This leads to the **rapid rolling movement of the eyeball** (hence the name rapid eye movement sleep). Unlike NREM sleep, the **thalamus is active** during REM sleep and sends signals (images, sounds, etc) that feed our dreams (Table 22.1).

PHYSIOLOGY OF SLEEP

The onset and maintenance of sleep involve complex neurochemical events in regions of the brain called the sleep centers situated in the hypothalamus. There are two important processes associated with sleep regulation, process C and process S. Process C is tasked with promoting sleep at night while process S is tasked with inducing sleep.

Process C

A normal human being is generally active during the daytime and goes to sleep at night. There is a **complex neurochemical process (process C)** that **promotes sleep at night** when the sun goes down and darkness sets in. It starts with perceiving the light during daytime via the light receptors (**melanopsin**) in the retina which send signals to the **suprachiasmatic nucleus (SCN)**. The suprachiasmatic nucleus acts as the **biological clock of the brain** whose primary function is to inhibit **melatonin** secretion from the pineal gland. The periodicity of the internal biological clock is slightly longer than 24 hours hence it needs to be reset every day to keep it tuned with the natural day-night periodicity (otherwise the process S becomes out of tune and starts promoting sleep during daytime after a few months). This mechanism of keeping the internal clock in tune with the natural clock is known as **entrainment**. SCN entrains the internal clock with a natural clock by receiving light stimulus from the retina and subsequently inhibiting the secretion of melatonin from the pineal gland during the daytime. When darkness sets in, this inhibitory effect is resealed with a subsequent increase in melatonin secretion from the pineal gland which acts on the sleep center in the hypothalamus to decrease sleep threshold and thereby promotes sleep at night, but it should be remembered that melatonin itself cannot induce sleep which is the function of process S.

Process S

Process S, also known as **homeostatic sleep drive**, is a neurochemical change that makes a person fall asleep after a period of awakening. It involves a gradual build-up of **sleep drive which creates pressure to fall asleep** and ultimately forces the person to go to sleep. Search for the chemical signal for homeostatic sleep drive has identified the chemical '**adenosine**' as the principal agent inducing sleep. During the daytime when the person is active, there is a breakdown of ATP leading to the accumulation of its end product 'adenosine'. So, adenosine gradually accumulates during the period of awakening and after reaching the threshold point it induces sleep by **acting on the 'ON' switch** of the sleep center.

The sleep center located in the hypothalamus consists of **ON** and **OFF** switches that induce sleep or promote wakefulness respectively. The **'ON'** switch has a certain threshold for shutting down the wakefulness-promoting center in the brain stem (the Reticular activating system). This threshold is reduced by the action of melatonin which promotes sleep at night and the threshold is broken by adenosine which induces sleep. There is a surge in the **neurotransmitter GABA** when the 'ON' switch is activated and it is this neurotransmitter that is responsible for decreasing the activities of the brainstem **RAS** and cerebral cortex. There are certain chemicals such as glutamate, noradrenaline, and histamine which act on the **'OFF'** switch and promote wakefulness.

SLEEP DISORDERS

Disorders of sleep can be categorized into **dyssomnias, parasomnias, and circadian sleep disorders**. Sleep disorders that affect timing, quality, and amount of sleep are known as dyssomnias and include insomnia and hypersomnia. Parasomnias include any behavioral disturbances occurring during sleep such as night terror, night walking (somnambulism), sleep paralysis, etc. Circadian sleep disorders are those that affect the tuning of sleep with day-night periodicity and include phase advanced sleep disorder, phase delayed sleep disorder and non-24-hour sleep disorder.

DYSSOMNIAS

Dyssomnia is the term applied to a group of sleep disorders that affect the **timing, quality, and/or quantity of sleep**. Insomnia is nothing but the decreased quantity of sleep or impairment in the quality of sleep. In most cases, insomnia is secondary to some underlying psychiatric disorders such as anxiety, depression, OCD, schizophrenia, substance withdrawal, etc. **Primary insomnia** is rare and may present with increased sleep latency or frequent awakening from sleep at night. This leads to a lack of freshness after sleep and a feeling of sleep and lethargy during the daytime. **Maintenance of sleep hygiene** frequently improves insomnia in most cases and medications are seldom needed. In case medications are necessary, **short-course benzodiazepines** (for 2-4 weeks) often improve the conditions. However, it should be kept in mind that benzodiazepines have abuse potential, and if given for a longer period then there is the possibility of tolerance. In cases where long-term medication therapy is needed for insomnia then non-benzodiazepine sedatives like **Z-group of drugs** (zolpidem, zopiclone, and zaleplon) or sedative antihistamines (cetirizine, diphenhydramine or promethazine) have better safety profile and are also efficacious.

Hypersomnias

An increase in the amount of sleep or daytime sleepiness may be due to certain primary conditions like cataplexy and **Kleine–Levin syndrome** or may be secondary to some psychiatric illness (atypical depression, substance intoxication, etc).

1. Idiopathic Hypersomnia

Idiopathic hypersomnia is a chronic debilitating condition presenting **excessive sleep** (more than 9 hours per day) with a lack of freshness after sleep. Most of them sleep excessively at night time without feeling fresh after sleep and an **irresistible desire to go to sleep again**. During the daytime, the patient always feels like going to sleep again with extreme lethargy, lack of clarity of thinking, poor motor coordination, and lack of energy for any activity. The patient faces problems in the workplace and in maintaining social and familial relationships due to excessive daytime sleepiness. It is thought to be due to decreased levels of **wakefulness-promoting chemicals** in the brain such as noradrenaline and histamine. Now researchers have also found increased sensitivity of GABA receptors to the sleep-inducing chemical GABA. These factors keep the sleep center in 'ON' mode leading to excessive sleepiness. Wakefulness-promoting agents like **modafinil and methylphenidate** can help keep the patient alert during the daytime but these agents lack good efficacy.

2. Narcolepsy

Narcolepsy is a condition characterized by excessive daytime sleepiness, sleep paralysis and vivid hallucinations which may or may not be associated with loss of muscle tone (cataplexy). These sudden bouts of sleep during the daytime can occur anytime, anywhere and sometimes the patient does not have any control over it. It is accompanied by sudden falls due to associated loss of muscle tone **(narcolepsy with cataplexy**) and the patient may sustain major injuries. They frequently experience sleep paralysis and vivid hallucinations while going to sleep or while waking from sleep (known as **hypnagogic** and **hypnopompic** hallucinations respectively). Narcolepsy is thought to be due to decreased levels of a chemical called **orexin B** involved in the regulation of sleep phases and the condition is heritable in some cases. Disturbances in the regulation of the sleep cycle result in sudden **intrusion of REM sleep** during awaken state leading to uncontrolled daytime sleepiness and loss of muscle control (cataplexy). Wakefulness-promoting agents like **modafinil, armodafinil,** and methylphenidate are standard medications used for controlling bouts of daytime sleep in narcolepsy.

3. Kleine–Levin Syndrome

Kleine-Levin syndrome is a rare condition characterized by **recurrent episodes of excessive sleep** lasting for weeks to months. The person may sleep for about 20 hours a day during the episodes. These episodes are often associated with cognitive impairment such as **clouding of consciousness** and behavioral problems like irritability**, excessive eating, or excessive sexual activities**. The onset of Klein–Levin syndrome often follows a viral infection, and viral damage to thalamic structures is often implicated as the basic pathology underlying this condition. There is no cure, but wakefulness-promoting agents like modafinil and armodafinil may improve daytime sleepiness although have no effects on cognitive and behavioral symptoms. Lithium may help decrease frequency and illness duration in some cases.

PARASOMNIAS

Parasomnias refer to **abnormal activities, behavior, emotions, perceptions, or dreams** while a patient is asleep**.** Parasomnias can **occur during NREM sleep or REM sleep**. One of the fundamental differences between parasomnia associated with REM sleep from that of NREM sleep is the **lack of bodily musculoskeletal activities** in parasomnias associated with **REM sleep**. This is due to paralysis of voluntary muscles during

REM sleep as a result of inhibitory signals from the cerebral cortex shutting down the reticular activating system. For example, somnambulism is characterized by waking up at night and walking here and there (musculoskeletal activities), hence somnambulism must occur during NREM sleep as it involves musculoskeletal activation. However, it should be remembered that **REM sleep behavior disorder is a notable exception** to this fundamental concept as it occurs due to the failure of higher centers to induce muscle atonia during REM sleep.

State Dissociation Hypothesis of Parasomnia

We have seen that awaken state, REM sleep, and NREM sleep are distinct behavioral states of human beings, but recent research has suggested that combinations of these states are possibly leading to unstable behavioral states characterized by abnormal activities and behavior in impaired consciousness. These dissociated states give rise to parasomnias.

REM Sleep Parasomnias

REM sleep behavior disorder is characterized by extreme bodily activities in REM sleep while the patient is dreaming. It occurs due to the failure of cerebral inhibitory signals in suppressing reticular activating systems and brainstem motor nuclei. Because of this, there is **lack of muscle atonia** that should be normally present during REM sleep. During REM sleep as the patients dream, they act out their dream with bodily activities. These patients may harm themselves or their bed partners.

Nightmare disorder involves experiencing **extremely horrific dreams** without any bodily activities. Nightmares are common in childhood but become less severe with an increase in age. The alpha-adrenergic blocking agent prazosin helps decrease horrific dreams to a great extent and should be prescribed in patients with problematic nightmare disorders.

Sleep paralysis occurs while the patient is going to sleep or waking up from sleep. The patient complains of an **inability to move his body parts and muscles** (except the eyes) even if he is fully awake and is out of sleep. This occurs due to the **prolongation of muscle atonia** even if the person is out of REM sleep. This condition is quite discomforting but does not cause any harm. Few persons with sleep paralysis often **experience vivid and scary visual hallucinations** (hypnagogic or hypnopompic hallucinations) like a ghost sitting on their chest. These patients may be scared of going to sleep again (avoidance behavior) leading to sleep deprivation. However, sleep deprivation can induce more severe sleep paralysis episodes with more fearful hallucinations initiating a vicious cycle. When treatment is needed, SSRIs such as fluoxetine or paroxetine and TCAs such as trazodone can help decrease both the frequency and severity of sleep paralysis.

NREM Sleep Parasomnias

Confusional arousal is a sleep disorder in which the patient **wakes up in the middle of deep sleep** looking visibly confused, sits on the bed for some time, looks here and there vacantly, and goes to sleep again. Some people in this condition may babble or speak incoherently (known as **somniloquy** or sleep talk). Confusional arousal is quite common in childhood and children show a lot of activities with groaning and may cry inconsolably. It goes with an increase in age and is rare in adulthood.

Somnambulism or **sleep walking** is a condition in which the person wakes up from sleep and begins to walk around the house without being conscious about their activities. Some may indulge in **complex activities** like unlocking the door and going outside, changing dresses, combing their hair, etc. All these activities occur in sleep without the person gaining full consciousness. Somnambulism occurs due to intrusion of the awakened state in deep slow-wave sleep **(N3 or phase 3 and phase 4).** When the patient is forced to wake-up from deep sleep due to this intrusion, the musculoskeletal system is activated without gaining consciousness. The person may roam outside meeting motor vehicular accidents or other inadvertent consequences. If a person is seen sleep-walking then he/she should not be awakened forcefully as it can make the person more confused and violent. Treatment includes night time benzodiazepines to prevent sleep disruption. The **tetracyclic antidepressant trazodone** also offers help to these patients.

Night terror or sleep terror is an NREM sleep disorder characterized by sudden waking from sleep with **extreme fear and screaming.** Such patients may suddenly try to escape from the room they are sleeping in and cause injury to themselves and others. A course of benzodiazepines and antidepressant trazodone may help mitigate night terror.

Other rare NREM sleep disorders include **sleep eating and sleep sex.** In sleep eating, the patient wakes up at night and eats foods without conscious knowledge. This may lead to significant weight gain and the patient has no clue regarding the cause. Sleep sex involves involvement in sexual behavior such as fondling, masturbation, intercourse, or sexual abuse without conscious knowledge which might invite serious medico-legal consequences.

Circadian Rhythm Sleep Disorders

Circadian rhythm sleep disorders arise due to dysfunction of the internal circadian clock or due to misalignment of the internal clock with the external day-night cycle. Accordingly, CRSDs are categorized into:

1. Arising due to **dysfunction of the internal circadian clock**
   - Advance sleep phase disorder
   - Delayed sleep phase disorder
   - Irregular sleep-wake rhythm
   - Free running disorder
2. Arising due to **misalignment with an external day-night cycle**
   - Jet lag
   - Shift work disorder

In the **advanced sleep phase disorder,** the person goes to bed early and wakes up early and these persons are known as **early larks**. This disorder is treated with **light therapy** given in the evening hours. In **delayed sleep phase disorder** the person goes to sleep at late night and wakes up late in the morning (known as a **night owl**). This disorder is treated by giving **melatonin in the evening hour** to induce sleep early. **Irregular sleep-wake disorder** arises due to **non-entrainment** of the internal biological clock with external cues which leads to a small drift in sleep-wake timing over a period of weeks to months ultimately leading to daytime sleep sleepiness and insomnia at night after a few months.

Shift work disorder arises due to non-conventional work schedules such as regular night duties which cause significant daytime sleepiness and chronic insomnia. **Jet lag** occurs due to rapid travel across time-zones leading to misalignment between internal circadian clocks with the external day-night cycle. These conditions are treated by giving **melatonin at night** and **exposure to bright light during the daytime**, alternatively, **modafinil or armodafinil** can be given to maintain daytime alertness and wakefulness.

ILLNESS ANXIETY DISORDER, FACTITIOUS DISORDER AND MALINGERING

ILLNESS ANXIETY DISORDER

Illness anxiety disorder or IAD presents with **excessive worry or fear** of having or developing a serious life-threatening medical illness. This fear or worry persists despite medical investigations revealing **no underlying serious medical illness**. This excessive worry or fear causes impairment in the the socio-occupational functioning of the person. As per DSM5, there might be an underlying medical illness but that cannot explain the amount of worry or fear associated with it. In contrast to somatic symptom disorder, these patients **do not complain about somatic symptoms**. DSM5 has introduced a paradigm shift and the diagnosis of the **hypochondriacal disorder** has been eliminated and merged under this condition.

The prevalence of IAD is found to be 0.1% in the general population. Onset is generally in late adolescent and generally worsens with age. There is no gender predominance and males and females are equally prone to develop IAD.

Clinical Presentation

Patients of illness anxiety disorder present with fear or worry of having or developing a serious medical illness. The worry or fear persists even after physical examination or laboratory investigations ruling out any underlying serious medical illness. They do not complain about any somatic symptoms or even if somatic symptoms are present, they are mild and are non-bothersome. Many patients have had multiple visits to general practitioners before coming to psychiatrists. However, they either disbelieve the laboratory findings or doubt the competency of a general practitioner in finding out the underlying illness. Many are very much eager to undergo any laboratory investigations to find out the underlying medical illness, even risky ones. These worries or fears about having or developing a medical illness cause significant impairment in the socio-economic functioning of the individual.

These patients can be categorized into the following types

1. **Care seeking type:** These patients pay multiple visits to medical professionals and are eager to go for any laboratory investigations to find out the underlying medical illness.
2. **Care-avoidant type:** They are very much anxious about any serious medical illness being revealed by laboratory investigations or physical examination. Because of this they generally avoid visiting health professionals.

Etiology

The exact etiology of IEDs has not been understood clearly. Persons who suffered from IED generally had a serious medical illness during childhood or have had a family member suffering from a serious medical illness. The amount of attention they got during childhood or their ailing family members were getting them prone to seek attention, albeit unconsciously (in contrast to a factitious disorder where attention-seeking behavior is fully conscious). Persons who are continuously seeking health-related information in articles or on the internet are also more prone to develop IAD. Unemployed or uneducated people are also at higher risk.

Pathophysiology

Persons with IAD generally have a **heightened perception of bodily sensations** and misinterpret them as symptoms of serious underlying medical illness. These persons also suffer from palpitation, increased breathing, and gastric discomfort due to **hyperarousal reaction** and they misinterpret them as symptoms of cardiological or respiratory illnesses. This misinterpretation of bodily sensations is primarily due to faulty cognition (thinking pattern) and ideas about medical illnesses.

Differential Diagnosis

Illness anxiety disorder is frequently confused with the following illnesses:

1. **Somatic symptom disorder**—these patients complain of troublesome somatic symptoms with excessive worry or preoccupation associated with it. These patients want their symptoms to be relieved rather than finding out the underlying illness.
2. **Factitious disorder**—these patients consciously induce, feign, or exaggerate physical or psychiatric symptoms mainly for some primary gain like attention or to deal with stress.
3. **Malingering**—these patients present as having a serious medical illness to avoid criminal or legal obligations or for monetary gain from insurance companies.

Complications

Illness anxiety disorder has a significant impact on the socio-occupational functioning of the individual. Apart from this, many undergo serious life-threatening medical investigations which can cause injury or death. Many develop depression and attempt or commit suicide.

Treatment

Treatment for illness anxiety disorder is primarily focused on helping the patient reduce health-related anxiety. Psychotherapy is the most effective therapeutic approach for patients who are willing to undergo therapy. A good rapport with an empathetic approach is imperative to get the patient into a trusting therapeutic relationship. Cognitive behavioral therapy is aimed at correcting faulty cognition and maladaptive thoughts present in these patients. Apart from CBT, supportive psychotherapy, and group therapy, mindfulness-based therapy also yields good results.

Few patients also respond to medications such as SSRIs, SNRIs, and TCAs. These patients get the best result from a combination of medications with psychotherapy.

FACTITIOUS DISORDER

Factitious disorder, also known as **Munchausen syndrome** or **hospital addiction,** is a rare psychiatric illness in which the patient presents himself as a sick patient for attention and care. The **sick role** is assumed by **inducing, feigning, or exaggerating physical or psychiatric symptoms**. They assume a sick role **to gain attention and care** from health professionals or gain pleasure by deceiving them. Factitious disorder is difficult to deal with condition by health professionals because of the inherent deceptive quality associated with it. Many patients become hostile when confronted with the diagnosis and avoid being treated for their true illness, although get repeatedly admitted by inducing or feigning an illness.

Factitious disorder is a rare psychiatric illness with a prevalence of less than 0.1 percent among psychiatric patients. Onset is generally in early adulthood and more common in men than in women.

Clinical Presentation

The assumption of a sick role by inducing, feigning, or exaggerating physical or psychiatric symptoms is the core feature of factitious disorder. This is done to get admitted to the hospital to **gain attention and care** from health professionals. They present to the clinics with symptoms that suggest a serious medical illness such as chest pain which has a good chance of hospital admission. Many patients also present with diarrhea, abdominal pain, arthralgia, excoriated skin, or infected wounds. These **symptoms are deliberately induced** by ingesting stalled food, injecting fecal matter into the skin to produce a wound, self-induced skin pricking, etc. Once admitted, many patients are more than eager to undergo risky procedures and laboratory investigations. They become hostile and quarrel with medical staff when discharge is planned or when confronted with the true nature of their illness. They generally take leave against medical advice and visit another hospital with new symptoms.

Etiology

The cause of the factitious disorder is mainly speculated to be due to abnormal psychological development. Many patients have had a difficult childhood with a history of abuse, torture, abandonment, etc. These patients try to seek the attention and care they lacked during their childhood. Patients with a history of a serious medical illness with early exposure to medical care are also at increased risk. This condition is considered to be a case of **behavioral addiction to medical health care**.

Complications

Patients with factitious disorders frequently undergo medical procedures such as explorative laparotomy which put the life of the patient at risk. Many also use risky methods to induce physical symptoms which can lead to serious medical illnesses. They also utilize the limited healthcare facility available. They are at increased risk of developing depression, substance abuse or self-harm, and suicidal behavior.

Treatment

Medications are prescribed only for comorbid psychiatric illnesses such as depression; otherwise, medications have no therapeutic benefit in these patients. Psychotherapy is the only effective treatment modality available.

The most difficult part is the unwillingness of the patient to be involved in the treatment protocol. Once the diagnosis is made, the person is taken into the treatment procedure without confrontation and without revealing the diagnosis. Individual psychotherapy helps in reducing factitious behavior.

MALINGERING

Malingering is the **falsification of physical or mental illness** by a person to gain some external **benefit.** The person may fake the illnesses to avoid trial, to gain monetary compensation, or to avoid work. However, it should be remembered that malingering is **not a psychiatric diagnosis**. Moreover, it is a diagnosis of exclusion and thorough evaluation and investigation by a specialist (from the field to which the clinical presentation belongs) should be done before making a diagnosis of malingering.

Etiology

Malingering is always associated with some underlying motive of **external gain**. Students malinger to avoid school, workers to avoid work with pay, and drug abusers to gain prescription medicines (benzodiazepines and opioids). However, malingering is most commonly seen in prisoners to avoid trial and conviction. Once the external gain is achieved the symptoms vanish and the malingerer stops complaining. Malingering is also seen more commonly in persons with antisocial and histrionic personality disorders.

History and Evaluation

Malingering is a diagnosis of exclusion. Therefore, a detailed history and meticulous examination must be carried out before giving a diagnosis. A malingerer presents **his idea of the illness**, hence, detailed questioning regarding the presenting illness makes the person uncomfortable and irritable at times. Because of their limited idea regarding the illness, meticulous history generally fishes out the truth. The patient may say yes to every question about the illness even without giving thought (for example, a patient malingering schizophrenia may reveal experiencing visual hallucinations which are not present in true cases of schizophrenia). Such behaviors point toward malingering.

During the evaluation, it is important to look into certain aspects when malingering is suspected. First of all the **referral pattern** may point toward malingering, for example when a lawyer sends an under-trial prisoner for evaluation, malingering should be strongly suspected. Secondly, **secondary gain** (external benefits) is always the underlying motive in all cases of malingering. This differentiates malingering from factitious disorder in which case the gain is primary (patient seeking care and attention as they are addicted to health care).

Even if malingering is suspected, the person should not be confronted. Such confrontations may lead to aggression, violence, or litigation.

Treatment

There is neither any treatment nor any cure for malingering. The malingerer stops complaining about the illness once his underlying motives are fulfilled.

PARAPHILIC DISORDERS

Paraphilic disorders are also known by the common name **'sexual perversions'**. These are sexual behaviors considered **deviations** from normal sexual behavior, however, are necessary to experience arousal and orgasm by the patient. As per DSM5, deviation from normal sexual behavior is considered a disorder only when it is **harmful and destructive** to the person himself, to his partner, or the greater community. Paraphilic disorders include a range of sexual behaviors which **involve aggression and victimization**. DSM5 mentioned pedophilia, frotteurism, fetishism, exhibitionism, voyeurism, sexual masochism, sexual sadism, and transvestism as paraphilic disorders.

The prevalence of paraphilic disorders is much more common in society than they are diagnosed in the clinic. Onset is generally in late adolescence or early adulthood and **men are more commonly affected** than women. A person generally has had multiple paraphilic disorders at different points in time during the course of the illness. **Pedophilia** is by far the most common type of paraphilic disorder.

Psychodynamic Theory of Paraphilia

According to **Freud's psychoanalytic theory**, paraphilia develops as a coping mechanism in persons with **non-resolved oedipal complex**. The **castration anxiety** persists due to non resolved oedipal complex and these persons indulge in deviant sexual behavior to vent the anxiety associated with fear of castration.

TYPES OF PARAPHILIC DISORDERS

The list of paraphilic disorders is exhaustive but DSM-5 has mentioned the following 8 paraphilias as paraphilic disorders because of their commonality and associated harm to the person or society at large.

1. **Pedophilia** is characterized by recurrent sexual urge and sexual involvement with children 13 years of age or younger over a period of 6 months or more. The perpetrator must be at least 16 years of age and must be 5 years older than the victim for a diagnosis.
   Pedophilia is the most common paraphilic disorder, most commonly seen in men and the victims can be male or female, or both. Paedophilia generally involves fondling of private parts of the child and oral sex, although penetrative sex can occur rarely. Pedophilia can be categorized into the following three types.
   - Sexually attracted to females
   - Sexually attracted to male
   - Sexually attracted toward both sexes
2. **Frotteurism** is the rubbing of the penis by a man against the body parts of a non-consenting woman to get sexual gratification. Some men also use their hands and legs to rub against an unsuspecting woman. It generally takes place in crowded places like markets, in queues, and in buses.
3. **Fetishism** is defined as getting sexual gratification by sexual involvement with nonsexual body parts or inanimate objects associated with the human body (shoes, stockings, etc).
4. **Exhibitionism** is characterized by exposing the genitals to a stranger or an unsuspecting person. Sexual gratification is achieved by showing genitals or by getting pleasure from the reaction of the opposite person such as fear, surprise, and disgust. Exhibitionism is carried out mainly by males toward unsuspecting females.
5. **Voyeurism** is the act of getting sexual gratification by observing an unsuspected person when she is naked, undressing, or involved in sexual activities. This action is accompanied by or followed by masturbation to orgasm. Voyeurism is almost always seen in males and the victims are females.
6. **Transvestism** is a paraphilic disorder in which the person gets sexual gratification by dressing in clothes of the opposite sex. Many females wear the dresses of males but to diagnose a case as transvestism the person must feel sexually aroused or excited while dressed in the clothes of the opposite sex.
7. **Sexual sadism** involves achieving sexual gratification by inflicting physical or psychological pain on the partner. The name has been derived from Marquis de Sade, a French military officer who used to commit violent crimes against his partners

during sexual intercourse. Few sadists rape and subsequently murder their partners and the condition is known as **'lust murder'.**

8. **Sexual masochism** is achieving sexual gratification by being abused or punished (physically or psychologically) by the partner during sexual intercourse. A specific type of sexual masochism is **asphyxiophilia** in which the person gets extreme sexual arousal by being smothered (or restricted from breathing by any means) by the partner.

Treatment of Paraphilic Disorders

There are multiple therapeutic approaches for the management of paraphilic disorders and are employed on a **case-to-case basis.**

1. **Pharmacotherapy:** Medications are used to decrease libido in patients who indulged in a repetitive sexual offense. Testosterone-decreasing agents such as **cyproterone acetate** and **medroxyprogesterone acetate** are used for this purpose. **Antipsychotics and antidepressants** are used to treat psychosis and depression comorbidity associated with paraphilic disorders.
2. **Cognitive behavioral therapy** is aimed at changing sexual thoughts and sexual behavioral patterns to make them socially acceptable. Insight-oriented psychotherapy helps the patient in being aware of daily events which make them not to act on their impulse and how to control them.
3. In extreme cases such as in regular sexual offenders and pedophiles, external control measures such as **imprisonment** are necessary.

SUMMARY

1. Neurodevelopment is a highly complex genetically programmed process consisting of neurulation (formation of neural tube), neurogenesis (production of neurons from the neuroepithelium), neural migration, axon guidance and synaptic pruning.
2. The central nervous system is divided into brainstem (which controls the basic neurological functions such as arousal, consciousness, thermoregulation and cardiorespiratory functions), limbic system (which controls the emotional functions) and cerebral cortex (which controls higher mental functions). Basal ganglia and cerebellum are involved in maintenance of posture and coordination of motor movements.
3. The neurotransmitter systems (peptide and monoamine neurotransmitters) have special roles in the causation of psychiatric illnesses. Peptide neurotransmitters consist of glutamate (the principal excitatory neurotransmitter) and GABA (the principal inhibitory neurotransmitter). Monoamine neurotransmitters consist of dopamine, serotonin, noradrenaline and histamine which are involved in modulation of neuronal excitation and inhibition and subsequent regulation of perception, cognition, emotion and action.
4. EEG is the process of measurement of cerebral neural activities by placing electrodes on the scalp. EEG is used in diagnosis of brain dysfunction (such as seizure) and damage (such as CVA and brain tumors) and in sleep studies.
5. The behavioral state of the human being is divided into wakefulness, NREM sleep and REM sleep. Disorders of sleep are classified as dyssomnias involving timing, quantity and quality of sleep and parasomnias which are defined as abnormal behaviors during sleep.
6. It is very important to differentiate between true illnesses and feigned illnesses (also known as malingering). It should be kept in mind that malingering is not a psychiatric diagnosis.
7. Paraphilias or sexual perversions are deviant sexual behaviors which are dangerous to the person involved or to the society at large. DSM-5 has mentioned 8 paraphilic disorders of clinical importance: pedophilia, frotteurism, fetishism, exhibitionism, voyeurism, sexual masochism, sexual sadism and transvestism.

BIBLIOGRAPHY

1. Ranabir Chakraborty, MJ Vijay Kumar, James P. Clement, Critical aspects of neurodevelopment, Neurobiology of Learning and Memory, 2021. Volume 180,2021,107415, ISSN 1074–7427.
2. Sadock, and Pedro Ruiz. Kaplan & Sadock. Synopsis of Psychiatry: Behavioral Sciences/ Clinical Psychiatry, 2015. Eleventh edition. Philadelphia: Wolters Kluwer.
3. Basinger H, Hogg JP. Neuroanatomy, Brainstem. [Updated 2021 May 8]. In: StatPearls [Internet]. Treasure Island (FL): StatPearls Publishing; 2022 Jan.
4. Javed K, Reddy V, Lui F. Neuroanatomy, Cerebral Cortex. [Updated 2021 Jul 31]. In: StatPearls [Internet]. Treasure Island (FL): StatPearls Publishing; 2022 Jan.
5. Degree of handedness and cerebral dominance. Keren L. Isaacs, William B. Barr, Peter Kim Nelson, Orrin Devinsky. Neurology Jun 2006;66 (12):1855.
6. Rajmohan V, & Mohandas, E. The limbic system. Indian Journal of Psychiatry, 2007;49(2): 132–139.
7. Bhattacharyya KB James Wenceslaus Papez, His Circuit, and Emotion. Annals of Indian Academy of Neurology, 2017;20(3):207–210.
8. Valenzuela CF, Puglia MP, & Zucca S. Focus on: neurotransmitter systems. Alcohol Research & health: the journal of the National Institute on Alcohol Abuse and Alcoholism, 2011; 34(1): 106–120.
9. Stahl, S. M., & Grady, M. M. Stahl's essential psychopharmacology: The prescribe guide, 2011. (4th ed.). Cambridge, UK; New York: Cambridge University Press.
10. Rayi A, Murr N. Electroencephalogram. [Updated 2022 May 15]. In: StatPearls [Internet]. Treasure Island (FL): StatPearls Publishing; 2022 Jan.
11. Nayak CS, Anilkumar AC. EEG Normal Waveforms. [Updated 2022 May 8]. In: StatPearls [Internet]. Treasure Island (FL): StatPearls Publishing; 2022 Jan.
12. Emmady PD, Anilkumar AC. EEG Abnormal Waveforms. [Updated 2022 May 8]. In: StatPearls [Internet]. Treasure Island (FL): StatPearls Publishing; 2022 Jan.
13. Institute of Medicine (US) Committee on Sleep Medicine and Research; Colten HR, Altevogt BM, editors. Sleep Disorders and Sleep Deprivation: An Unmet Public Health Problem. Washington (DC): National Academies Press (US); 2006. 2, Sleep Physiology.
14. Borbély AA, Daan S, Wirz-Justice A, Deboer T. The two-process model of sleep regulation: a reappraisal. J Sleep Res. 2016 Apr;25(2):131–43.
15. Carley DW and Farabi SS. Physiology of Sleep. Diabetes spectrum: a publication of the American Diabetes Association, 2016;29(1):5–9.
16. Abad VC and Guilleminault, C. Diagnosis and treatment of sleep disorders: a brief review for clinicians. Dialogues in clinical neuroscience, 2003;5(4):371–388.
17. Karna B, Gupta V. Sleep Disorder. [Updated 2021 Nov 20]. In: StatPearls [Internet]. Treasure Island (FL): StatPearls Publishing; 2022 Jan.
18. Kim MJ, Lee JH, & Duffy JF. Circadian Rhythm Sleep Disorders. Journal of clinical outcomes management: JCOM, 2013;20(11):513–528.
19. Shreekantiah Umesh and Shamshul Haque Nizamie . Indian J Hum Genet. 2014 Apr-Jun; 20(2): 120–128.
20. Kumar V, Abbas AK, & Aster JC. Robbins Basic Pathology, 2017. (10th ed.). Elsevier - Health Sciences Division.
21. French JH, Hameed S. Illness Anxiety Disorder. [Updated 2022 Apr 28]. In: StatPearls [Internet]. Treasure Island (FL): StatPearls Publishing; 2022.
22. Carnahan KT, Jha A. Factitious Disorder. [Updated 2022 May 1]. In: StatPearls [Internet]. Treasure Island (FL): StatPearls Publishing; 2022.
23. Alozai Uu, McPherson PK. Malingering. [Updated 2022 Jun 21]. In: StatPearls [Internet]. Treasure Island (FL): StatPearls Publishing; 2022 Jan.
24. McManus MA, Hargreaves P, Rainbow L, Alison LJ. Paraphilias: definition, diagnosis, and treatment. F1000Prime Rep. 2013 Sep 2;5:36.

Index

A

B

C

D

E

F

G

N

O

P

R

S

T

U

V

W

Z